MRI of the Abdomen with CT Correlation

MRI of the Abdomen with CT Correlation

Editors

Richard C. Semelka
Associate Professor
Department of Radiology
and Clinical Director
Magnetic Resonance Services
University of North Carolina at Chapel Hill
Chapel Hill, North Carolina

J. Patrick Shoenut
Medical Projects Coordinator
University of Manitoba
and Research Associate
Department of Medicine
St. Boniface General Hospital Research Centre
Winnipeg, Manitoba
Canada

Raven Press New York

Raven Press, Ltd., 1185 Avenue of the Americas. New York, New York 10036

Made in the United States of America

Library of Congress Cataloging-in-Publication Data

MRI of the abdomen with CT correlation/editor, Richard C. Semelka, J. Patrick Shoenut.
p. cm.
Includes bibliographical references and index.
ISBN 0-7817-0019-1
1. Abdomen–Magnetic resonance imaging. 2. Abdomen—Tomography.
I. Semelka, Richard C. II. Shoenut, J. Patrick
[DNLM: 1. Abdomen—radiography. 2. Gastrointestinal Diseases—diagnosis. 3. Magnetic Resonance Imaging. 4. Tomography, X-Ray Computed. WI 900 M939 1992]
RC944.M655 1992
617.5′507′548—dc20
DNLM/DLC
for Library of Congress 92-48523
CIP

The material contained in this volume was submitted as previously unpublished material, except in the instances in which credit has been given to the source from which some of the illustrative material was derived.

Great care has been taken to maintain the accuracy of the information contained in the volume. However, neither Raven Press nor the editors can be held responsible for errors or for any consequences arising from the use of the information contained herein.

9 8 7 6 5 4 3 2 1

To our families

Contents

Contributing Authors

Howard M. Greenberg, M.D. *Associate Professor, Department of Radiology, University of Manitoba, Health Science Center, 820 Sherbrook Street, Winnipeg, Manitoba, Canada R2H 2A6.*

Mervyn A. Kroeker, M.D. *Associate Professor, Department of Radiology, University of Manitoba, 409 Tache Avenue, Winnipeg, Manitoba, Canada R2H 2A6.*

Gerhard A. Laub, Ph.D. *Director, Magnetic Resonance Research and Development, Siemens Medical Systems, Iselin, New Jersey 08830.*

Allan B. Micflikier, M.D. *Associate Professor, Department of Medicine, University of Manitoba, 409 Tache Avenue, Winnipeg, Manitoba, Canada R2H 2A6.*

Richard C. Semelka, M.D. *Associate Professor, Department of Radiology, and Clinical Director, Magnetic Resonance Services, University of North Carolina at Chapel Hill, Chapel Hill, North Carolina 27599.*

J. Patrick Shoenut, B.Sc. *Medical Projects Coordinator, University of Manitoba, and Research Associate, Department of Medicine, St. Boniface General Hospital Research Centre, 351 Tache Avenue, Winnipeg, Manitoba, Canada R2H 2A6.*

Richard Silverman, M.D. *Assistant Professor, Department of Surgery, University of Manitoba, 409 Tache Avenue, Winnipeg, Manitoba, Canada R2H 2A6.*

Clifford S. Yaffe, M.D. *Assistant Professor, Department of Surgery, University of Manitoba, 409 Tache Avenue, Winnipeg, Manitoba, Canada R2H 2A6.*

Preface

This book provides a compendium of MR images of various abdominal disease processes. It demonstrates the tremendous current diagnostic capability of this modality using optimized techniques on standard MR systems. High-quality CT images are used as reference in order to highlight the strengths of MRI by comparing MR images to the current "gold standard" for abdominal imaging. Since the inception of MRI as a clinical tool in the early 1980s, the expectation has been that MRI would, ultimately, surpass the diagnostic capabilities of CT. This superiority has been established in the central nervous system and musculoskeletal system. We believe that this book illustrates that abdominal MRI has also fulfilled this expectation.

Acknowledgments

The editors thank Terrance P. Madden, BSc. for preparation of the manuscript and St. Boniface General Hospital Research Foundation, Milton Lautatzis, M.D., Charles B. Higgins, M.D., Hedvig Hricak, M.D., Donna L. Semelka, M.D., Suzanne La Plante, M.Sc., Gyan P. Sharma, M.D., and Robert E. Kohrman, Ph.D. for their support.

MRI of the Abdomen
with
CT Correlation

CHAPTER 1

Physics of Magnetic Resonance: Sequences Tailored for Abdominal Magnetic Resonance Studies

Gerhard A. Laub and Richard C. Semelka

Comprehensive description of the physics of magnetic resonance imaging (MRI) is contained in many larger magnetic resonance (MR) textbooks. The purpose of this chapter is to describe the physics behind sequences optimized for abdominal studies and the theoretical methodology behind sequence modification and optimization.

The challenges of abdominal MRI primarily relate to compensation and avoidance of image artifacts. The most severe artifact is respiration-induced ghosting artifact from the motion of subcutaneous abdominal fat; however, bowel peristalsis, chemical shift, and blood flow artifacts also cause problems. Other limitations of conventional MRI include relatively low spatial resolution, limited contrast resolution, and the lack of an established suitable oral contrast agent.

The two most common approaches to compensate for respiratory artifact are averaging of multiple acquisitions and reordering of the phase-encoding table according to the respiratory cycle (1). More recently, additional techniques have been used in clinical practice to address respiratory artifacts:

1. Frequency-selective fat suppression (fatsat) removes the signal intensity (SI) of abdominal fat and thereby diminishes most of the ghosting artifacts (2,3).
2. Breath-hold imaging avoids respiratory artifacts (4,5).
3. Snapshot imaging allows the acquisition of images in a second or less and is basically breathing independent (6–9).
4. A modification of spin echo imaging termed *rapid acquisition with relaxation* (RARE) acquires several lines of data per repetition time (TR) interval, which decreases imaging time for spin echo studies by approximately fourfold (10–12). This time saving can be translated into higher spatial resolution, faster imaging, or both.

G. A. Laub: MR Research, Siemens Medical Systems, Iselin, New Jersey 08830.

R. C. Semelka: Department of Radiology and Magnetic Resonance Services, University of North Carolina at Chapel Hill, Chapel Hill, North Carolina 27599.

FREQUENCY-SELECTIVE FAT SUPPRESSION

This technique relies on the inherent frequency shift of fat and water protons. Although frequency shift in Hertz increases with field strength, this technique can be used on midfield (0.5T) MR systems. The basic design for this sequence uses a frequency-selective excitation pulse, which selectively excites protons at the frequency of fat. The created magnetization is immediately spoiled by a gradient pulse. A spin echo sequence then acquires data from only water protons. The sequence design is illustrated in Fig. 1.

The advantages of fatsat include (a) decrease in ghosting artifact, (b) removal of chemical shift artifact, (c) improvement of the dynamic range of signal intensities of intraabdominal tissues, and (d) increased conspicuity of enhancement with gadopentetate dimeglumine (Gd-DTPA) by removal of the competing high signal intensity of fat (2,3,13,14).

The major limitation of fat suppression using frequency-selective radiofrequency (RF) pulses is spatially inhomogeneous suppression of fat due to a variation of the main magnetic field within the imaging volume. The most critical factors to maximize uniformity of suppression are a good shim status of the magnetic field and

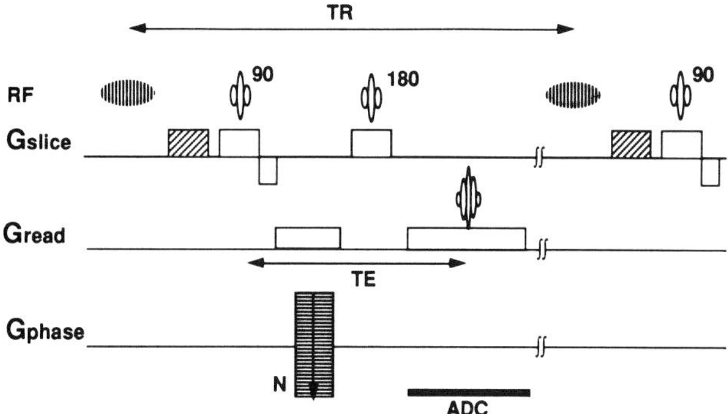

FIG. 1. Spin echo sequence with frequency selective preparation pulse for fat saturation. G, gradient; n, phase encoding steps; ADC, analog digital converter.

adjustment of the chemically selective excitation pulse to the spectral frequency of lipids (14). Currently, adjustment of the chemically selective pulse is routinely performed; however, shimming the main (Bo) magnetic field is not as commonly performed. Our practice is to optimize the homogeneity of the main magnetic field by manual adjustment of the shim currents on each patient. The base line shim currents, selected from a menu of shim settings, are specified to anatomical location and patient size (e.g., large liver). Certain factors, such as the presence of ferromagnetic surgical implants, disturb the homogeneity of the magnetic field and may make fat suppression unusable.

BREATH-HOLD IMAGING

Three general categories of fast imaging techniques are in common clinical practice: rapid acquisition spin echo (RASE) (4), spoiled gradient echo sequences [e.g., fast low-angle shot (FLASH) or spoiled GRASS] (5,15,16), and magnetization-prepared snapshot gradient echo (e.g., TurboFLASH) (5–8) techniques.

Rapid Acquisition Spin Echo

The RASE technique is a spin echo sequence that uses a 128 × 256 matrix and half Fourier data reconstruction to shorten data acquisition to a breath-hold period (4). A short echo time (TE) is recommended to maximize signal-to-noise ratio (SNR) and the number of sections acquired. Currently, an TE of 8 msec is achievable (5). The SNR of RASE is lower than that of FLASH, it acquires fewer sections per breath-hold, and it has lower spatial resolution (5). As spin echo sequences generally are much less sensitive to local magnetic field inhomogeneities, this technique would be most applicable in circumstances in which magnetic susceptibility may limit the quality of FLASH images (e.g., studies on patients with ferromagnetic surgical clips).

Fast Low-Angle Shot Technique

Our preferred breath-hold sequence is a FLASH technique. It has (a) good inherent SNR; (b) good spleen-liver contrast (good T1-weighting); (c) multislice acquisition permitting the acquisition of 14 sections in a 19-second breath-hold, which is sufficient to perform whole-organ coverage of liver or kidneys; (d) robust image quality; and (e) good spatial resolution (5,16). Figure 2 illustrates the sequence design of FLASH. Critical factors are the use of a high flip angle to maximize SNR and T1-weighting and a short TE (5,16). In our experience and that of Taupitz et al., 80° is an optimal flip angle (16). The shortest TE with fat and water in phase is also critical. A short TE maximizes the number of sections acquired per acquisition, maximizes SNR, and minimizes susceptibility artifacts. Our results and those of Taupitz et al. suggest that 4.5 msec is the optimal TE at 1.5T (5,16). At other field strengths fat and water are in phase at a different echo time. As an example, at 1.0T a TE of 6 msec is the first echo with fat and water in phase.

The advantage of a spoiled gradient echo technique is that images possess true T1-weighting. This is unlike nonspoiled techniques, such as FISP or gradient recalled acquisition at steady state (GRASS), which retain transverse magnetization and generate images with T1/T2* information (Fig. 3). For a given TR the SNR is higher for these sequences, but image contrast is generally less useful than with spoiled sequences because of the retention of T2* information. For example, liquid in a cystic structure, such as the bladder, is bright on FISP or GRASS images, rather than being dark as on T1-weighted spin echo or FLASH images. This results in confusing information, particularly when Gd-DTPA is also employed. A major advantage of the multisection FLASH sequence is the ability to acquire Gd-DTPA-enhanced images of an entire organ in a serial dynamic fashion.

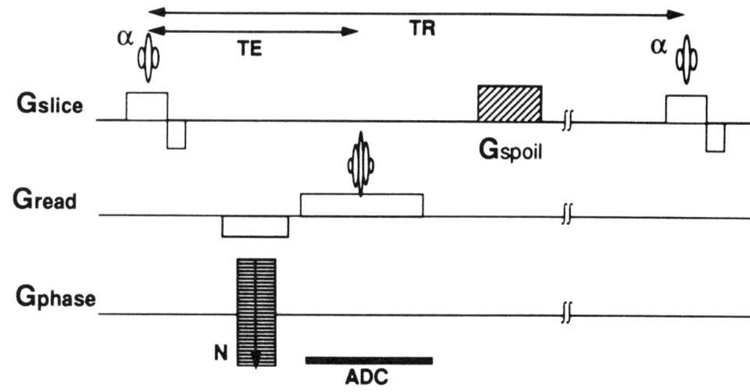

FIG. 2. Typical sequence diagram of a FLASH sequence. A spoiler pulse Gspoil (or RF spoiling) is used to destroy transverse magnetization before the application of the next RF pulse.

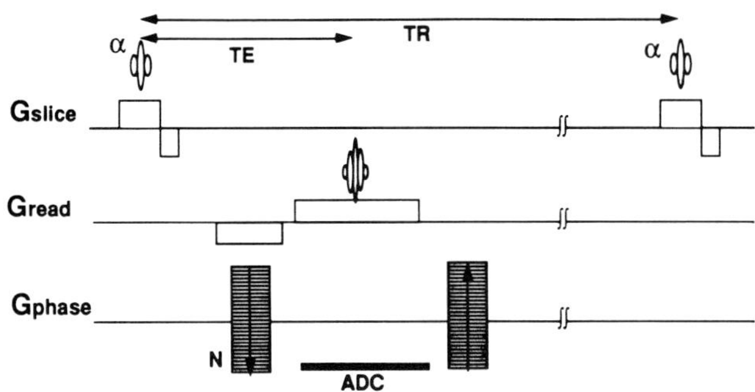

FIG. 3. Typical sequence diagram of an FISP sequence. Transverse magnetization is maintained by the application of a phase encode rewinder gradient.

Snapshot Gradient Echo

Magnetization-prepared snapshot gradient echo imaging (e.g., TurboFLASH) can acquire data within 1 second or less and generates images that are breathing independent (5–9). This technique is therefore ideal in patients who are noncooperative. The TurboFLASH technique consists of a two-step process: a preparation period that determines the contrast in the resulting images and an acquisition period that is used to acquire the raw data of the image. Spatial resolution is mostly determined by the number of lines used within the acquisition period. In most of the clinical applications of TurboFLASH, the preparation period involves a 180° inversion pulse followed by a variable wait time during which the magnetization recovers. In this case a T1-weighted image will be produced according to the amount of magnetization recovery, which depends on the T1 relaxation time. The data acquisition period consists of a series of gradient echoes (Fig. 4). Typically, pulse repetition times as short as 9 msec can be used; this will result in a data acquisition time of about 1 second for a 128 × 256 image matrix.

Problems with this technique are particularly related to T1 relaxation during the acquisition of the data. In other words, the longitudinal magnetization changes when scanning K-space, which has some effects on the resulting tissue contrast and also causes a lower spatial resolution. If rapid sequential section acquisition is performed with this technique, a variation of tissue SI is usually observed. This latter problem arises because the sequence is not in steady state and can be overcome with sufficient time between sections (approximately 3 seconds) to allow tissue relaxation. Modification of this technique such as three-dimensional (3D) data acquisition (17,18), reordering the phase encoding table (7), segmenting K-space (19), and combining reordered phase table and segmented K-space (20) have been performed to improve sequence performance.

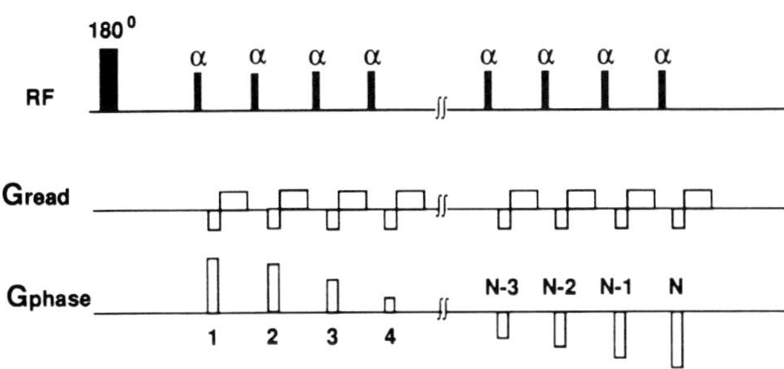

FIG. 4. TurboFLASH sequence diagram. A 180° pulse is used to create T1 contrast.

RAPID ACQUISITION WITH RELAXATION ENHANCEMENT

The recently developed RARE sequence has shown tremendous potential for examining the central nervous system (10–12) and the pelvis (21,22). The advantage of RARE is that it results in T2-weighted images with scan times up to 16 times faster than conventional spin echo (SE) sequences. This offers the possibility of acquiring T2-weighted SE images in a breath-hold. Alternatively, the shorter scan time can be used to acquire high-resolution abdominal images with multiple averages in several minutes. The basic idea of RARE is to create multiple echoes by using a series of 180° refocusing pulses. Each echo is phase encoded separately, which results in a faster scanning of K-space as compared to conventional spin echo imaging, where only one line in K-space is scanned per TR interval. The time savings depends on the number of echoes used per TR interval and is usually on the order of 4 to 16 echoes.

The advantage of RARE is that it is a T2-weighted sequence that results in a fourfold decrease in imaging time compared with regular spin echo. The underlying basis for the technique is the acquisition of multiple lines of data for each TR; these lines are combined into one image with an effective TE of the echo acquired at low spatial frequency (Fig. 5).

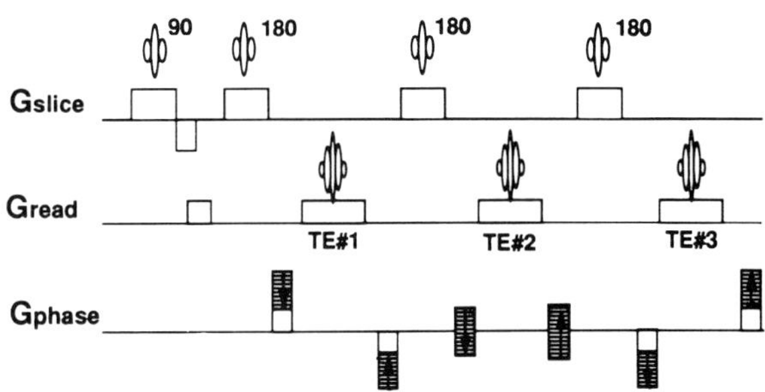

FIG. 5. Typical Turbo SE sequence diagram. Three echoes are used to scan K-space. Central Fourier lines will determine image contrast. In the case shown, central Fourier lines are measured by Echo #2.

One of the greatest advantages of RARE may be the ability to generate images of higher spatial resolution (512 × 512 matrix) compared to the usual matrix of 128 or 192 × 256. This permits the detection of smaller lesions. Increasing the number of lines of data sampled per TR interval reduces the length of the sequence to approximately 21 seconds for a 128 × 256 matrix, which permits data acquisition during a breath-hold period. The clinical usefulness of these modified techniques has not been evaluated.

Other minor modifications are useful to improve image quality. These include the use of superior and inferior saturation pulses to saturate the signal of flowing blood and a rectangular field of view (FOV).

SATURATION PULSES

Spatially selective saturation pulses improve the image quality of abdominal studies by removing the flow artifact created by the pulsatile motion of blood. The vessels targeted are the inferior vena cava (inferior saturation pulse) and the aorta (superior saturation pulse). As in the implementation of fat suppression, the sequence uses an additional RF pulse, which in this case is spatially selective instead of frequency selective. As a result, the number of slices that can be measured during one TR interval is reduced. This is of particular concern in breath-hold FLASH techniques where TR is limited (such that the scan time does not exceed typically 20 seconds). Therefore, this technique is generally recommended in combination with spin echo sequences. Whether to use saturation pulses with gradient echo sequences is a matter of preference. Edelman et al. advocated using saturation pulses on the FLASH sequence (15). In our opinion, however, the cost of using saturation pulses [which is the reduction of sections acquired per acquisition (in our case 14 sections are reduced to 7 sections)] is too great a sacrifice for the benefit. We consider the need to acquire images encompassing the entire liver in the capillary phase of enhancement too great to sacrifice the number of sections acquired. To use the liver as an example, if we need to exclude lesions from the left lobe of the liver we will follow the immediate postcontrast FLASH sequence with a FLASH sequence with frequency and phase encoding directions swapped to remove flow artifact from the left lobe (23).

RECTANGULAR FIELD OF VIEW

The size of a pixel is given by the length of the FOV divided by the number of pixels measured in this particular direction. There is a tradeoff in the choice of number of lines used in a sequence; a larger number of lines will improve the spatial resolution at the cost of scan time, which is given by TR multiplied by the number of lines. Likewise, a smaller number of lines will result in a shorter scan time at the cost of spatial resolution. The ability to have a different length of the FOV in read and phase encode directions provides a powerful tool in tailoring the sequence variables (number of lines, pixel size) to the anatomical needs. As the FOV is different in read and phase encode directions, it is referred to as *rectangular FOV*. On our system this can be stepped by 1/8 increments from 4/8 to full FOV. In practice 3/4 rectangular FOV generally conforms to the cross-sectional dimensions of most patients' abdomens while maintaining sufficient signal to noise ratio (SNR).

The application of rectangular FOV permits a decrease in study time with maintenance of spatial resolution. As SNR typically decreases with shorter scan times (assuming a constant pixel size), it is necessary to compromise between rectangular FOV and rectangular pixels. We apply a 128 × 256 measurement matrix with a 3/4 rectangular FOV. The relative pixel size for this case is 1.5 × 1.0, which means that the length of an individual pixel in the phase encode direction is 1.5 times larger than the length in readout direction. Because of the larger pixels, the SN is increased by 50%, which otherwise would require more than twice the scan time.

NEW DIRECTIONS

The future directions for MR of the abdomen lie in two basic areas: (a) faster data acquisition to improve spatial resolution, temporal resolution, or both and (b) organ- and/or tissue-specific contrast agents. Future directions for contrast agents will be discussed by organ system in the following chapters.

At present T1-weighted images have good spatial and temporal resolution with the FLASH sequence. Breath-hold T2-weighted images could benefit from considerable improvement. Echo planar imaging (EPI) produces reasonably good quality T2-weighted images in less than 1 second. EPI has stringent requirements on the gradient system and cannot be routinely used on standard MR systems (24–26). Modifications of imaging acquisition trains, such as combined gradient and spin echo RARE sequences (GRASE or FLARE) and other image train schemes, are currently being investigated to generate T2-weighted images in a breath-hold (27–30). Other necessary modifications are further improvements in magnetic field homogeneity and improved table incrementation to facilitate the study of larger volumes of tissue along the z-axis.

REFERENCES

1. Bailes DR, Gilderdale DJ, Bydder GM, Collins AG, Firmin DN. Respiratory ordered phase encoding (ROPE): a method for reducing respiratory motion artifacts in MR imaging. *J Comput Assist Tomogr* 1985;9:835–838.

2. Semelka RC, Chew W, Hricak H, Tomei E, Higgins CB. Fat saturation MR imaging of the abdomen. *AJR* 1990;155:1111–1116.
3. Mitchell DG, Vinitski S, Saponaro S, Tasciyan T, Burk DL Jr, Rifkin MD. Liver and pancreas: improved spin-echo T1 contrast by shorter echo time and fat suppression at 1.5T. *Radiology* 1991;178:67–71.
4. Mirowitz SA, Lee JKT, Brown JJ, Eilenberg SS, Heiken JP, Perman WH. Rapid acquisition spin-echo (RASE) MR imaging: a new technique for reduction of artifacts and acquisition time. *Radiology* 1990;175:131–135.
5. Semelka RC, Simm FC, Recht M, Deimling M, Lenz G, Laub GA. T1-weighted sequences for MR imaging of the liver—comparison of three techniques for single breath whole volume acquisition at 1.0T and 1.5T. *Radiology* 1991;180:629–635.
6. Haase A. Snapshot FLASH MRI: applications to T1, T2, and chemical-shift imaging. *Magn Reson Med* 1990;13:77–89.
7. Holsinger AE, Riederer SJ. The importance of phase encoding order in ultra-short TR snapshot MR imaging. *Magn Reson Med* 1990;16:481–488.
8. Holsinger-Bampton AE, Riederer SJ, Campeau NG, Ehman RL, Johnson CD. T1-weighted snapshot gradient-echo MR imaging of the abdomen. *Radiology* 1991;181:25–32.
9. Jakob PM, Haase A. Scan time reduction in snapshot FLASH MRI. *Magn Reson Med* 1992;24:392–396.
10. Hennig J, Naureth A, Friedburg H. RARE imaging: a fast imaging method for clinical MR. *Magn Reson Med* 1986;3:823–833.
11. Mulkern RV, Wong STS, Winalski C, Jolesz FA. Contrast manipulation and artifact assessment of 2D and 3D RARE sequences. *Magn Reson Imaging* 1990;8:557–566.
12. Jones KM, Mulkern RV, Mantello MT, et al. Brain hemorrhage: evaluation with fast spin-echo and conventional dual spin-echo images. *Radiology* 1992;182:53–58.
13. Semelka RC, Hricak H, Stevens SK, Finegold R, Tomei E, Carroll PR. Combined gadolinium-enhanced and fat saturation MR imaging of renal masses. *Radiology* 1991;178:803–809.
14. Semelka RC, Kroeker MA, Shoenut JP, Kroeker R, Yaffe CS, Micflikier AB. Pancreatic disease: prospective comparison of CT, ERCP, and 1.5T MR imaging with dynamic gadolinium enhancement and fat suppression. *Radiology* 1991;181:785–791.
15. Edelman RR, Siegel JB, Singer A, Dupuis K, Longmaid HE. Dynamic MR imaging of the liver with Gd-DTPA: initial clinical results. *AJR* 1989;153:1213–1219.
16. Taupitz M, Hamm B, Speidel A, Deimling M, Branding G, Wolf K-J. Multisection FLASH: method for breath-hold MR imaging of the entire liver. *Radiology* 1992;182:73–79
17. Mugler JP III, Brookeman JR. Three-dimensional magnetization-prepared rapid gradient-echo imaging (3D MP RAGe). *Magn Reson Med* 1990;15:152–157.
18. DeLange EE, Mugler JP III, Bertolina JA, Gay SB, Janus CL, Brookeman JR. Magnetization prepared rapid gradient-echo (MPRAGE) MR imaging of the liver: comparison with spin-echo imaging. *Magn Reson Imaging* 1991;9:469–476.
19. Edelman RR, Wallner B, Singer A, Atkinson DJ, Saini S. Segmented TurboFLASH: method for breath-hold MR imaging of the liver with flexible contrast. *Radiology* 1990;177:515–521.
20. Chien D, Atkinson DJ, Edelman RR. Strategies to improve contrast in TurboFLASH imaging: reordered phase encoding and K-space segmentation. *JMRI* 1991;1:63–70.
21. Smith RC, Reinhold C, Lange RC, McCauley TR, Kier R, McCarthy S. Comparison of conventional and fast spin-echo body coil MR imaging of the female pelvis. *Radiology* 1991;181(p):168.
22. Francis IR, Steiner RM, Herfkens RJ, Jain K, Glover GH. T2-weighted fast spin-echo MR imaging of the pelvis. *Radiology* 1991;181(p):169.
23. Silverman PM, Patt RH, Baum PA, Teitelbaum GP. Ghost artifact on gradient-echo imaging: a potential pitfall in hepatic imaging. *AJR* 1990;154:633–634.
24. Stehling MK, Howseman AM, Ordidge RJ, et al. Whole-body echo-planar MR imaging at O.5T. *Radiology* 1989;170:257–263.
25. Stehling MK, Charnley RM, Blamire AM, et al. Ultrafast magnetic resonance scanning of the liver with echo-planar imaging. *Br J Radiol* 1990;63:430–437.
26. Saini S, Stark DD, Rzedzian RR, Pykett IL, Rummeny E, Hahn PF, Wittenberg J, Ferrucci JT Jr. Forty-millisecond MR imaging of the abdomen at 2.0T. *Radiology* 1989;173:111–116.
27. Feinberg DA, Oshio K. GRASE (Gradient and spin-echo) MR imaging a new fast clinical imaging technique. *Radiology* 1991;181:597–602.
28. Oshio K, Feinberg DA. GRASE (Gradient and spin-echo) imaging: a novel fast MRI technique. *Magn Reson Med* 1991;20: 344–349.
29. Jones RA, Rinck PA. Snapshot imaging using a FLARE sequence. *Magn Reson Med* 1991;21:282–287.
30. Norris DG. Ultrafast low-angle RARE: U-FLARE. *Magn Reson Med* 1991;17:539–542.

CHAPTER 2

General Considerations for Conducting Abdominal Magnetic Resonance Imaging Examinations

Richard C. Semelka and J. Patrick Shoenut

The great variety of sequences available in modern MRI poses a daunting problem of which to use and of how many sequences are enough when performing an abdominal MR study. As a general principle it would seem prudent to limit abdominal studies to 1 hour and preferable to keep studies to approximately ½ hour of total magnet time. We limit examinations to ½ hour in the majority of studies by imaging one anatomical region or organ. In addition we use a standard protocol to study the majority of organs (1–5). We use T2-weighted sequences only when examining the liver (6). The essential sequences used are T1-weighted breath-hold FLASH, T1-weighted fat-suppressed spin echo (T1FS), and a T2-weighted sequence, usually fat-suppressed spin echo (T2FS). Additional or alternative sequences include T1-weighted TurboFLASH, T1-weighted RASE, and T2-weighted high-resolution RARE. Table 1 summarizes the imaging variables of these sequences as we use them. Our standard imaging protocol includes an initial T1-weighted FLASH sequence in the transverse plane. These images are used as a scout to center the organ of interest to the 0 position along the z-axis of the magnet. A shim current setting selected from the shim table is manually adjusted to maximize the homogeneity of the magnetic field for fat-suppressed sequences. The RF transmitter is then adjusted to ensure accurate selection of the lipid peak for the suppression scheme. T1-weighted fat suppression is then performed. If the liver is to be specifically studied, a T2-weighted sequence is performed as either T2-weighted fat suppression or high-resolution T2-weighted RARE. A repeat FLASH sequence of the liver may be needed if the region examined with the initial FLASH sequence did not include the entire liver. Gadopentetate dimeglumine is hand-injected as a bolus over a 5-second span with the patient positioned in the bore of the magnet. Normal saline is flushed through the line for 3 seconds. Imaging commences with a FLASH sequence concurrent with the completion of the normal saline flush, followed immediately by fat-suppressed T1-weighted spin echo at 40 seconds and a delayed FLASH at 10 minutes. If the presence of liver lesions is under investigation, a repeat FLASH sequence is added between the immediate postcontrast FLASH and the fat-suppressed spin echo sequences. Table 2 summarizes the imaging protocols used.

The majority of patients are able to cooperate with this imaging protocol; however, certain patients are unable to cooperate for a number of reasons. The major difficulty is the inability to suspend respiration during the 19-second breath-hold. Several options exist; if patients are cooperative but cannot suspend respiration for 19 seconds, then the FLASH sequence is modified (TR and/or phase encoding steps are reduced). If patients are uncooperative but sedate, substitution with a T1-weighted conventional, non-breath-hold spin echo is effective. If patients are uncooperative and agitated, a breathing-independent snapshot technique such as TurboFLASH may be useful.

Regarding T2-weighted sequences for studying the liver, our preferred method is to use T2-weighted fat-suppressed spin echo because chemical shift artifact

R. C. Semelka: Department of Radiology and Magnetic Resonance Services, University of North Carolina at Chapel Hill, Chapel Hill, North Carolina 27599.

J. P. Shoenut: University of Manitoba and Department of Medicine, Saint Boniface General Hospital, Winnipeg, Manitoba R2H 2A6.

TABLE 1. *MR imaging variables of 512 × 512 RARE, T2FS, RASE, TurboFLASH, FLASH and spin echo*

Variable	RARE	T2FS	RASE	TurboFLASH	FLASH	Spin echo
No. of sections	11	13	12	12	14	14
Section thickness (mm)	10	10	9.6	10.0	9.6	9.6
Intersection gap (%)	30	20	20	20	20	20
Matrix[a]	512 × 512	192 × 256	128 × 256[b]	128 × 128	128 × 256	192 × 256
FOV	350	350	350	350	350	350
Resolution (mm)	.7 × .7	2.1 × 1.4	2.7 × 1.4	2.7 × 2.7	2.7 × 1.4	2.1 × 1.4
TR (msec)	3500	2300	240	6.5[c]	130	500
Time between inversion pulses (sec)				1.13		
TE (effective) (msec)	90	70	8	3.5	4.5	15
Bandwidth (Hz/pixel)	78	78	195	355	355	130
Flip angle			90°	180° [d], 8°	80°	90°
No. of acquistions	3	2	1	1	1	4
No. echo[e]	3	1	1	1	1	1
Imaging time (sec)	516	668	22	15	19	288

[a] All sequences used 3/4 rectangular field of view.
[b] Half-Fourier reconstruction.
[c] Time between alpha pulses.
[d] 180° inversion flip angle with a nonselective inversion pulse and inversion time = 300 msec.
[e] Number of echoes combined to form one image.
FOV, field of view; TR, repetition time; TE, echo time; RARE, rapid acquisition with relaxation; T2FS, T2-weighted fat-suppressed spin echo; RASE, rapid acquisition spin echo; FLASH, fast low-angle shot.

(CSA) is removed and high-SI fat surrounding liver is attenuated. Both CSA and high-SI fat create problems for the detection of small subcapsular lesions, which fat suppression obviates (Fig. 1)(7,8). The drawbacks of fat suppression include the need for more experienced operators and the greater set-up time for the sequence because of the shimming involved. In many cases the added benefit of detection of a subcapsular lesion may not outweigh these drawbacks. High-resolution RARE has several attractive features including a matrix size (512 × 512) equivalent to computed tomographic images, minimal chemical shift, and low-SI blood vessels because gradient moment refocusing is not used (Fig. 2)(8).

Gd-DTPA is a nonspecific extracellular contrast agent that rapidly equilibrates in the interstitial space. There is a relatively rapid equilibration of contrast material in the interstitial space of focal lesions and surrounding normal tissue, which reduces lesion conspicuity. This occurs over a 1- to 2-minute period. Foley et al. described three phases of contrast enhancement in dynamic contrast-enhanced CT of the liver: the injection (perfusion) phase, the nonequilibrium phase, and the equilibrium phase (9,10). The initial images of dynamic contrast-enhanced CT are usually acquired in a mixed perfusion/early nonequilibrium phase. Image acquisition in the equilibrium phase results in decreased lesion detection on computed tomographic images, and the same is true of MR images. This explains why Gd-DTPA-enhanced conventional (3½-minute duration) T1-weighted spin echo is a poor sequence for liver lesion detection; the majority of data are acquired at 1 to 3 minutes, in the equilibrium phase. On serial dynamic Gd-DTPA-enhanced FLASH, it is possible to acquire images encompassing the entire liver in distinct phases of enhancement including the perfusion phase, the nonequilibrium phase, the equilibrium phase (interstitial phase), and the washout phase (6). The selection of sequence timing at 1 second, 45 seconds, 90 seconds, and 10 minutes postcontrast corresponds to these phases. The following features are used to deter-

TABLE 2. *Imaging protocols for the liver and other organs*

Liver	Liver and other organs[a]	Organ[a]
TurboFLASH	FLASH (organ)	FLASH
FLASH	T1FS (organ)	T1FS[b]
T2	FLASH (liver) Gd-DTPA	Gadolinium injection
Gadolinium injection	T2 (liver)	FLASH (1 sec)
FLASH (1 sec)	Gadolinium injection	T1FS (30 sec)
FLASH (45 sec)	FLASH (liver, 1 sec)	FLASH (10 min)
FLASH (90 sec)	FLASH (liver, 45 sec)	
FLASH (10 min)	T1FS (organ, 90 sec)	
	FLASH (liver and organ, 10 min)	

[a] Organ = pancreas, kidney, adrenal glands, or bowel.

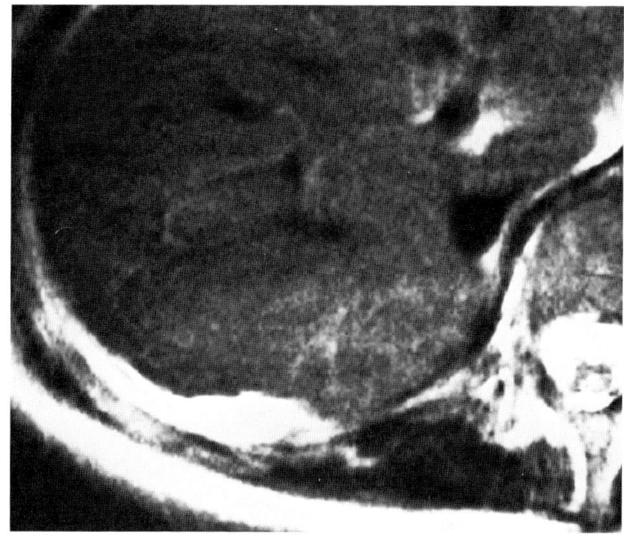
A

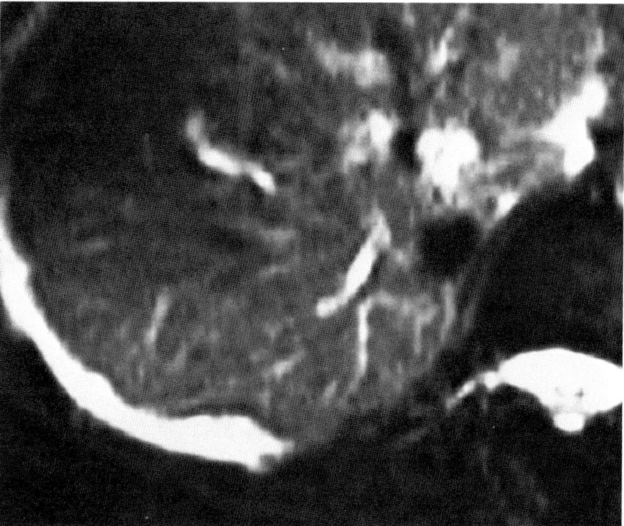
B

FIG. 1. Subcapsular metastases. T2 (512 × 512) RARE (**A**) and T2FS (**B**) images in a 64-year-old woman with subcapsular liver metastases from colon cancer. Subcapsular metastases are more conspicuous on the T2FS image because of the removal of the competing high SI of fat. Reprinted with permission from ref. 8.

mine the adequacy of timing of the perfusion phase images: (a) arciform enhancement of the spleen, (b) high corticomedullary difference of the kidneys, (c) enhancement of the pancreas (greater than background fat), and (d) enhancement of portal veins and lack of enhancement of hepatic veins (Fig. 3). This series of postcontrast images is useful for both detection and characterization of liver lesions. Other abdominal organs are usually best studied in either the perfusion or the interstitial phase of contrast enhancement rather than with a serial dynamic examination. Organs that may contain non-organ deforming lesions, such as the liver and the spleen, require imaging in the perfusion phase of enhancement (5,6). Imaging in the perfusion phase is helpful in kidney studies to assess the vascularity of mass lesions and the relative renal blood flow between kidneys. Dynamic imaging is important when imaging the pancreas in cases of islet cell tumors, may be important is assessing necrosis in acute pancreatitis or fibrosis in chronic pancreatitis, and is occasionally helpful for accentuating pancreatic adenocarcinoma. Imaging in the interstitial phase of enhancement is helpful to detect presence of disease in thin-walled viscera. The small and large bowel, gallbladder, and bile ducts are examples (3,4). They are best examined in the interstitial phase to allow Gd-DTPA to accumulate in the interstitial space. This permits im-

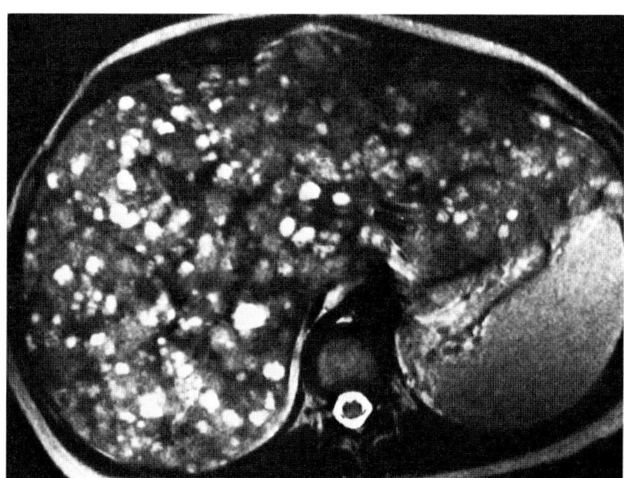
A

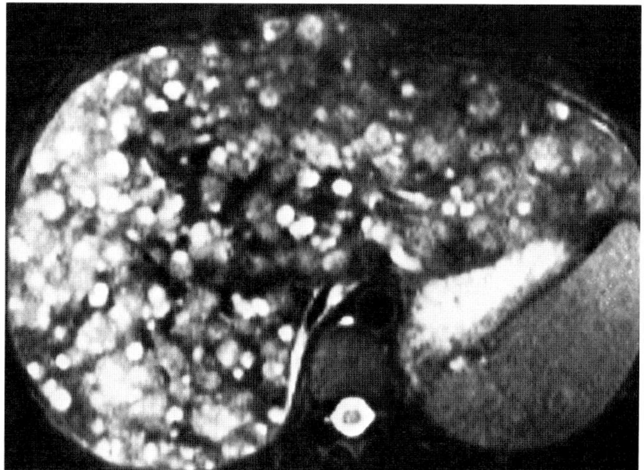
B

FIG. 2. Liver metastases. T2FS (**A**) and T2 (512 × 512) RARE (**B**) images in a 33-year-old woman with liver metastases from gastrinoma. Good image quality is apparent in both images. The high resolution of the RARE image provides greater lesion sharpness than does the T2FS image. Reprinted with permission from ref. 8.

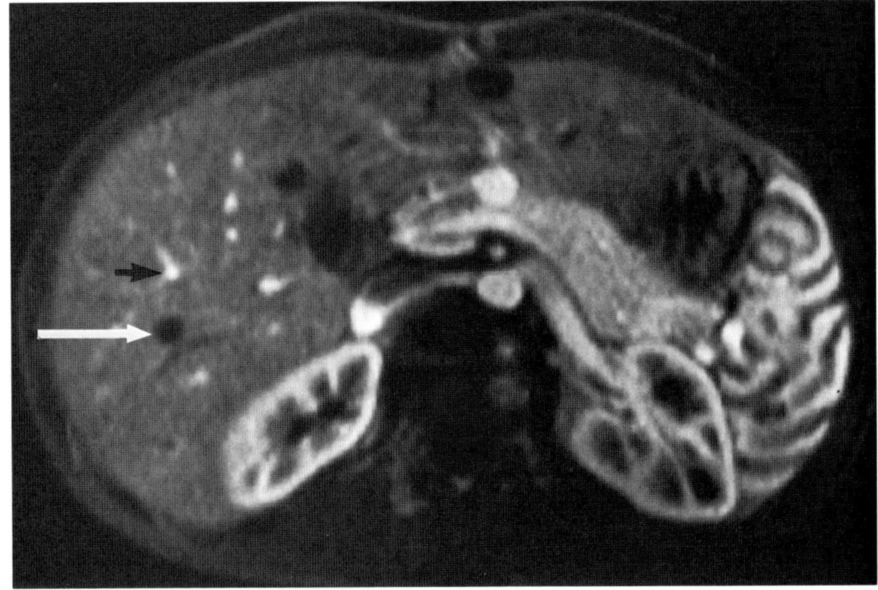

FIG. 3. Normal abdomen, perfusion phase of enhancement. The following features are present: arciform enhancement of the spleen, high corticomedullary difference of the kidneys, enhancement of the pancreas greater than that of the background fat, and enhancement of portal veins (*black arrow*) and lack of enhancement of hepatic veins (*white arrow*).

proved conspicuity of diseased tissue. In these hollow viscera it is often essential to combine fat suppression with Gd-DTPA enhancement to improve the conspicuity of increased enhancement by removing the competing high SI of adjacent fat. The interstitial phase of enhancement is also important for the investigation of renal mass lesions because accumulation of Gd-DTPA in the tubules of renal cortex is greater and more uniform than in the interstitial space of renal tumors. Table 3 summarizes the phases of contrast enhancement that provide the most diagnostic information for various abdominal organs.

COMPUTED TOMOGRAPHIC TECHNIQUE

The CT technique commonly used employs dynamic intravenous 60% iodinated contrast administration in combination with oral administration of a dilute iodinated or barium solution with images acquired during rapid contiguous table incrementation (5,6). The typical volume of intravenous contrast material is 150 ml, which we administer at a rate of 2 ml/sec for 25 seconds and 1 ml/sec for 100 seconds as a dynamic biphasic machine-powered injection. As recommended by Foley, scanning is initiated 45 seconds after the start of contrast administration (9,10). This basic technique is used for all abdominal studies. Section thickness and the timing of administration of oral contrast agent are varied depending on the region examined. CT is limited by the large volume of intravenous contrast agent administered and the relatively long period necessary to acquire a full data volume. A 2-second scan time with a 6-second interscan delay on modern third generation CT scanners requires about 2 minutes to image the entire liver with 1-cm contiguous incremental CT sections. Disagreement exists as to the optimal contrast administration technique because of the timing difficulty (monophasic or biphasic), the rate of administration, and controversy over when to initiate scanning in relation to contrast injection (11). A major strength of CT is the use of an oral contrast agent, which provides uniform enhancement of bowel. A typical volume of oral contrast agent is 500 to 1,000 ml, and the timing of administration depends on what segment of the bowel requires optimal opacification.

TABLE 3. *Phase of contrast enhancement essential to study abdominal organs*

Dynamic enhancement	Interstitial enhancement	Dynamic and interstitial enhancement
Liver	Bowel	Kidneys
Spleen	Gallbladder	Adrenals (?)
Pancreas	Bile ducts	
(islet cell tumors)		

COMPUTED TOMOGRAPHY VS MAGNETIC RESONANCE IMAGING

Advantages of CT over MRI include greater spatial resolution, uninterrupted contiguous incremental image acquisition encompassing large imaging volumes (i.e., the abdomen and pelvis), short scanning time of individual sections, consistent image quality, and an oral contrast agent with uniform appearance throughout all segments of bowel (12).

Advantages of MRI over CT include a safer imaging procedure, a safer contrast agent (Gd-DTPA), higher conspicuity for the presence or absence of contrast enhancement, higher whole-volume temporal resolution for Gd-DTPA-enhanced studies (using a FLASH sequence), and higher contrast resolution (using a Gd-DTPA-enhanced fat-suppressed spin echo sequence) (1–6). MR cannot replace CT as a technique for general screening of the entire abdomen at present. MRI is superior to CT in imaging studies limited to specific organ systems such as the liver, spleen, pancreas, and kidneys. MRI is approximately equivalent to CT in evaluating the adrenal glands but has a limitation in achieving uniform fat suppression due to the close proximity of the adrenal glands to the lungs. The substantial magnetic susceptibility differences between lung and abdomen in the same shimming volume make accurate shimming difficult in this location. MRI is probably superior to CT in evaluating inflammatory bowel disease (IBD) (3). The ability of MRI to image other types of bowel abnormalities is currently under investigation. The role and the type (positive or negative) of oral contrast agents used in MR studies have yet to be established.

REFERENCES

1. Semelka RC, Shoenut JP, Kroeker MA, MacMahon RG, Greenberg HM. Renal lesions: controlled comparison between CT and 1.5T MR imaging with nonenhanced and gadolinium-enhanced fat-suppressed spin-echo and breath-hold FLASH techniques. *Radiology* 1992;182:425–430.
2. Semelka RC, Kroeker MA, Shoenut JP, Kroeker R, Yaffe CS, Micflikier AB. Pancreatic disease: prospective comparison of CT, ERCP, and 1.5T MR imaging with dynamic gadolinium enhancement and fat suppression. *Radiology* 1991;181:785–791.
3. Semelka RC, Shoenut JP, Silverman R, Kroeker MA, Yaffe CS, Micflikier AB. Bowel disease: prospective comparison of CT and 1.5T pre and postcontrast MR imaging with T1-weighted fat-suppressed and breath-hold FLASH sequences. *JMRI* 1991; 1:625–623.
4. Semelka RC, Shoenut JP, Kroeker MA, Hricak H, Minuk GY, Yaffe CS, Micflikier AB. Bile duct disease: prospective comparison of ERCP, CT, and 1.5T MRI using pre and post contrast breath-hold FLASH and fat suppression. *Gastrointest Radiol* 1992; 17:347–352.
5. Semelka RC, Shoenut JP, Lawrence PH, Greenberg HM, Madden TP, Kroeker MA. Spleen: dynamic enhancement patterns on gradient-echo MR images enhanced with gadopentetate dimeglumine. *Radiology* 1992;185:479–482.
6. Semelka RC, Shoenut JP, Kroeker MA, Greenberg HM, Simm FC, Minuk GY, Kroeker R, Micflikier AB. Focal liver disease: comparison of dynamic contrast-enhanced CT and T2-weighted fat-suppressed, FLASH, and dynamic gadolinium-enhanced MR imaging at 1.5T. *Radiology* 1992;184:687–694.
7. Semelka RC, Hricak H, Bis KG, Werthmuller WC, Higgins CB. Liver lesion detection: comparison between excitation-spoiling fat suppression and regular spin echo at 1.5T. *Abdom Imaging* 1993;18:56–60.
8. Semelka RC, Shoenut JP, Kroeker RM. T2-weighted imaging of focal hepatic lesions: a comparison of variations of RARE sequence and fat-suppressed conventional spin echo. *JMRI* (*in press*).
9. Foley WD. Dynamic hepatic CT. *Radiology* 1989;170:617–622.
10. Foley WD, Berland LL, Lawson TL, Smith DF, Thorsen MK. Contrast enhancement technique for dynamic hepatic computed tomographic scanning. *Radiology* 1983;147:797–803.
11. Walkey MM. Dynamic hepatic CT: how many years will it take 'til we learn? *Radiology* 1991;181:17–24.
12. Chezmar JL, Rumanicik WM, Megibow AJ, Hulnick DH, Nelson RC, Bernardino ME. Liver and abdominal screening in patients with cancer: CT versus MR imaging. *Radiology* 1988;168:43–47.

CHAPTER 3

The Liver

Richard C. Semelka, J. Patrick Shoenut, Howard M. Greenberg, and Allan B. Micflikier

NORMAL ANATOMY

The liver, the largest organ in the abdomen, is divided into right and left hepatic lobes, each of which comprises two segments. The right lobe is divided into anterior and posterior segments, and the left lobe is divided into medial and lateral segments. The caudate lobe is a separate, smaller lobe that derives its arterial supply from both the right and the left hepatic arteries and has venous drainage directly into the inferior vena cava.

The separation into right and left lobes is defined by the middle hepatic vein superiorly and by the gallbladder fossa inferiorly. The division of the right lobe into anterior and posterior segments is defined by the right hepatic vein. The division of the left lobe into medial and lateral segments is defined superiorly by the left hepatic vein and inferiorly by the fissure for the ligamentum teres.

A more recent nomenclature (1) divides the liver into segments based on portal venous supply and hepatic venous drainage. This technique is a classification refinement introducing a plane to create superior and inferior subsegments of the anterior and posterior segments of the right lobe defined by the right portal vein and another plane to create anterior and posterior subsegments of the lateral segments of left lobe defined by the left hepatic vein.

R. C. Semelka: Department of Radiology and Magnetic Resonance Services, University of North Carolina at Chapel Hill, Chapel Hill, North Carolina 27599.

J. P. Shoenut: University of Manitoba and Department of Medicine, Saint Boniface General Hospital, Winnipeg, Manitoba R2H 2A6.

H. M. Greenberg: Department of Radiology, University of Manitoba, Winnipeg, Manitoba R2H 2A6.

A. B. Micflikier: Department of Medicine, University of Manitoba, Winnipeg, Manitoba R2H 2A6.

The liver contains three fissures: (a) the interlobar fissure, (b) the fissure for the ligamentum teres (left intersegmental fissure), and (c) the fissure for the ligamentum venosum. The interlobar fissure is an incomplete fissure, occasionally identified on lower tomographic sections of the liver situated in the plane of cleavage defined by the gallbladder fossa. The fissure for the ligamentum teres has a vertical orientation and contains the ligamentum teres which is a continuation of the falciform ligament. The fissure for the ligamentum venosum has a transverse orientation and is present at the level of contact between the lateral segment of the left lobe and the caudate lobe.

The vascular anatomy of the liver includes the hepatic arterial system, the portal venous system, and the hepatic venous system. Intrahepatic portal triads include branches of the portal vein, hepatic arteries, and bile ducts. Those structures are situated in the central portion of lobes and segments. Hepatic veins are located between segments and are not accompanied by other structures. Figure 1 illustrates anatomical landmarks in the normal liver. The anatomy of the biliary tree and gallbladder is described in Chapter 4.

MR TECHNIQUE

The essential sequences used to image the liver are T1-weighted sequences, T2-weighted sequences (for lesion detection), and dynamic serial post-Gd-DTPA-enhanced images (for lesion characterization) (2). The FLASH sequence is optimal as a T1-weighted sequence and is also used for serial postcontrast images (2–6). Additional sequences that may be useful are out-of-phase FLASH images (to detect fatty liver) and Gd-DTPA-enhanced fat-suppressed images (to evaluate the biliary tree). Adequate T1-weighting on MR images can be assessed by comparing the signal intensities of the liver and

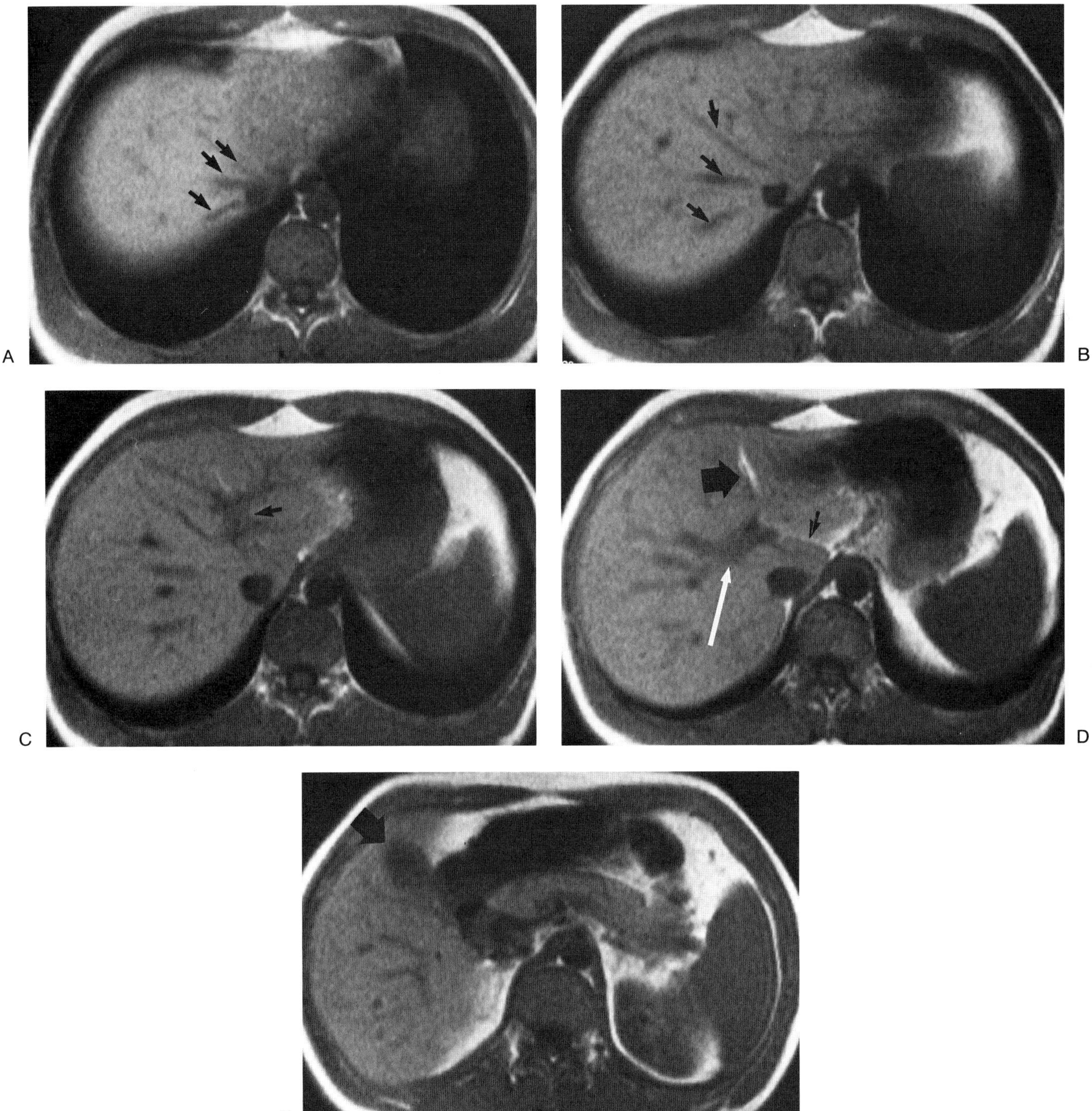

FIG. 1. Anatomical landmarks of the normal liver from cranial to caudal sections. In the superior aspect of the liver, the right, middle, and left hepatic veins (*arrows*) enter the inferior vena cava (**A,B**). The left portal vein (*arrow*) is apparent on a more caudal section (**C**). Immediately inferior, the fissure for the ligamentum teres (*large arrow*), the fissure for the ligamentum venosum (*black arrow*), and the right portal vein (*white arrow*) are identified (**D**). More inferiorly, the gallbladder (*large arrow*, **E**) is identified; it lies in the fossa between the right and left hepatic lobes.

spleen; the liver should be relatively bright and the spleen relatively dark. On T2-weighted images adequate T2-weighting is determined by the presence of a relatively bright spleen and a relatively dark liver. This rule is effective only if there is no iron deposition in the reticuloendothelial system. Iron deposition lowers the signal intensities of spleen and liver, with the SI of the spleen usually affected to a greater extent.

DISEASES OF THE HEPATIC PARENCHYMA

Benign Mass Lesions

Cysts

Hepatic cysts are common lesions and are frequently multiple. Most simple cysts are congenital and are believed to arise from aberrant bile ducts or congenital obstruction caused by inflammatory hyperplasia. Cysts are more frequently found in female patients, with a relative incidence of 4:1. Cysts are homogeneous, well-defined lesions showing a sharp margin with liver and are usually oval, although slight variations are common (7). Occasionally, cysts are so closely grouped that they resemble a multicystic mass. Because cysts have long T1 and T2 values, they are low in SI on T1-weighted images and high in SI on T2-weighted images and they retain SI on longer TE (e.g., 120 msec) T2-weighted images. Cysts do not enhance with Gd-DTPA on MR images (Fig. 2). In some circumstances images must be acquired up to 10 minutes after intravenous contrast administration to ensure that lesions are cysts and not poorly vascularized metastases, which show gradual enhancement (Fig. 3). An advantage of MRI over CT in the characterization of cysts is that on Gd-DTPA-enhanced MR images, cysts

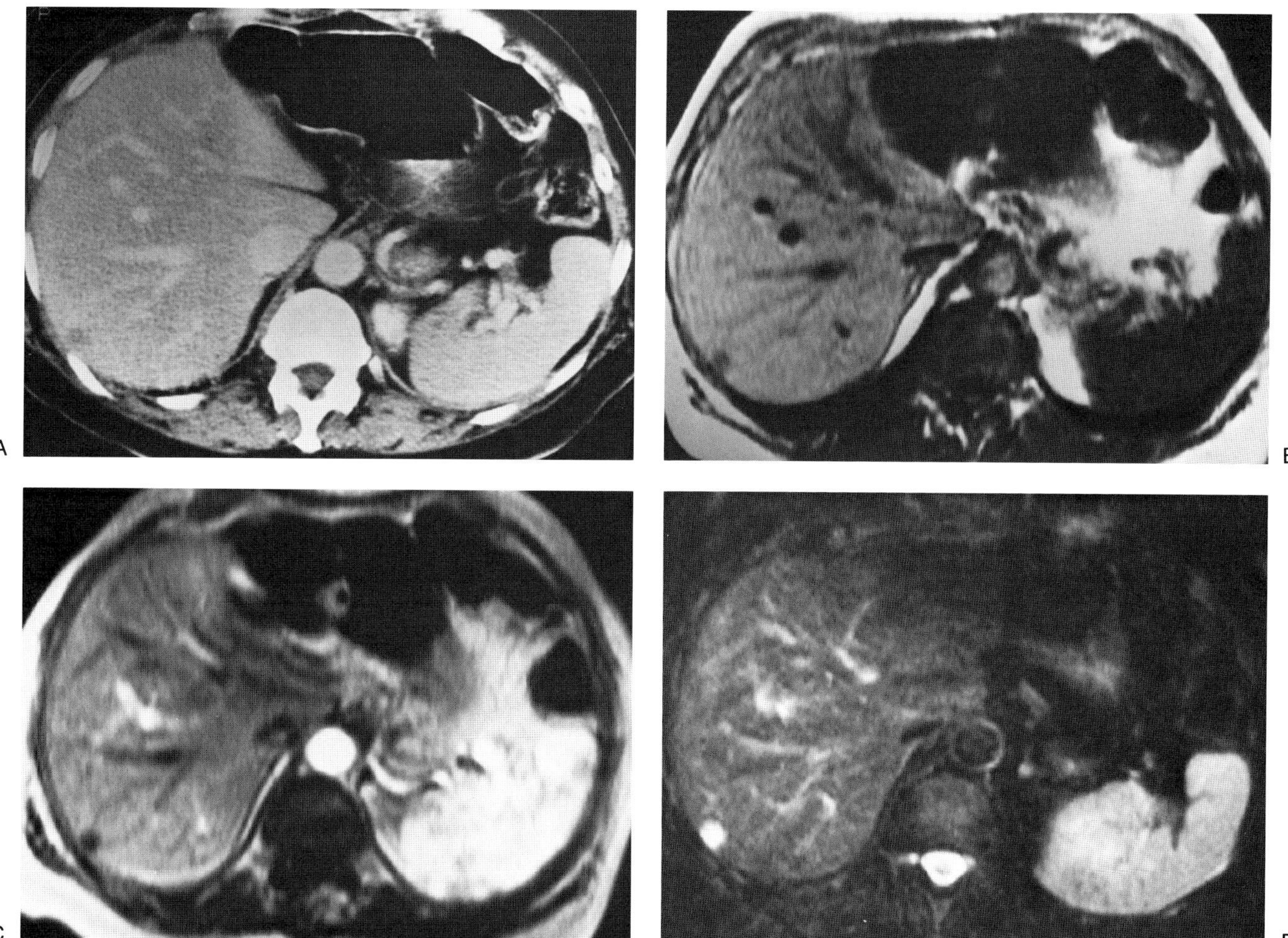

FIG. 2. Liver cyst. Dynamic contrast-enhanced CT (**A**), FLASH (**B**), 1-second postcontrast FLASH (**C**), and T2FS (**D**) images show a 6-mm liver cyst in the posterior segment of the right lobe in a 69-year-old woman. The greatest conspicuity of this lesion is on the T2FS image. The Gd-DTPA-enhanced FLASH image most reliably characterizes the lesion as cystic by the signal void and the sharp margin. Reprinted with permission from ref. 2.

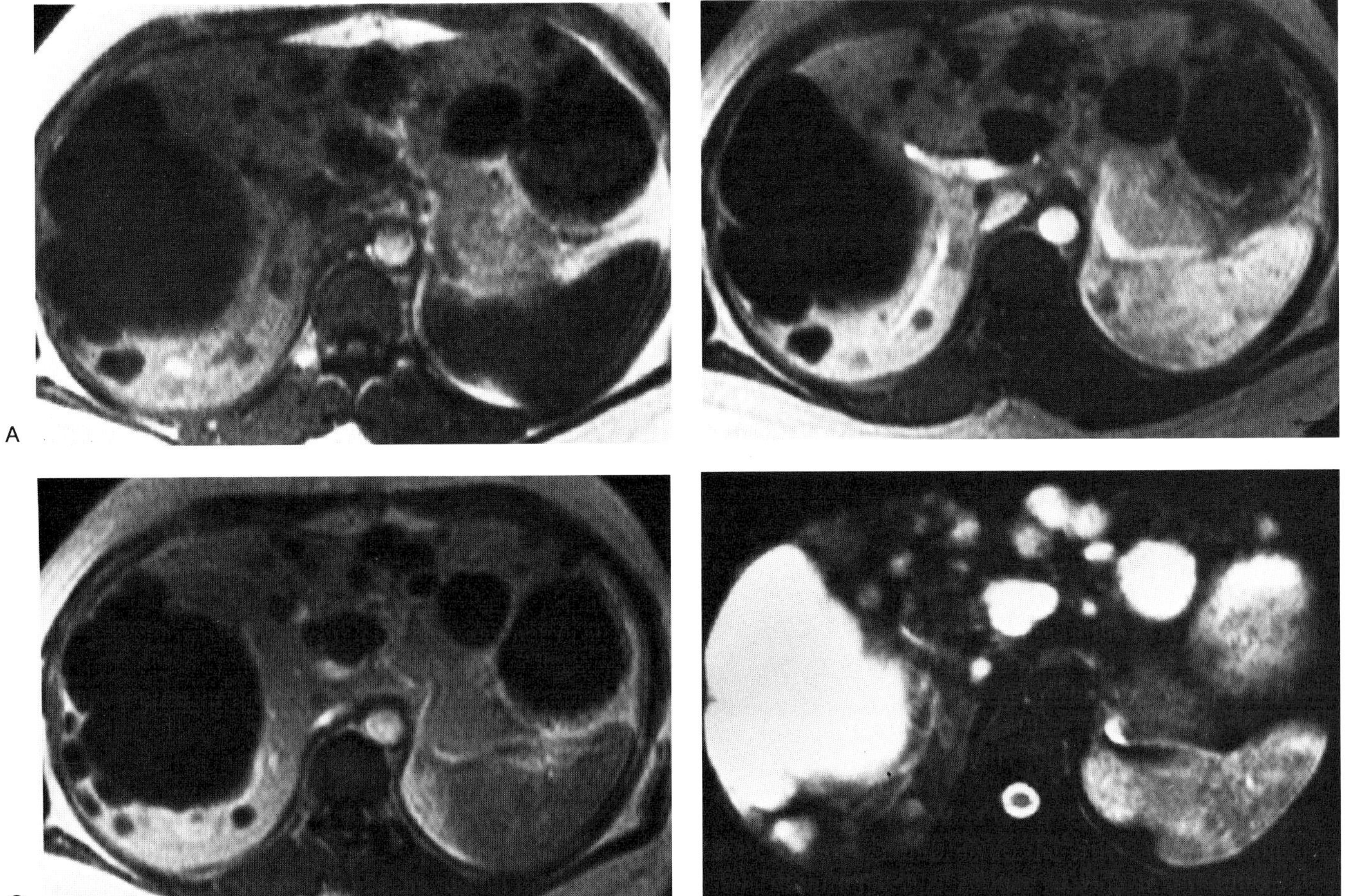

FIG. 3. Multiple liver cysts. FLASH (**A**), 1-second postcontrast FLASH (**B**), 10-minute postcontrast FLASH (**C**), and T2FS (**D**) images show multiple liver cysts in a 34-year-old woman. Multiple lesions are present throughout all segments of the liver. The lack of contrast enhancement and the lack of change in size or shape of all liver lesions on later postcontrast images confirm that these lesions are cysts.

are signal void (virtually black), whereas cysts on contrast-enhanced CT images are a light gray in attenuation. MRI is particularly valuable when lesions are small and the patient has a known primary malignant neoplasm.

Foregut cysts are rare congenital cysts with a pathognomonic MRI appearance. Foregut cysts are located at the anterosuperior margin of the liver and are iso- or hyperintense on T1-weighted and hyperintense on T2-weighted images and do not enhance with Gd-DTPA (8) (Fig. 4).

Hemangiomas

Hemangiomas rarely manifest clinically and are usually detected in the investigation of other disease (9). Hemangiomas are more frequent in female patients. The great majority of these lesions are cavernous hemangiomas, but rarely they may be capillary. Hemangiomas have long T1 and T2 values so they are low in SI on T1-weighted images and high in SI on T2-weighted images, with maintenance of SI on longer TEs (e.g., 120 msec) (10,11). Hemangiomas have a well-defined lobular border with liver (10,11). Hemangiomas typically enhance in a peripheral globular fashion on dynamic serial contrast-enhanced CT or MR images, with slowly progressive complete or nearly complete fill-in of the entire lesion at 10 minutes (Fig. 5)(12,13).

A globular enhancement pattern is the most characteristic of the enhancement features (14). Large "giant" hemangiomas frequently have central scars that do not enhance (Fig. 6). Choi et al. reported on 10 patients with giant hemangiomas. All of the tumors had a central region of nonenhancement consistent with a central scar on delayed contrast-enhanced CT images (15). Another variation in enhancement pattern seen in hemangiomas is that contrast enhancement may spread at a fairly rapid rate; complete enhancement may occur at 1 to 2 minutes. Very small lesions (<1 cm) may enhance completely on initial postcontrast images; in these circum-

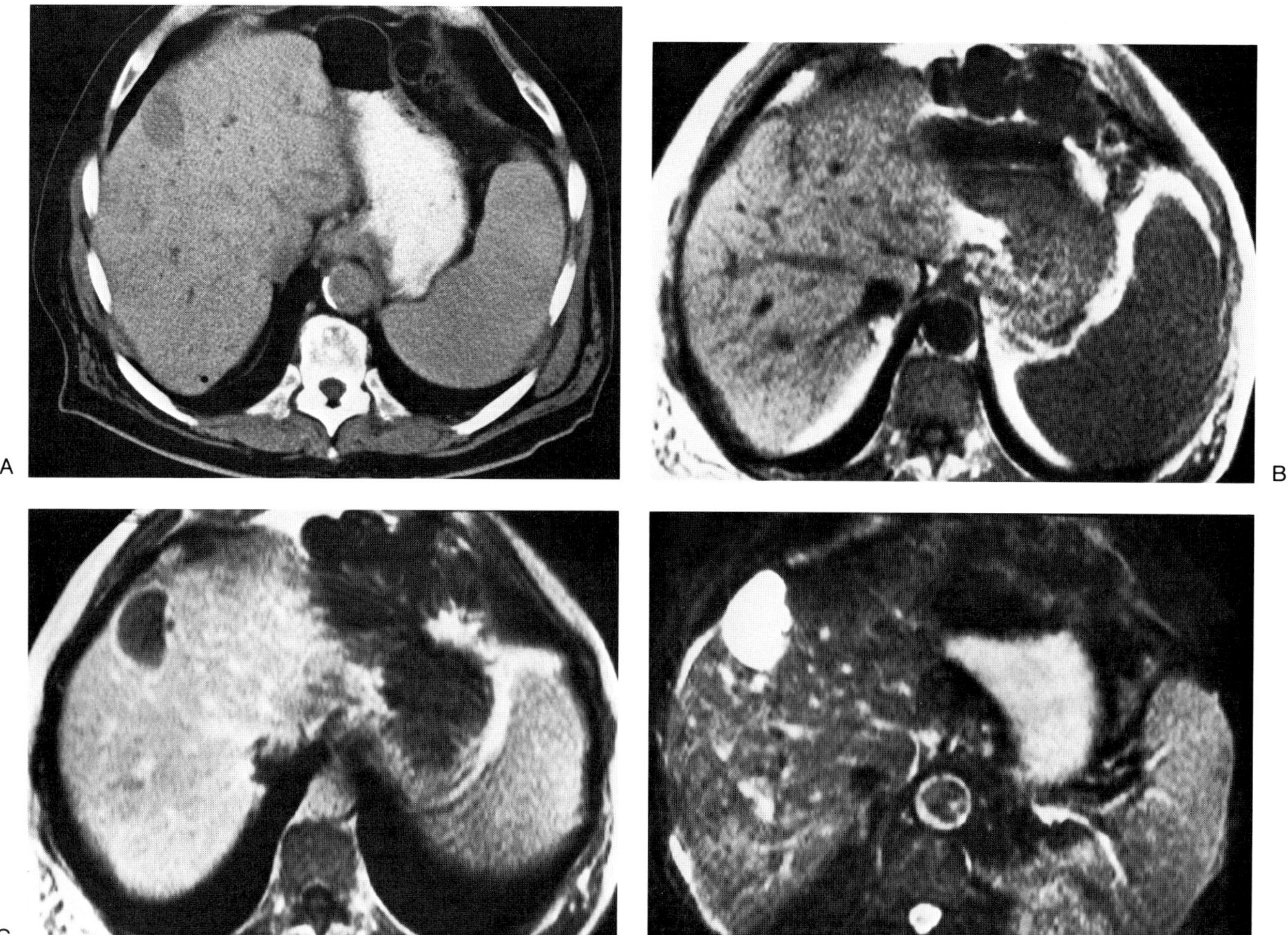

FIG. 4. Intrahepatic foregut cyst. Contrast-enhanced CT (**A**), FLASH (**B**), 90-second Gd-DTPA-enhanced FLASH (**C**), and T2FS (**D**) images of a 76-year-old man with a foregut cyst. The typical location at the anterosuperior margin of the liver, the isointense SI of the lesion on the FLASH image, and the lack of contrast enhancement are pathognomonic features. Enhancement of the wall of the cyst is apparent on the Gd-DTPA-enhanced image (C).

stances the observation that these lesions are very high in SI on T2-weighted images provides complementary information.

Advantages of MRI over CT in the evaluation of hemangiomas include (a) the ability to image the entire liver in the same phase of contrast enhancement, which is helpful when multiple lesions are present, and (b) higher contrast resolution such that lesions are comparatively brighter in surrounding liver than in comparable CT images (Fig. 5).

Hepatic Adenomas/Focal Nodular Hyperplasia

Most hepatic adenomas (90%) are found in young adult women (16,17). These lesions have a strong association with the use of birth control pills. Adenomas are derived from hepatocytes. Adenomas usually are homogeneous lesions, which may on occasion undergo central necrosis when the tumor is large. These tumors do not possess a true capsule, but a pseudocapsule of compressed normal liver is not uncommon. Adenomas may hemorrhage in up to 50% of cases, and a malignant potential is present (17). In an uncommon entity, adenomatosis, more than ten adenomas are present. This condition is not related to the use of birth control pills and has a higher incidence of hemorrhage and malignant transformation (17).

Focal nodular hyperplasia (FNH) is frequently found in adult women; however, 10% to 20% of these cases occur in men (17). The origin of FNH is unknown, but a vascular malformation is suspected. FNH frequently possesses a central scar and is characterized by the presence of Kupffer cells, which are not present in adenomas. FNH is not related to the use of birth control pills. FNH does not seem to have malignant potential, and hemorrhage is very rare (17).

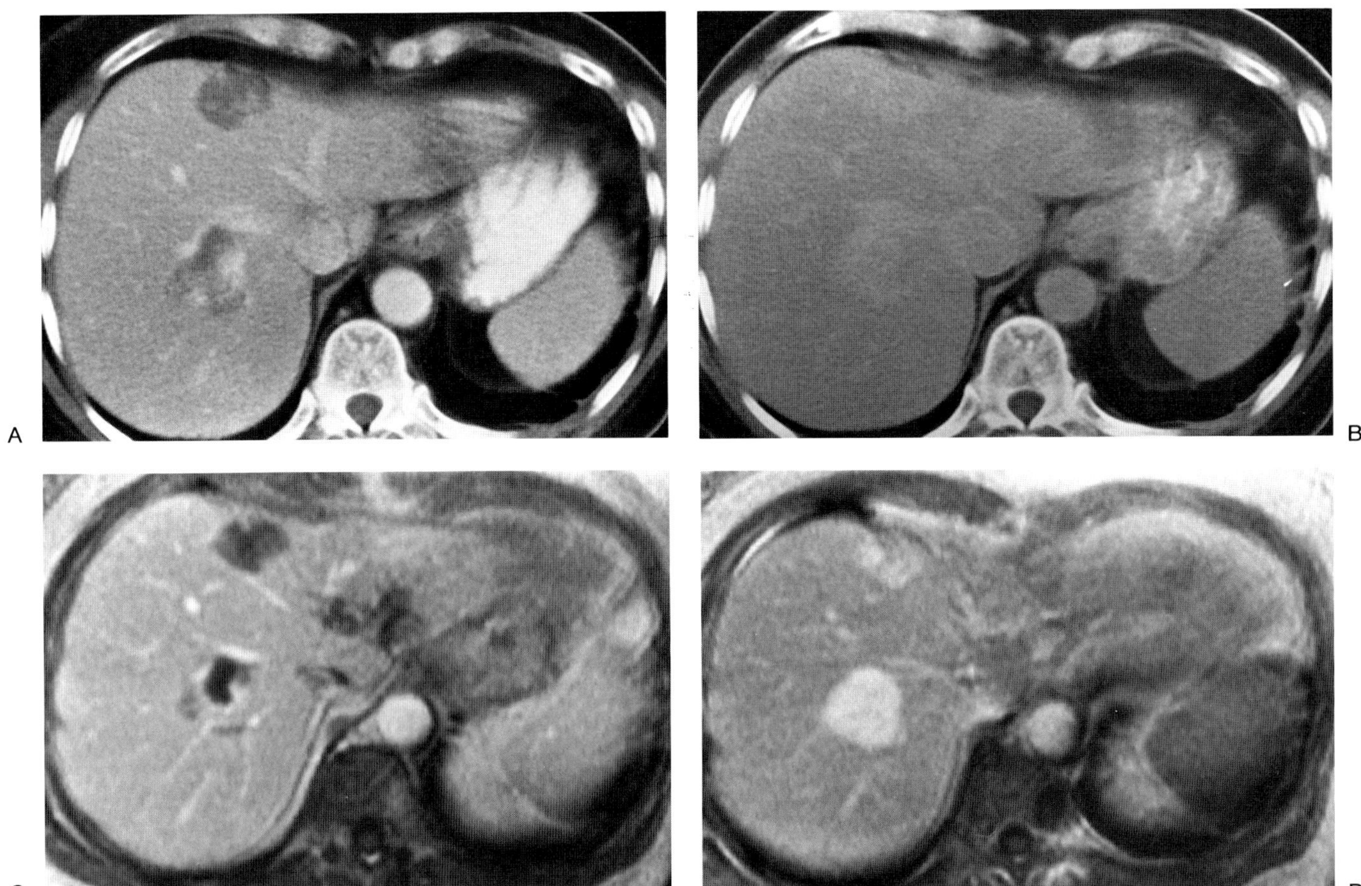

FIG. 5. Hemangioma. Forty-five-second (**A**) and 10-minute (**B**) contrast-enhanced CT and 45-second (**C**) and 10-minute (**D**) Gd-DTPA-enhanced FLASH (130/4.5/80°) images in a 65-year-old woman with two hemangiomas, one in the right lobe and the second in the medial segment of the left lobe of the liver. The peripheral fill-in pattern to a homogeneous, slightly hyperdense lesion is apparent on the CT images. Similar findings are apparent on MRI, in which low-SI lesions fill in to homogeneous high SI. Note the higher relative signal compared to liver of these lesions on the late MR images compared to CT images. Reprinted with permission from ref. 2.

There is variability in the SI of adenomas/FNH relative to liver on T1- and T2-weighted images, but these lesions consistently have a SI not much different from that of normal liver (18) (in distinction to the great difference observed between hemangiomas and liver on T2-weighted images). The most common pattern observed is slight hypointensity on T1-weighted images and slight hyperintensity on T2-weighted images (18). The pathognomonic feature of these lesions is that they have an intense uniform blush on immediate postcontrast images and fade to isointensity rapidly (typically at 45 seconds postcontrast) (19–21). The central scar may remain low in SI on the dynamic images, but delayed enhancement is typical. Figure 7 illustrates an example of an uncomplicated adenoma, and Fig. 8 illustrates FNH. The appearance of these lesions is similar.

Adenomas/FNH are on occasion isointense with liver on all sequences, including dynamic postcontrast images. Lesions identified on CT images as >2 cm hypodense masses which are isointense on all MR sequences are usually adenomas/FNH. There does not seem to be a consistent MR feature that permits distinction between adenomas and FNH. Although uncommon, the presence of a pseudocapsule and internal hemorrhage are features more in keeping with adenomas (Fig. 9), whereas a central scar is more suggestive of FNH. Vilgrain et al. reported on the MR appearance of 48 lesions of FNH in 37 patients (22). In 20 of these lesions, a central hyperintense scar was identified on T2-weighted images, whereas 7 lesions had a hypointense scar. The SI of the scar presumably reflects the age of the scar; scars of more recent origin have a higher SI. A pseudocapsule was also observed in six lesions. The presence of Kupffer cells in FNH and their absence in adenomas may suggest a role for iron oxide particulate contrast agent, which could distinguish these tumors on the basis of contrast uptake by FNH and not by adenomas, analogous to a scintigraphic technetium sulfur colloid study.

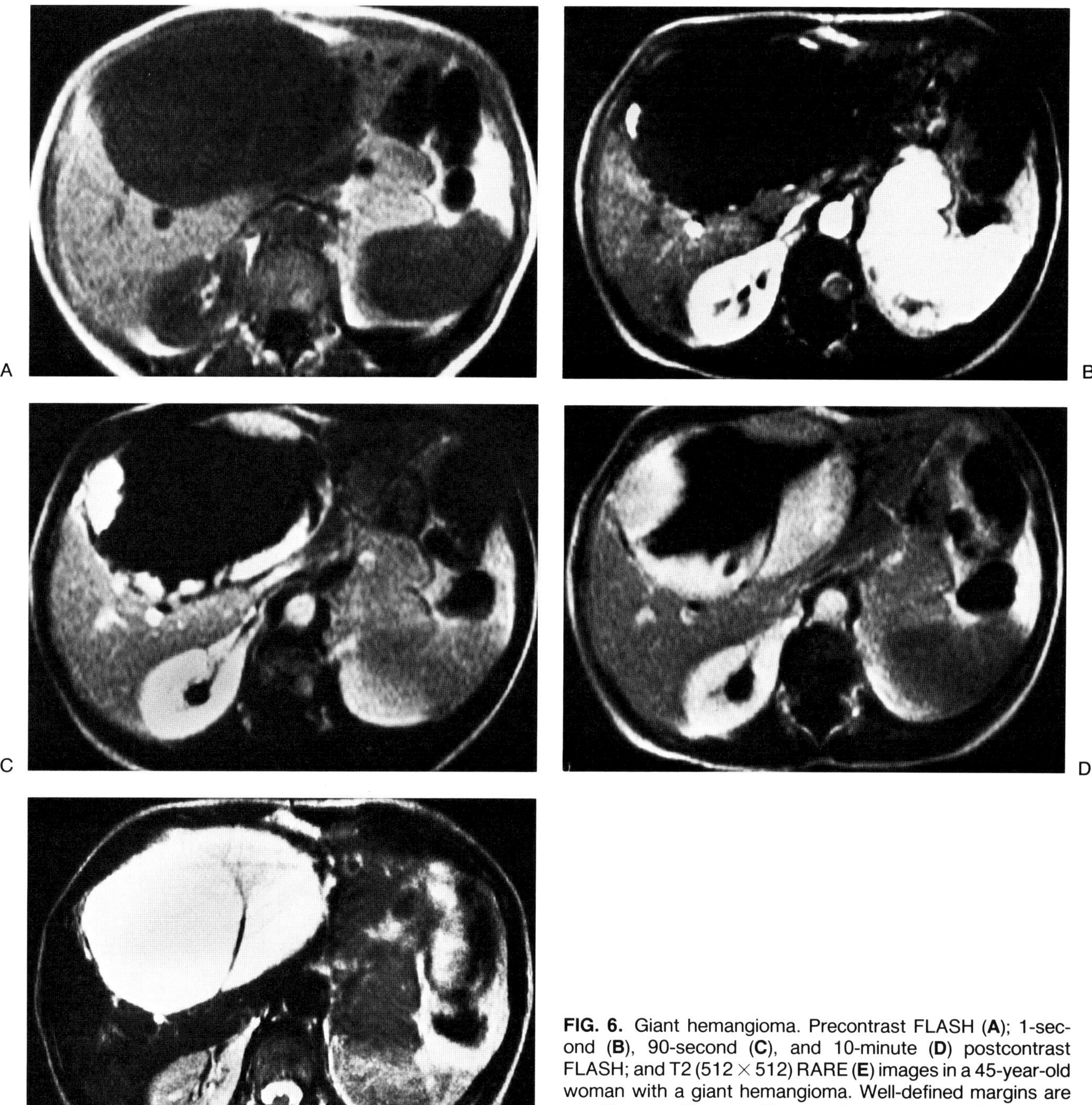

FIG. 6. Giant hemangioma. Precontrast FLASH (**A**); 1-second (**B**), 90-second (**C**), and 10-minute (**D**) postcontrast FLASH; and T2 (512 × 512) RARE (**E**) images in a 45-year-old woman with a giant hemangioma. Well-defined margins are identified on all images. The peripheral globular enhancement pattern confirms the diagnosis. The lack of complete enhancement at 10 minutes is typical for giant hemangiomas.

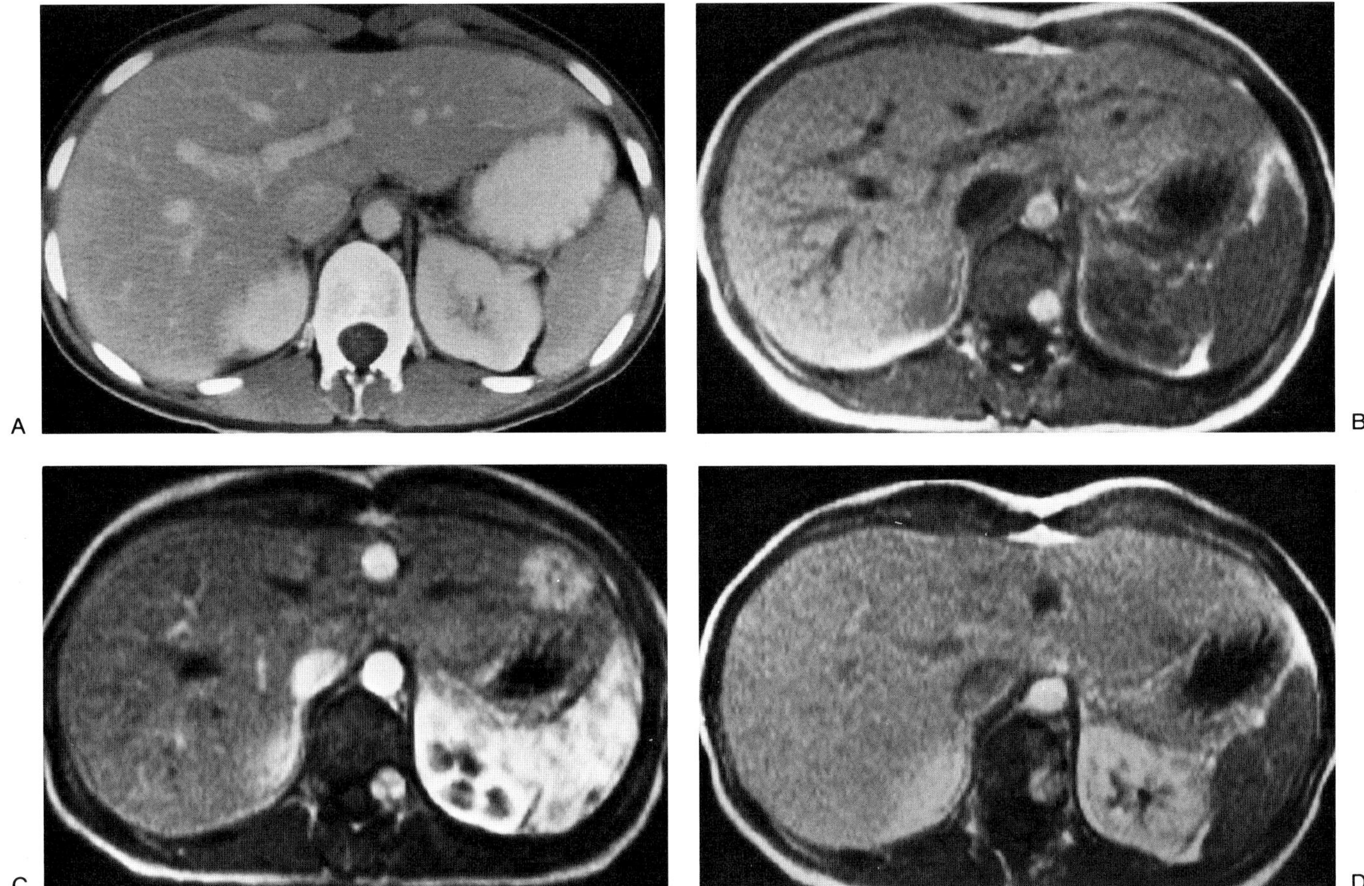

FIG. 7. Hepatic adenoma. Dynamic contrast-enhanced CT (**A**), FLASH (**B**), 1-second postcontrast FLASH (**C**), and 90-second postcontrast FLASH (**D**) images in a 27-year-old woman with biopsy-proven hepatic adenoma. A subtle, hypodense, 3-cm lesion is present in the lateral segment of the left lobe of the liver on the CT image (A), which is slightly more conspicuous on the precontrast FLASH image (B). The lesion exhibits transient, uniform high SI 1 second after contrast enhancement (C), which fades to isointensity on later images (D). Reprinted with permission from ref. 2.

Malignant Tumors

Liver Metastases

Liver metastases are the most common malignant lesions of the liver. A common indication for CT or MR examination of the liver is to exclude liver metastases in patients with a known primary malignancy. It is critical that imaging investigations both detect and characterize liver lesions (23–26). Detection involves identification of the presence of lesions and the segmental extent of liver involvement (24). It is generally accepted that with some neoplasms (e.g., colorectal) patient survival can be improved by partial hepatectomy if metastases are localized to three or fewer segments (27–33). There is no universal agreement as to whether MRI is superior to CT in the evaluation of the liver; however, a number of reports have shown MRI to be superior to CT (2,34–36). In addition, greater incremental improvement in MRI compared with CT is expected.

An imaging protocol including both T2-weighted sequences and T1-weighted whole-liver breath-hold imaging with serial postcontrast images permits both good detection (T2-weighted images) and characterization (serial postcontrast FLASH images) (Fig. 10). We compared dynamic contrast-enhanced CT with MRI using T2-weighted fat-suppressed, FLASH, and dynamic serial postcontrast FLASH images in 73 patients with clinically suspected liver disease (2). Lesion detection was greatest with T2FS (272 lesions), and detection with Gd-DTPA-enhanced FLASH (244 lesions) was statistically greater than with CT (220 lesions) and FLASH (219) (p<.03). Correct lesion characterization was greatest with Gd-DTPA-enhanced FLASH (236 lesions) (p<.01), followed by CT (199 lesions), FLASH (164 lesions), and T2FS (144 lesions). The importance of characterization is that patients with known primary malignant neoplasms may have small hepatic lesions that are not infrequently benign cysts or hemangiomas. Jones et al. reported the detection of small (<15 mm) lesions in 254 of

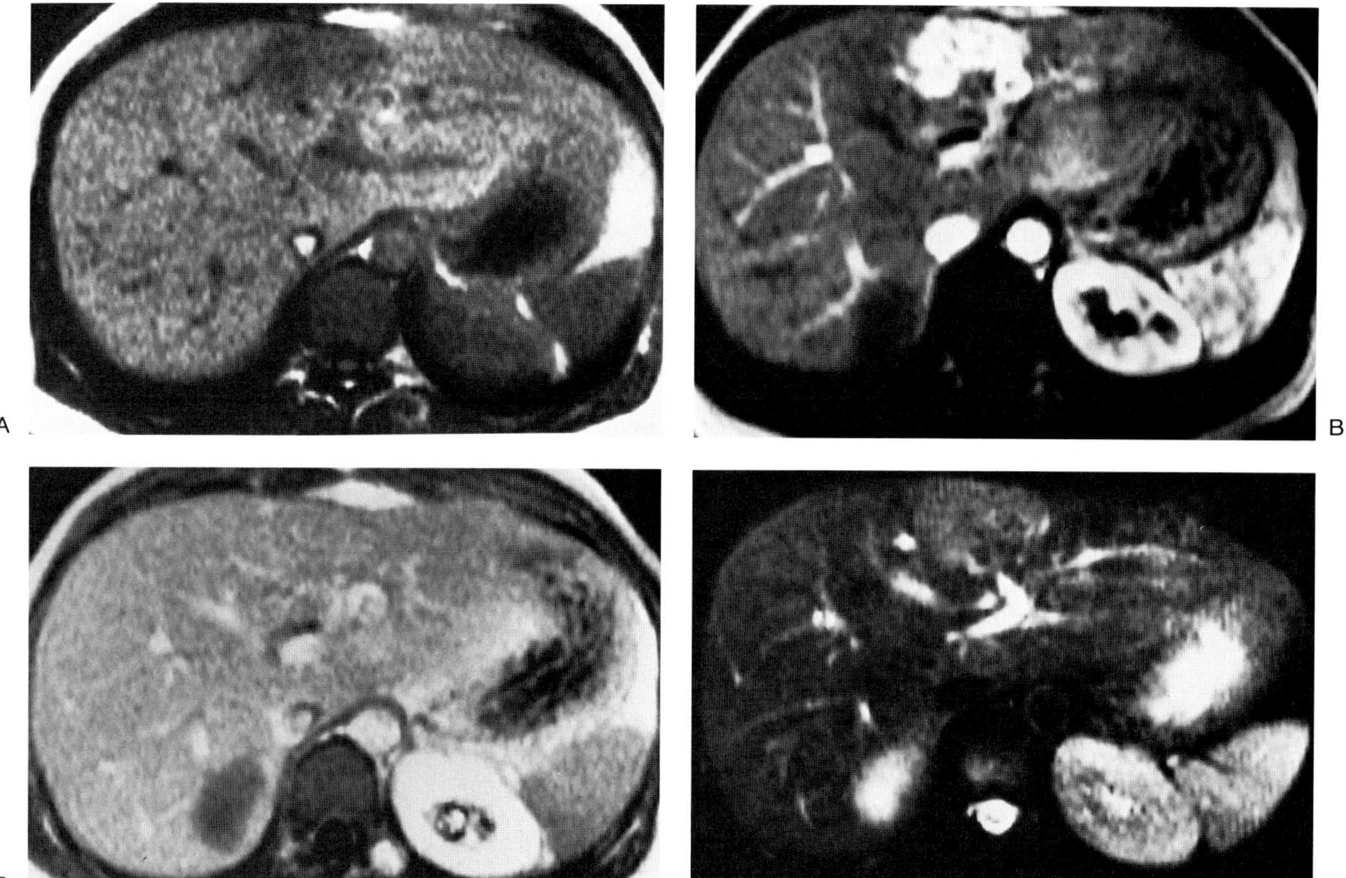

FIG. 8. Focal nodular hyperplasia. Precontrast FLASH (**A**), 1-second (**B**) and 90-second (**C**) postcontrast FLASH, and T2FS (**D**) images in a 42-year-old woman with FNH. The lesion is mildly hypointense on the T1-weighted image (A) and hyperintense on the T2-weighted image (D). The characteristic enhancement pattern is apparent with intense initial enhancement (B), which fades rapidly to isointensity (C).

1,454 patients who underwent CT examination (37). The majority of patients (82%) with liver lesions had a known primary tumor, and yet lesions in 51% of these patients were benign lesions. Patients may have a variety of lesions that can be multiple and scattered throughout the liver; the whole organ coverage of MRI per acquisition permits optimal evaluation of the entire liver with serial contrast enhancement.

Metastases vary substantially in appearance on T1- and T2-weighted images (34). Borders are usually irregular but may be sharp. Lesion shape is frequently irregular but may be oval. In general, metastases are low in SI on T1-weighted images and modestly high in SI on T2-weighted images. Some metastases, particularly vascular metastases from islet cell tumors, pheochromocytoma, and renal cell cancer or necrotic metastases, can be high in SI on T2-weighted images, which may make distinction from hemangiomas difficult (10).

Metastases do not have the classic enhancement patterns of benign lesions (i.e., no enhancement, as seen with cysts; peripheral globular enhancement, as seen with hemangiomas; or transient immediate postcontrast blush, as seen with FNH or adenomas). The most common enhancement pattern is heterogeneous enhancement.

Hypovascular metastases can mimic cysts on early images. At 10 minutes, however, lesion borders become indistinct and lesions appear smaller because of peripheral enhancement (Fig. 11).

Dynamic serial Gd-DTPA-enhanced MR images are essential for lesion characterization in patients with known vascular primary tumors. Vascular metastases from renal or bowel cancer tend to enhance with a thick, irregular rim, which may gradually fill in. The lack of globular enhancement and the presence of peripheral washout of contrast distinguish these lesions from hemangiomas (Fig. 12). Vascular metastases from islet cell tumor tend to enhance with a uniform ring pattern, which may fade on more delayed images (Fig. 13). This appearance is better shown on MR than CT images because of the higher sensitivity of MR for Gd-DTPA and better temporal resolution for dynamic acquisition. In

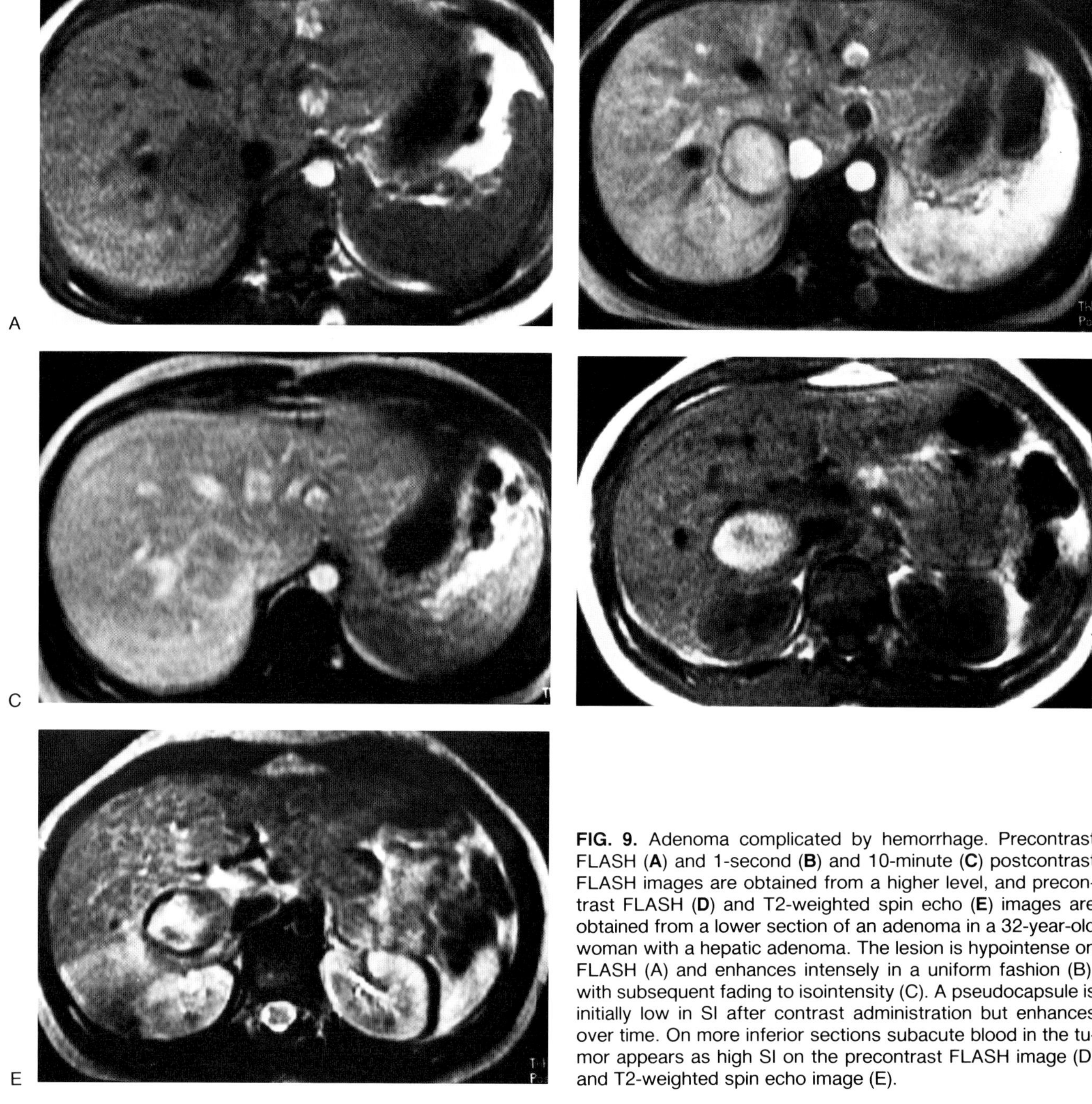

FIG. 9. Adenoma complicated by hemorrhage. Precontrast FLASH (**A**) and 1-second (**B**) and 10-minute (**C**) postcontrast FLASH images are obtained from a higher level, and precontrast FLASH (**D**) and T2-weighted spin echo (**E**) images are obtained from a lower section of an adenoma in a 32-year-old woman with a hepatic adenoma. The lesion is hypointense on FLASH (A) and enhances intensely in a uniform fashion (B), with subsequent fading to isointensity (C). A pseudocapsule is initially low in SI after contrast administration but enhances over time. On more inferior sections subacute blood in the tumor appears as high SI on the precontrast FLASH image (D) and T2-weighted spin echo image (E).

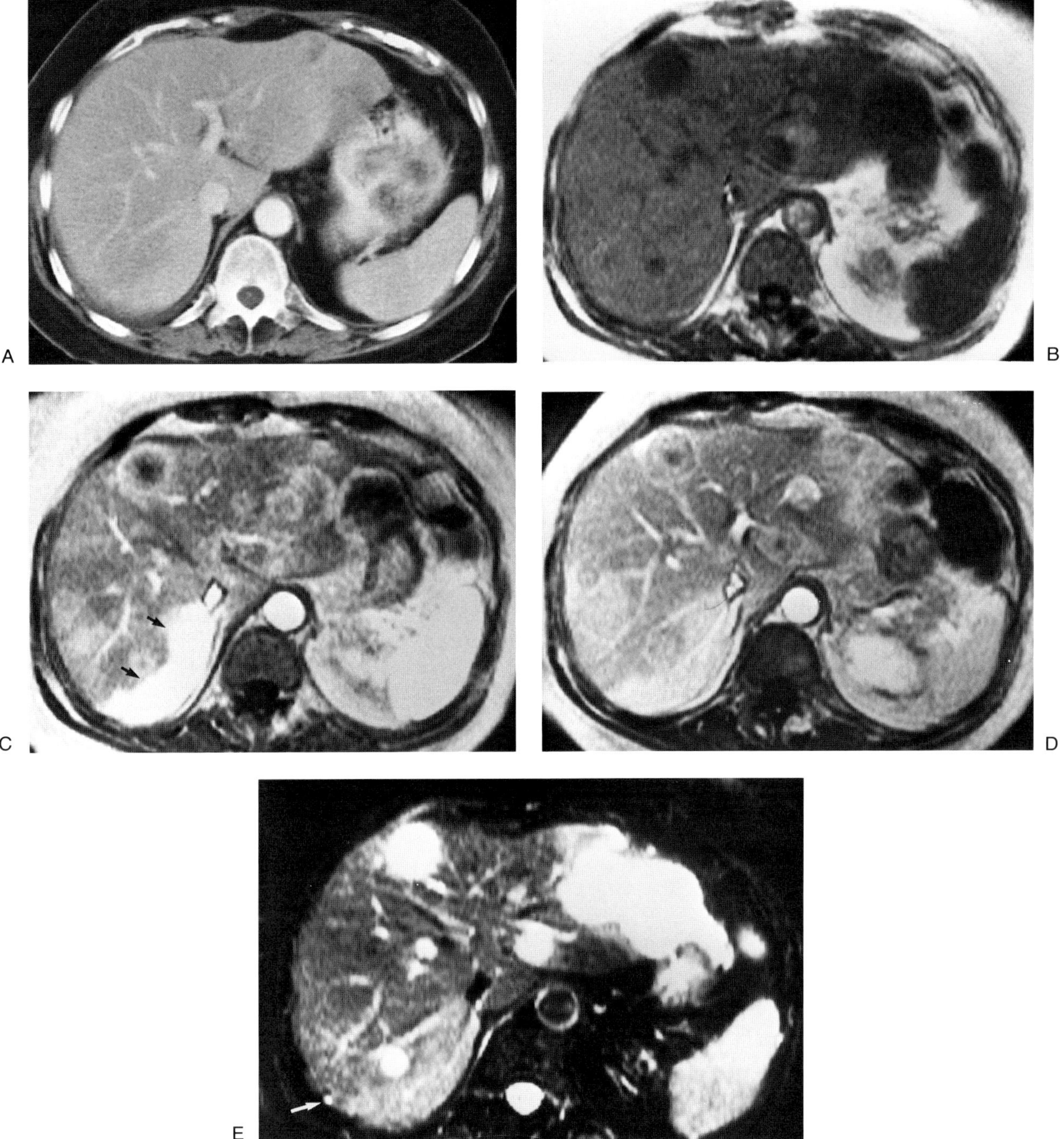

FIG. 10. Hepatic metastases. Dynamic contrast-enhanced CT (**A**), FLASH (**B**), 1-second (**C**) and 90-second (**D**) postcontrast FLASH, and T2FS (**E**) images in a 79-year-old woman with hepatic metastasis from colon cancer. The CT images (A) show the fewest lesions. The precontrast FLASH images (B) show slightly more lesions than does CT. Heterogeneous contrast enhancement with a target-like appearance is apparent on postcontrast FLASH images (C,D). Additionally, transient high SI of a focus of liver in the right lobe (*arrows*) on the 1-second postcontrast FLASH image (C) is apparent and becomes more isointense on subsequent images. T2-weighted fat-suppressed spin echo images (E) show the greatest number of lesions, with lesions as small as 3 mm identified (*arrow*). Reprinted with permission from ref. 2.

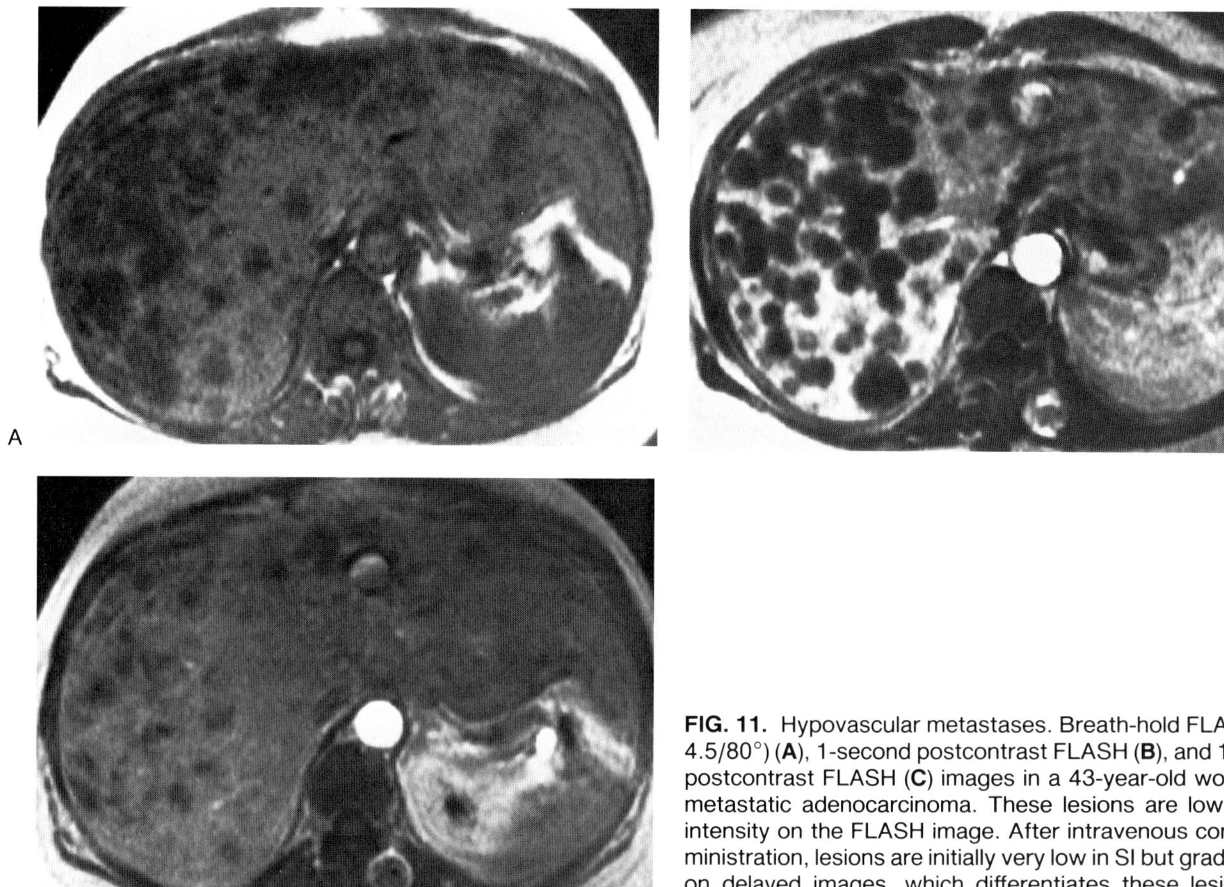

FIG. 11. Hypovascular metastases. Breath-hold FLASH (130/4.5/80°) (**A**), 1-second postcontrast FLASH (**B**), and 10-minute postcontrast FLASH (**C**) images in a 43-year-old woman with metastatic adenocarcinoma. These lesions are low in signal intensity on the FLASH image. After intravenous contrast administration, lesions are initially very low in SI but gradually fill in on delayed images, which differentiates these lesions from cysts.

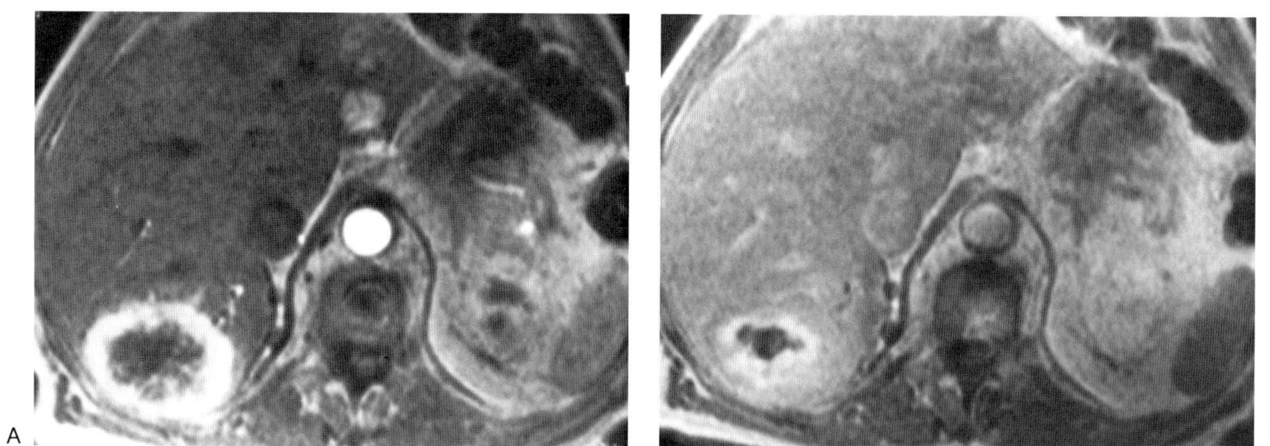

FIG. 12. Hypervascular metastases. One-second (**A**) and 10-minute (**B**) postcontrast FLASH (130/4.5/80°) images in an 86-year-old man with liver metastases from renal cancer. Intense peripheral enhancement present on early images superficially resembles the enhancement pattern of a hemangioma. Late postcontrast images show an irregular peripheral washout of contrast agent by the lesion, demonstrating that this lesion is a metastasis and not a hemangioma. Reprinted with permission from ref. 2.

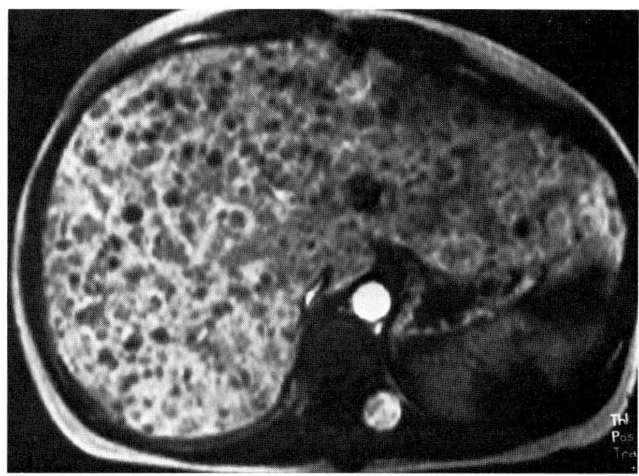

FIG. 13. Hypervascular islet cell metastases. One-second postcontrast FLASH image in a 35-year-old woman with gastrinoma liver metastases. Thin, uniform, ring-like enhancement is apparent.

lesions with ring enhancement, features that are more consistent with malignant lesions than with hemangiomas are (a) uniformity of the thickness of the ring, (b) a jagged or serrated internal margin of the ring rather than a lobular margin, and (c) peripheral washout of the ring with the presence of more central enhancement.

Transient enhancement is observed in small vascular metastases. In these lesions immediate postcontrast imaging is particularly critical (Fig. 14).

There are a variety of unusual MR appearances of metastatic lesions. Metastases can undergo hemorrhage, which may result in differing high- and low-SI lesions on T1- and T2-weighted images. Metastases that have a high content of fibrous tissue can be isointense on T2-weighted images. In these cases T1-weighted images are necessary for detection (Fig. 15). Melanoma metastases usually are a mixture of high- and low-SI lesions because of the paramagnetic property of melanin (38) (Fig. 16).

Lymphoma

Lymphomatous involvement of the liver occurs most frequently in patients with non-Hodgkin's lymphoma. Lesions are typically low in SI on T1-weighted images, minimally high in SI on T2-weighted images, and low in SI on Gd-DTPA-enhanced images and may possess a high-SI rim (Fig. 17).

Hepatocellular Carcinomas

Hepatocellular carcinoma (HCC) is the most common primary malignant neoplasm of the liver and occurs most frequently in male patients. In North America HCC tends to arise in a previously damaged liver, most commonly in patients with alcoholic cirrhosis, chronic active hepatitis, or hemochromatosis. HCC occurs as a solitary lesion in approximately 50% of cases, is multifocal in 20%, and is diffuse in 30% of cases (39). An uncommon type of HCC is the fibrolamellar HCC. This tumor is unusual in that it occurs in younger patients who are frequently female, without underlying cirrhosis (40,41). This tumor grows slowly and has a better prognosis than other forms of HCC (40,41).

On MR images, HCCs can have a variety of SI patterns on T1- and T2-weighted images. The most frequent appearance is low SI on T1-weighted images and moderately high SI on T2-weighted images. HCCs are frequently vascular and enhance in a heterogeneous fashion (39). Hypovascular HCCs are, however, common. Lesion size and number are usually best seen on T2-weighted images (42). Tumor margins with liver are best shown on T2-weighted images and frequently are poorly shown on dynamic contrast-enhanced CT or MR images (Fig. 18). A characteristic feature of HCC is tumor extension into portal or hepatic veins (Fig. 19). This feature is observed in <50% of cases (43). A pseudocapsule may be seen in HCC but is not as frequently observed in North America as in Asian countries (43). An unusual imaging feature of HCC is that, on occasion, these tumors may show low SI on T2-weighted images, which may be related to fibrosis (Fig. 20). Fat and copper accumulation in HCCs may result in high SI on T1-weighted images (44,45).

Cholangiocarcinomas

Cholangiocarcinoma is described in greater detail in Chapter 4. Peripheral cholangiocarcinoma is an uncommon form of the tumor and bears mentioning with focal mass lesions of the liver as it frequently presents as a hepatic mass lesion.

GENERAL LIVER DISEASES

Cirrhosis

Cirrhosis is a result of chronic injury of the liver; in North America cirrhosis is most frequently secondary to alcoholic liver disease. Chronic hepatitis caused by drugs, viruses, or unknown factors is a distant second in frequency. The histological changes in cirrhosis include hepatocyte destruction, alteration of normal hepatic architecture, fibrosis, and regenerating nodules. Cirrhosis presents with a spectrum of appearances on CT and MR images ranging from a normal appearance to an irregularly shaped, shrunken liver with splenomegaly, ascites, and varices (46). The diagnosis of cirrhosis is suggested

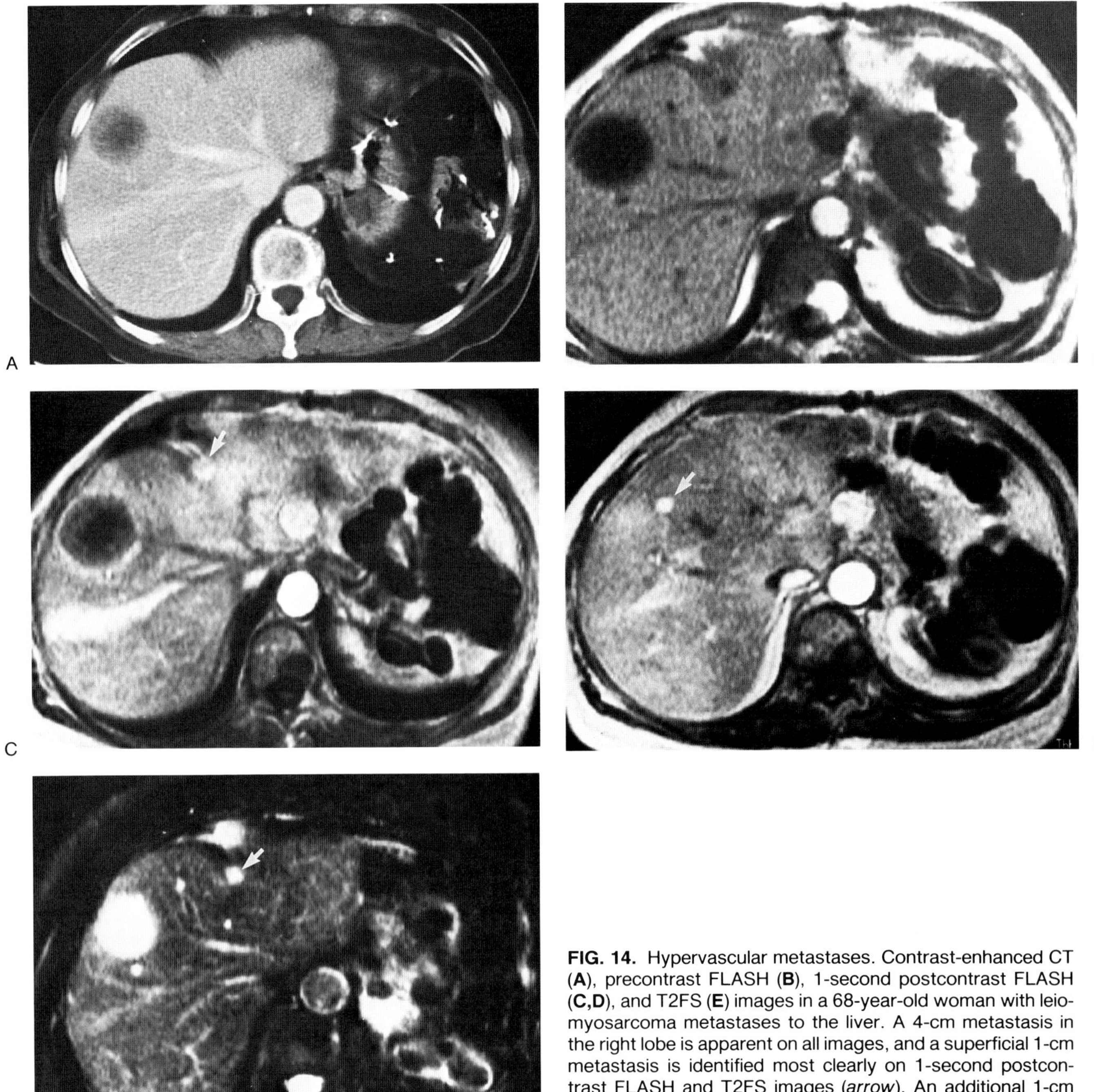

FIG. 14. Hypervascular metastases. Contrast-enhanced CT (**A**), precontrast FLASH (**B**), 1-second postcontrast FLASH (**C,D**), and T2FS (**E**) images in a 68-year-old woman with leiomyosarcoma metastases to the liver. A 4-cm metastasis in the right lobe is apparent on all images, and a superficial 1-cm metastasis is identified most clearly on 1-second postcontrast FLASH and T2FS images (*arrow*). An additional 1-cm enhancing metastasis on a more inferior section is identified only on the 1-second postcontrast FLASH image (D, *arrow*).

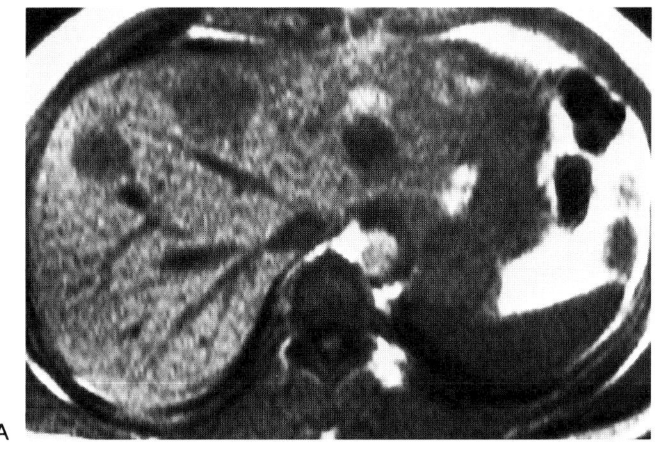
A

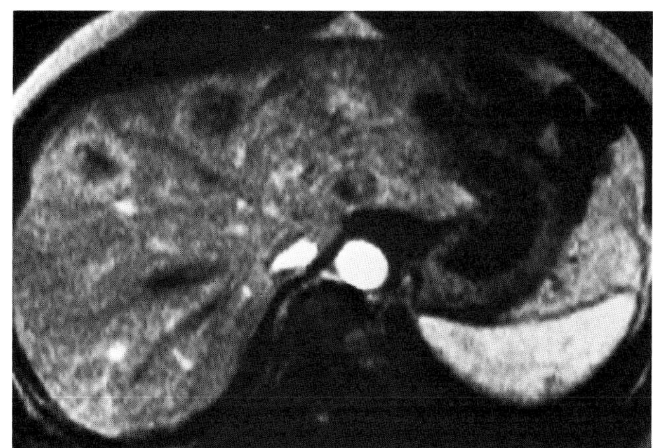
B

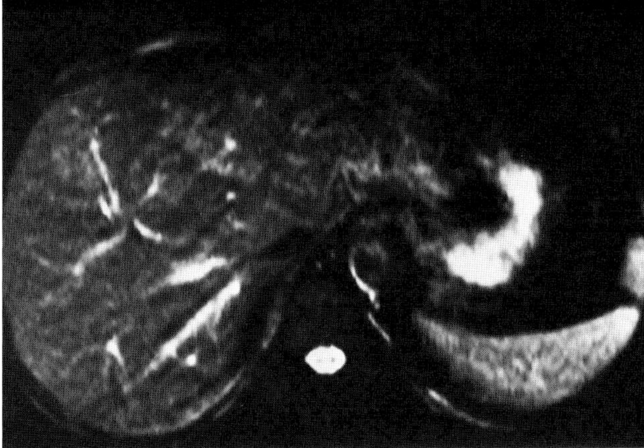
C

FIG. 15. Fibrous metastases. Precontrast FLASH (**A**), 1-second postcontrast FLASH (**B**), and T2FS (**C**) images in a 48-year-old man with carcinoid metastases to the liver. Lesions are well seen on precontrast FLASH images and demonstrate peripheral ring enhancement on Gd-DTPA-enhanced images, which is typical for neuroendocrine tumor metastases. Lesions are, however, poorly seen on T2-weighted images because of their fibrous composition.

on MR images when the liver contour is nodular and irregular. Selective hypertrophy of the caudate lobe and atrophy of the right lobe are more specific changes of cirrhosis (Fig. 21). Regenerating nodules are occasionally identified as focal regions that are low in SI on T1- and T2-weighted images. Areas of fibrosis can be appreciated as linear structures low in SI on T1-weighted images and high or low in SI on T2-weighted images, depending on the age of the granulation tissue. In the acute phase, fibrotic tissue demonstrates enhancement with Gd-DTPA (Fig. 22). Associated features of portal hypertension include the presence of ascites, splenomegaly, and enlarged portosystemic collaterals (varices).

Budd-Chiari syndrome is an unusual form of chronic liver damage which occurs secondary to hepatic venous thrombosis or thrombosis of the suprahepatic inferior vena cava (IVC) (47,48). In the acute phase hepatomegaly is due to venous obstruction. Eventually, in the chronic phase, the liver becomes shrunken and irregular. Frequently, the caudate lobe is substantially enlarged and multiple varices develop. The absence of hepatic veins or thrombosis of the suprahepatic IVC confirms the diagnosis (Fig. 23).

Hemochromatosis

Hemochromatosis results from increased iron deposition in the liver. This occurs either as a primary process (idiopathic hemochromatosis) or as a process secondary to hemolytic anemias or multiple blood transfusions. Primary hemochromatosis is usually genetic and inherited in an autosomal recessive manner. Men are affected 10 times more frequently than women, and presentation occurs usually between the fourth and sixth decades. The underlying abnormality is increased absorption of iron and increased deposition in the tissues (frequently liver, pancreas, and heart).

The great sensitivity of T2-weighted images to iron deposition in the liver has long been recognized. As the iron load increases, the loss of signal intensity on T1-weighted images is appreciated because of extreme T2 shortening. The concentration of excess iron in the liver has been shown to correlate with T2 calculations (49).

Siegelman et al. have shown that primary hemochromatosis can be distinguished from secondary forms by the distribution of SI decrease (50). In primary hemochromatosis, iron deposition in the liver occurs

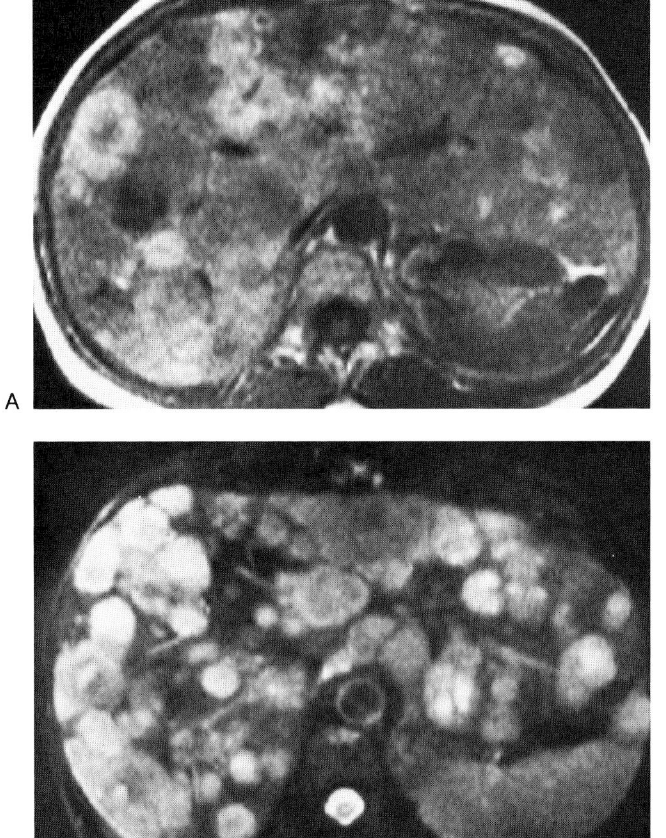

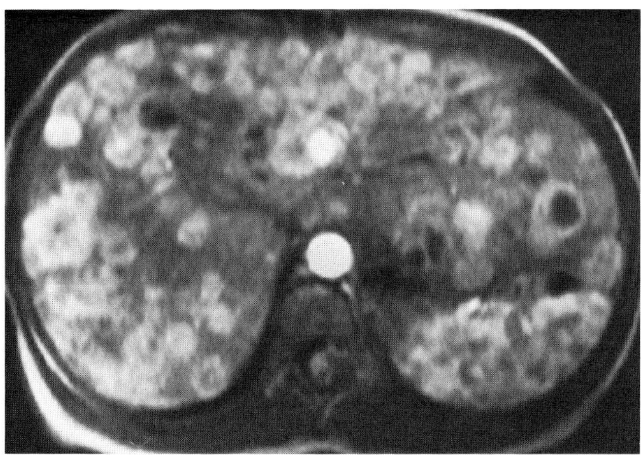

FIG. 16. Melanoma metastases. FLASH (**A**), 1-second postcontrast FLASH (**B**) and T2FS (**C**) MR images in a 66-year-old woman with melanoma liver metastases. A varied population of high- and low-SI metastases are apparent on T1- and T2-weighted images due to the paramagnetic property of melanin. Ring-like enhancement is apparent on the immediate postcontrast images reflecting the hypervascular nature of these lesions.

mainly in hepatocytes; in patients with secondary hemochromatosis, however, iron deposition is in the reticuloendothelial system. Patients with primary hemochromatosis may have SI decrease in the pancreas due to diffuse iron deposition in organ systems and uncommonly have SI decrease of the spleen. Patients with reticuloendothelial system (RES) iron overload almost invariably have a diminished SI of the spleen (Fig. 24).

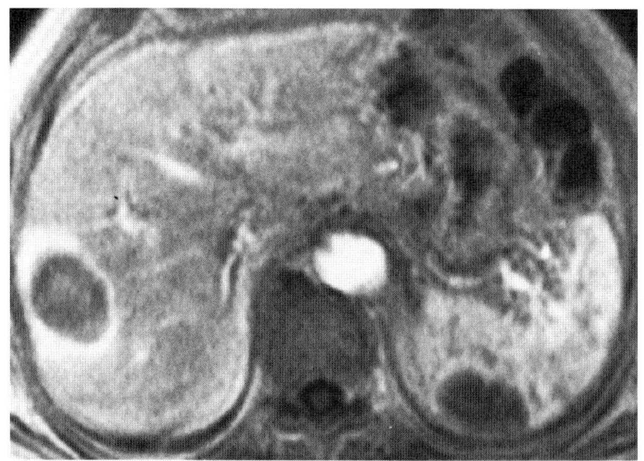

FIG. 17. Non-Hodgkin's lymphoma. Deposits of non-Hodgkin's lymphoma are present in the liver and spleen of a 54-year-old man. Lymphomatous deposits in the liver typically enhance poorly with contrast. Rim enhancement is relatively common.

Fatty Infiltration

Fatty infiltration of the liver occurs from excessive deposition of triglycerides. It is a nonspecific response to cell injury and is seen in a variety of conditions including obesity, alcohol consumption, steroid use, diabetes, intravenous parenteral nutrition, Cushing's disease, and radiation changes.

Areas of fatty infiltration are generally not demonstrated on standard T1- and T2-weighted spin echo sequences. Modified MR sequences that exploit the frequency shift between fat and water protons (excitation-spoiling fat saturation techniques) or the phase-cycling of fat and water (out-of-phase techniques) have been shown to be sensitive to the presence of fatty infiltration (51,52) (Fig. 25). Regions of focal fatty infiltration may be difficult to distinguish from focal hepatic mass lesions. A distinguishing feature is that the margins of focal fatty infiltration usually are linear, rather than rounded, corresponding to a vascular territory (53,54). It has also been observed on dynamic Gd-DTPA-

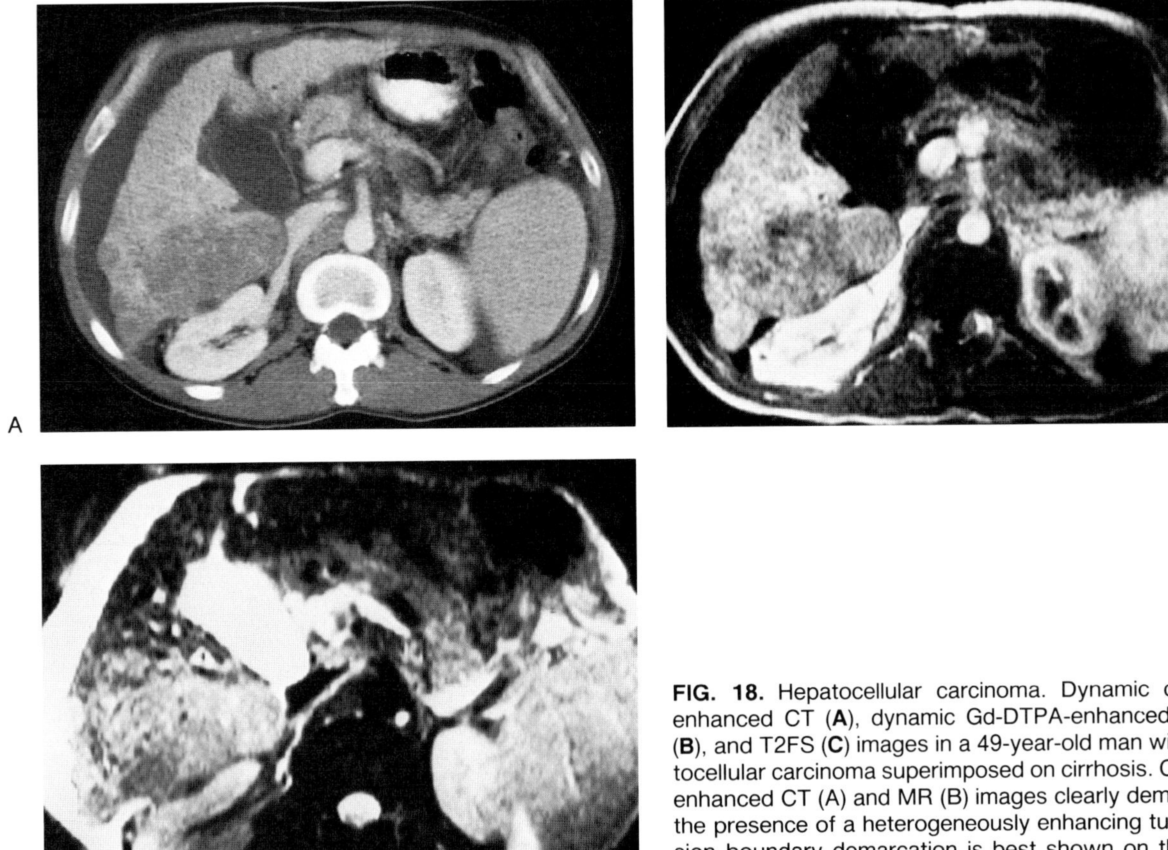

FIG. 18. Hepatocellular carcinoma. Dynamic contrast-enhanced CT (**A**), dynamic Gd-DTPA-enhanced FLASH (**B**), and T2FS (**C**) images in a 49-year-old man with hepatocellular carcinoma superimposed on cirrhosis. Contrast-enhanced CT (A) and MR (B) images clearly demonstrate the presence of a heterogeneously enhancing tumor. Lesion boundary demarcation is best shown on the T2FS image (C). Reprinted with permission from ref. 2.

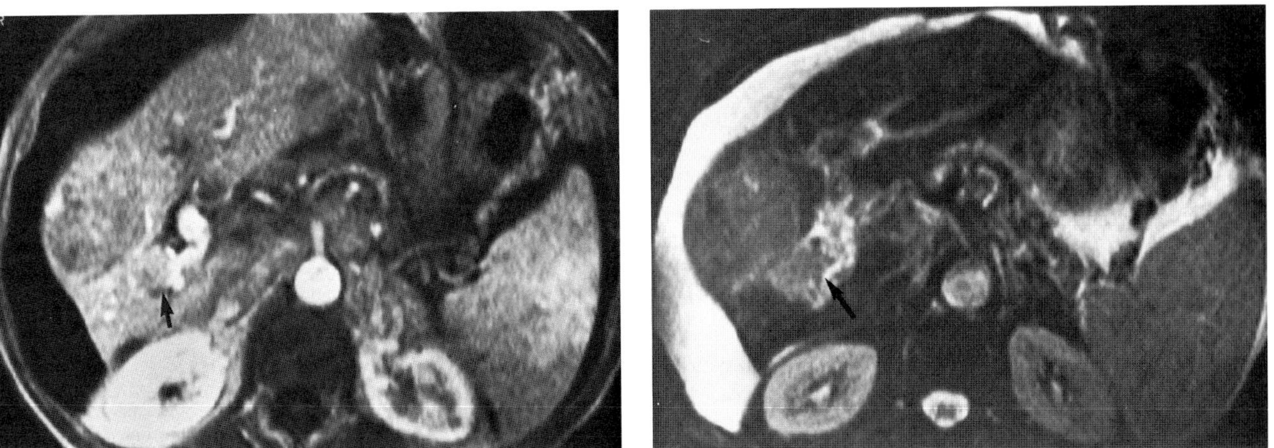

FIG. 19. Hepatocellular carcinoma with portal venous extension. One-second postcontrast FLASH (**A**) and T2FS (**B**) images in a 72-year-old man with HCC. A large mass is identified in the right lobe of the liver, with extension of tumor thrombus (*arrow*) into an expanded right portal vein. On the 1-second postcontrast FLASH image (A), increased SI in the right portal vein renders clear demonstration of the thrombus.

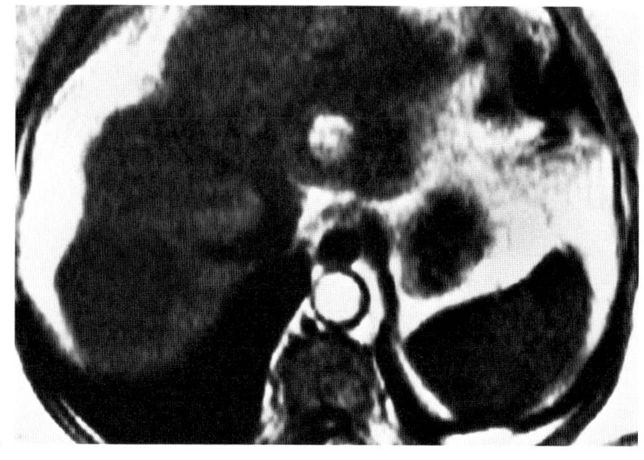

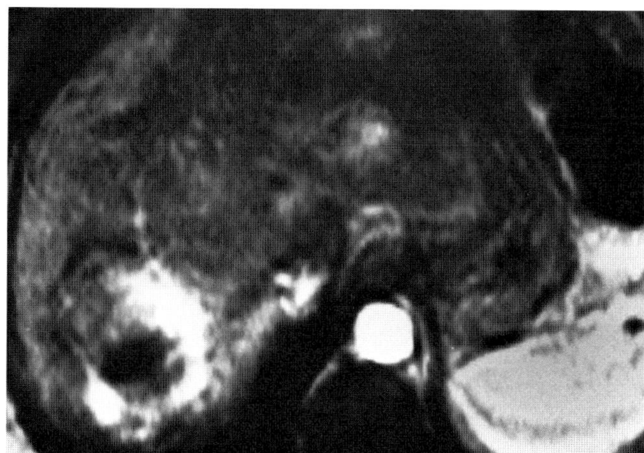

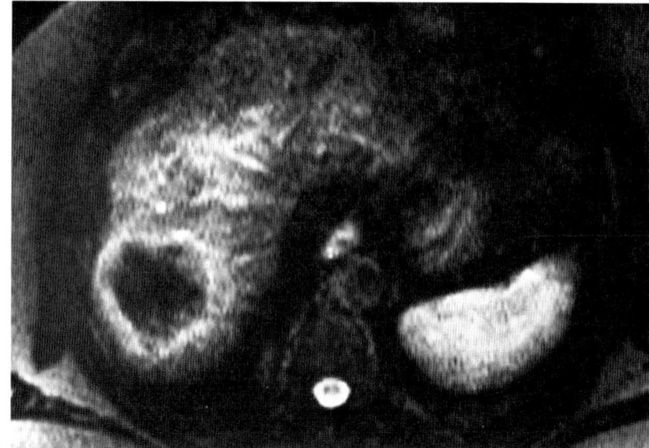

FIG. 20. Hepatocellular carcinoma. Precontrast FLASH (**A**), 1-second postcontrast FLASH (**B**), and T2FS (**C**) images in a 69-year-old man with HCC. The tumor is low in SI centrally with a high-SI pseudocapsule on the T2FS image (C). The tumor shows heterogeneously increased enhancement on postcontrast images (B).

enhanced FLASH images that areas of transient diminished enhancement correspond to low-attenuation defects on CT images (2) (Fig. 26). It is uncertain at present whether these findings represent fatty infiltration or another process.

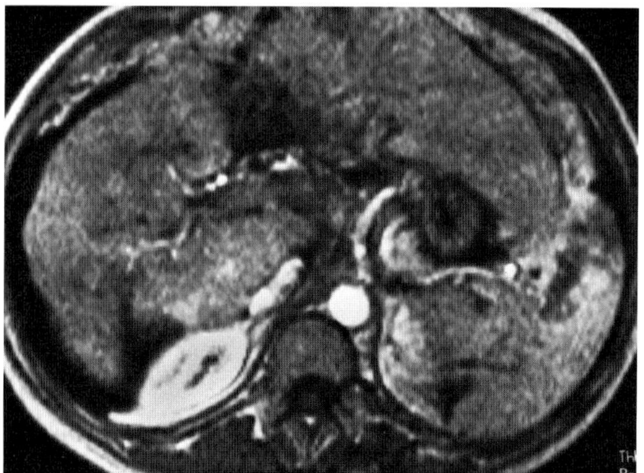

FIG. 21. Cirrhosis. One-second postcontrast FLASH image in a 46-year-old woman with cirrhosis. Selective atrophy of the right lobe and hypertrophy of the caudate lobe are characteristic of cirrhosis. Ascites, which is also present, is a feature of associated portal hypertension.

Heterogeneous Enhancement

Transient heterogeneous enhancement of liver has been observed on dynamic contrast enhancement CT, CT arterial portography, and dynamic Gd-DTPA enhancement MR images. Processes that interfere with hepatic blood flow can result in transient diminished or increased hepatic enhancement (Fig. 27). Congestive heart failure is not frequently associated with generalized transient heterogeneous hepatic enhancement (55). The mechanisms behind increased attenuation are not known, but several factors are probably involved. Transient heterogeneous enhancement has also been observed in individuals with elevated liver enzymes and patchy areas of decreased attenuation on CT images (Fig. 28).

INFECTIOUS DISEASES

Abscesses

Pyogenic Abscesses

Patients with pyogenic abscesses are typically very ill. Predisposing conditions, such as recent surgery, Crohn's

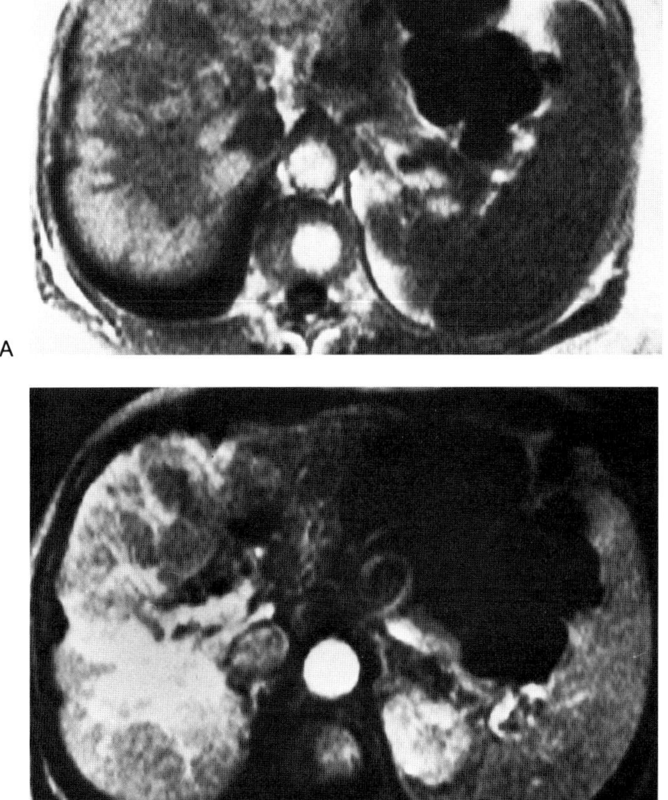

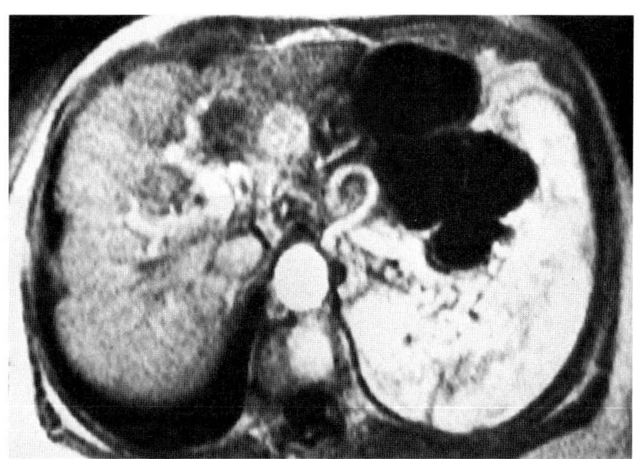

FIG. 22. Cirrhosis with prominent scarring. Precontrast FLASH (**A**) and 1-second (**B**) and 10-minute (**C**) postcontrast FLASH images in a 77-year-old woman with cirrhosis. Large, irregular, linear low-SI densities are identified on the FLASH image, which initially demonstrate isointense enhancement (B) and become progressively hyperintense over time (C) after contrast administration. This appearance is consistent with acute granulation tissue. Splenomegaly, which is also present, is a feature of portal hypertension.

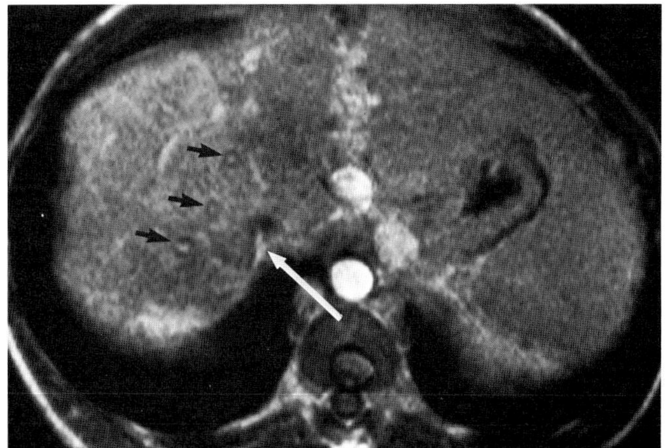

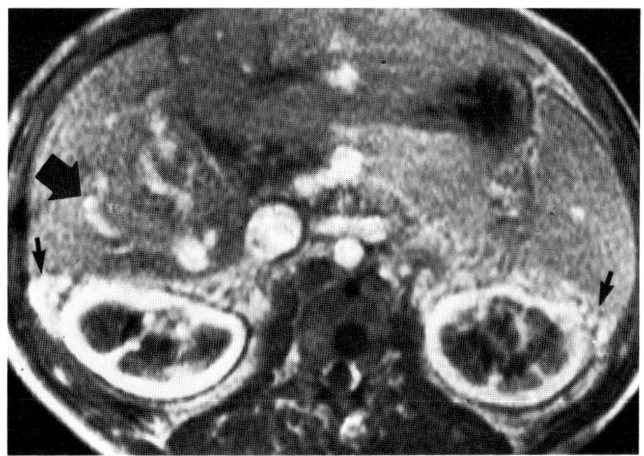

FIG. 23. Budd-Chiari syndrome. One-second postcontrast FLASH images from cranial (**A**) and caudal (**B**) sections of the liver of a 48-year-old man with Budd-Chiari syndrome. At the anatomical level of hepatic vein entry into the IVC, no normal hepatic veins are identified. A solitary, diminutive vessel is seen entering the IVC (*white arrow*). Vessels that possess a low-SI halo are present (A, *black arrows*). At a more inferior level, large, tortuous abnormal vessels are present in the right lobe of the liver (B, *large arrow*). Prominent varices are present throughout the abdomen (B, *black arrows*).

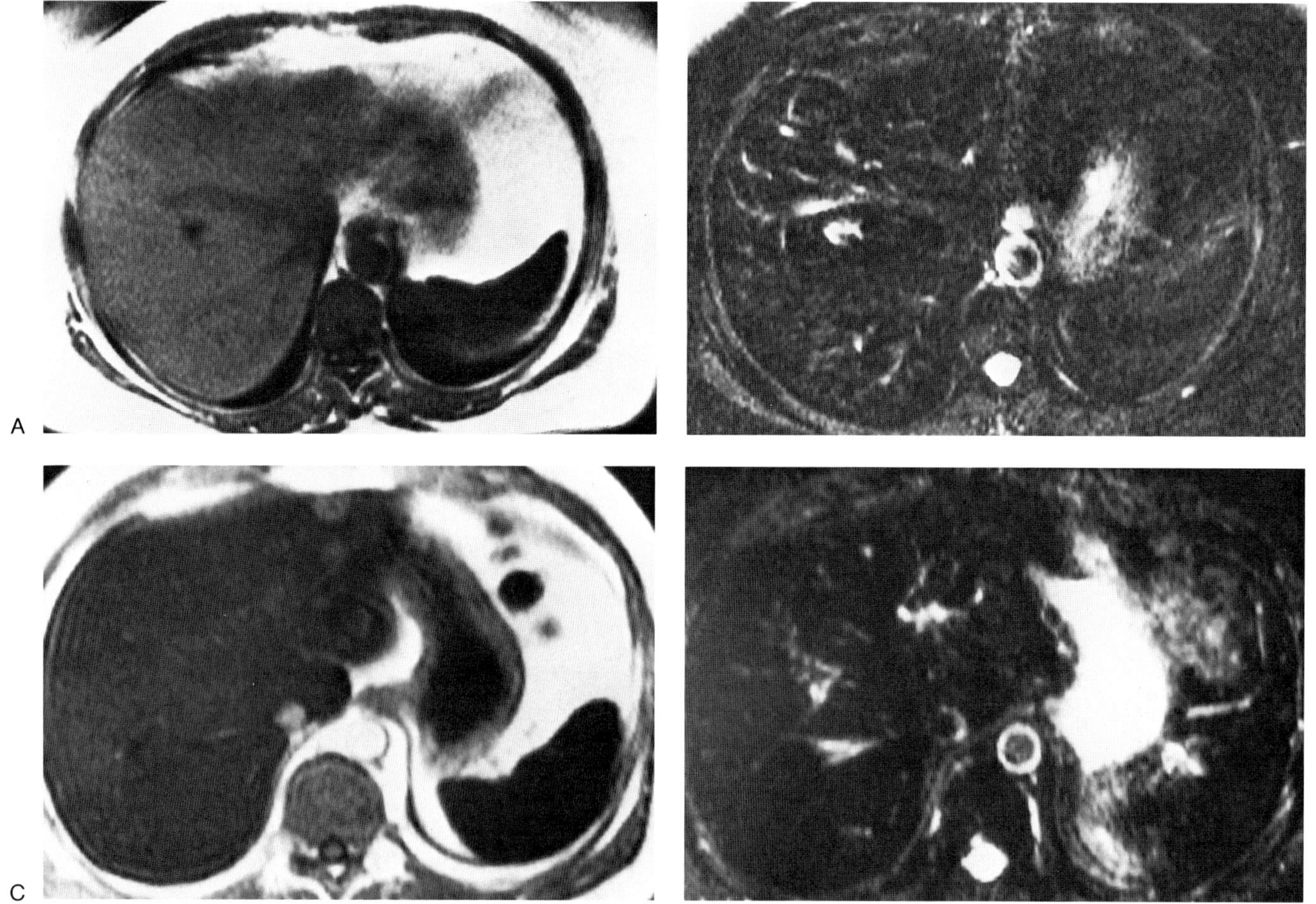

FIG. 24. Hemochromatosis. Precontrast FLASH (**A**) and T2FS (**B**) images in a 64-year-old woman with acute myelogenous leukemia. This patient had received multiple blood transfusions within 1 year of examination with MR imaging, resulting in iron deposition in the RES. Slightly diminished SI is present in the liver and spleen on the T1-weighted images (A). Dramatic loss of SI is present on the T2-weighted images (B), rendering the SI of the liver and spleen comparable to background noise. Precontrast FLASH (**C**) and T2FS (**D**) in a 43-year-old man demonstrate substantial loss of SI of the liver and spleen on both T1- and T2-weighted images, which corresponds to a high concentration of iron deposition in the RES.

disease, and diverticulitis, are usually present (56). Characteristic contrast-enhanced CT or MR findings are low-attenuation lesions with an enhancing capsule and a peripheral rim of low attenuation/SI (Fig. 29). The higher sensitivity of MRI to Gd-DTPA suggests that dynamic enhanced MRI may be a useful technique in patients in whom distinction between simple cysts and multiple abscesses cannot be made on the basis of CT examination. Other lesions may mimic the appearance of hepatic abscesses. Uncommonly, liver metastases may demonstrate typical features of an abscess (Fig. 30).

Nonpyogenic Abscesses

Amebic Abscesses

Amebic abscess occurs in patients who live in or have traveled to tropical climates. Presenting features include pain, fever, weight loss, nausea and vomiting, diarrhea, and anorexia (57). Lesions are usually solitary, and there is a tendency for lesions to invade the diaphragm, with the development of an empyema (58). Lesions are encapsulated, and increased enhancement of the capsule is usually apparent, providing differentiation from liver cysts (Fig. 31).

Echinococcal Disease

Echinococcus granulosus is the causative organism for hydatid cysts and is the form of *Echinococcus* found in North America. The classic appearance is an intrahepatic encapsulated multicystic lesion with daughter cysts arranged peripherally within the larger cyst. Satellite cysts located exterior to the fibrinous membrane of the main hepatic cyst occur. Kalovidouris et al. reported an

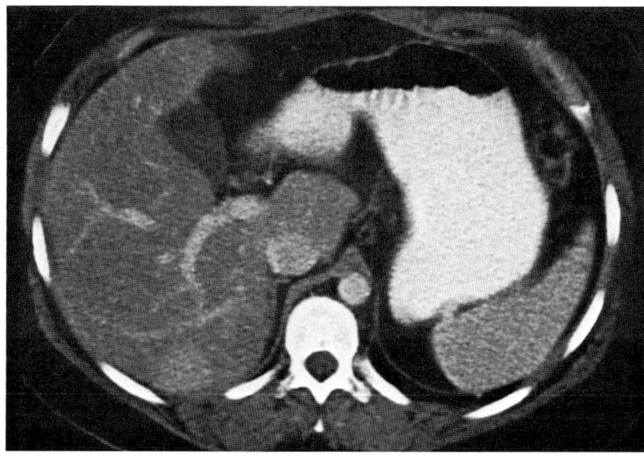
A

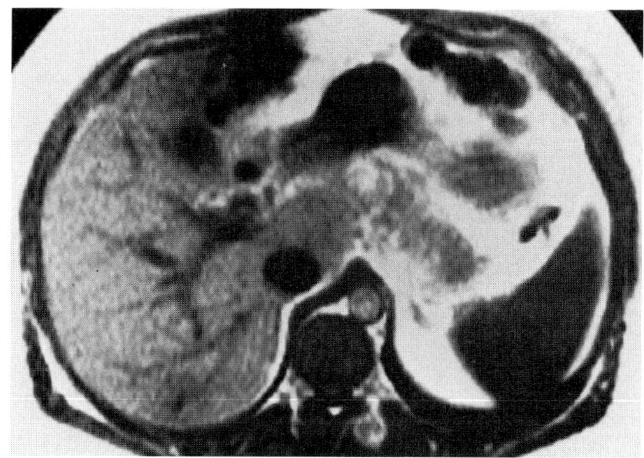
B

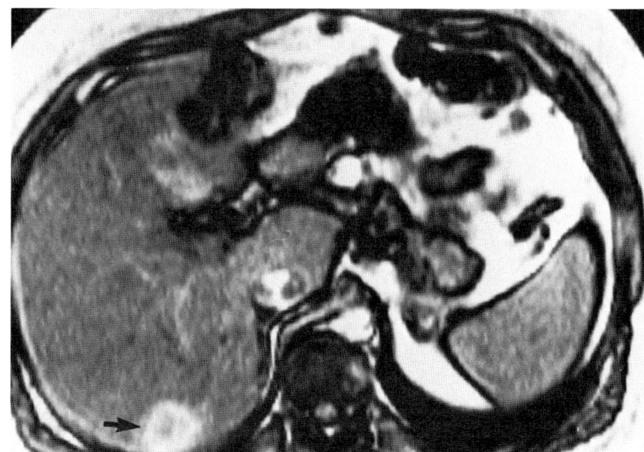
C

FIG. 25. Fatty infiltration. Contrast-enhanced CT (**A**) and in-phase (**B**) and out-of-phase (**C**) FLASH images in a 32-year-old woman with hepatic adenoma (*black arrow*). The liver has decreased attenuation on the CT image, consistent with fatty infiltration. On the in-phase FLASH image, the liver has a normal SI with a low-SI focal mass lesion. The out-of-phase FLASH image demonstrates diminished SI of the liver, rendering the liver lower in SI than the liver lesion and the spleen; this causes a reverse in the liver-lesion contrast. A phase cancellation artifact is also apparent on the out-of-phase image as a black line surrounding abdominal organs. This artifact arises from cancellation of the signal intensity of fat and water protons in the same voxel.

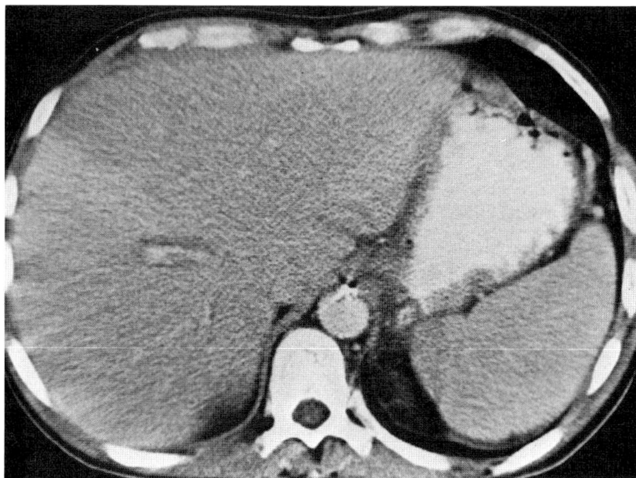
A

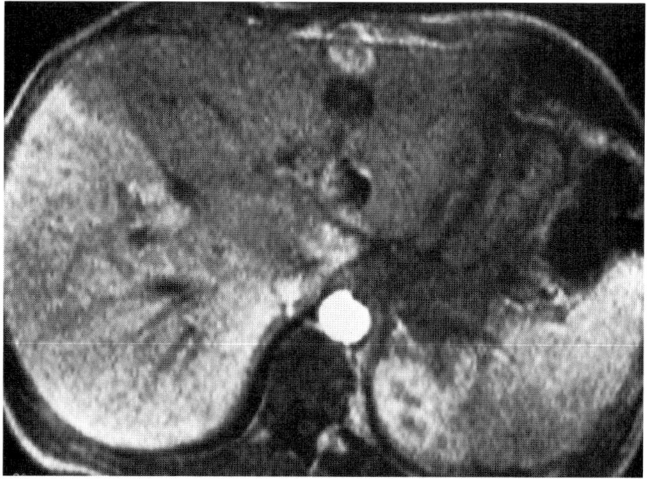
B

FIG. 26. Fatty infiltration of the left lobe of the liver shown by contrast-enhanced CT (**A**) and 1-second postcontrast FLASH (**B**) images in a 45-year-old man with acute pancreatitis and focal fatty infiltration of the liver. Subtle diminished attenuation of the left lobe is identified on the CT image, compatible with fatty infiltration. Greater conspicuity of diminished SI of the left lobe is apparent on the MR image.

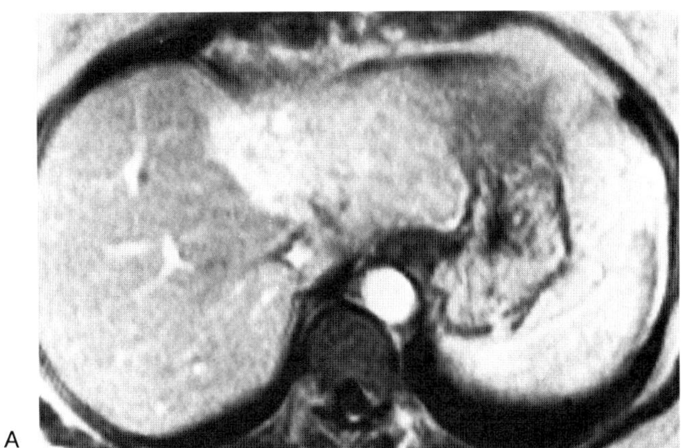

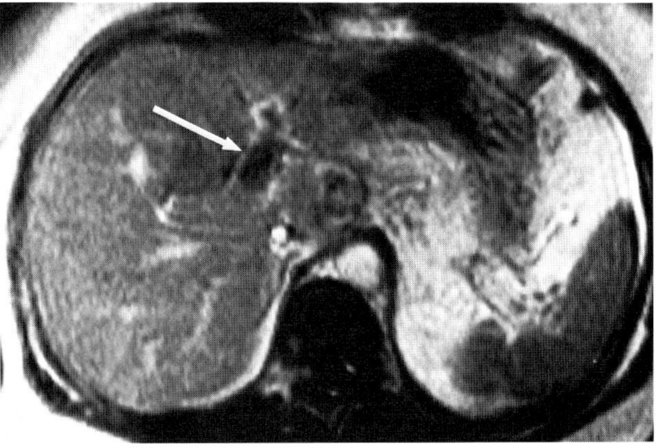

A B

FIG. 27. Heterogeneous enhancement on 1-second (**A**) and 10-minute (**B**) postcontrast FLASH images in a 66-year-old women with liver metastases and left portal vein thrombus from bowel cancer. Transient increased enhancement of the left lobe of the liver is identified on the immediate postcontrast FLASH image, which returns to isointensity on later images. Tumor thrombus in the left portal vein is clearly shown on the 10-minute postcontrast image (B, *white arrow*).

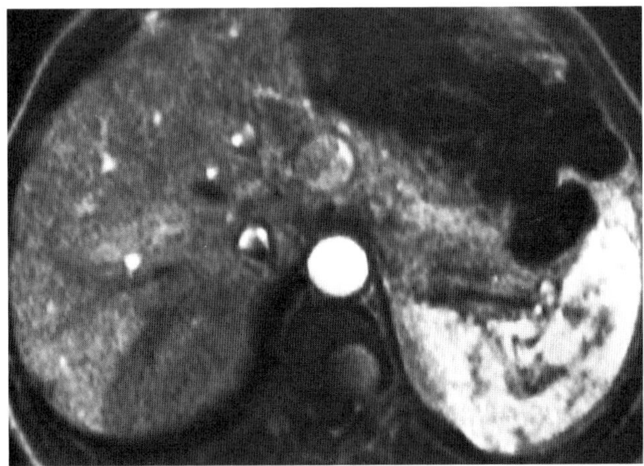

FIG. 28. Heterogeneous enhancement. One-second FLASH image in a 46-year-old man with liver enzyme abnormalities demonstrates heterogeneous enhancement of the liver.

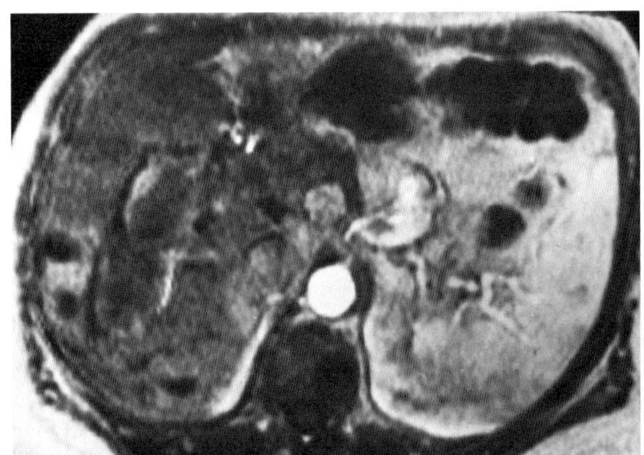

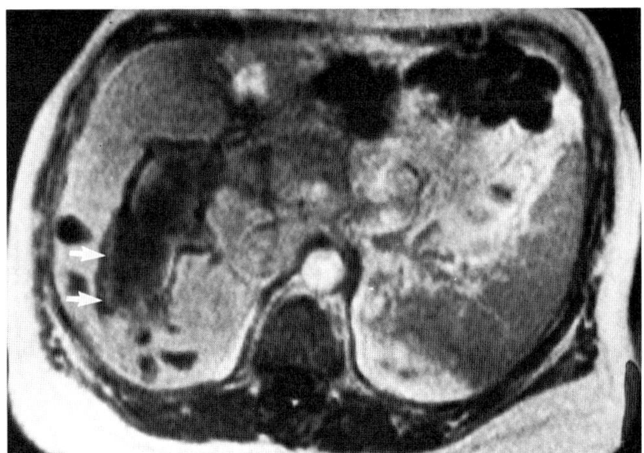

A B

FIG. 29. Liver abscess. One-second postcontrast FLASH (**A**) and 10-minute postcontrast FLASH (**B**) images in a 64-year-old woman with hepatic cirrhosis and superimposed hepatic abscesses. An irregular signal-void cavity in the right lobe of the liver is associated with several small signal-void lesions (A); there is also increased enhancement of adjacent liver consistent with inflammatory changes. On the delayed image an enhancing rim (*arrows*) is compatible with an abscess capsule.

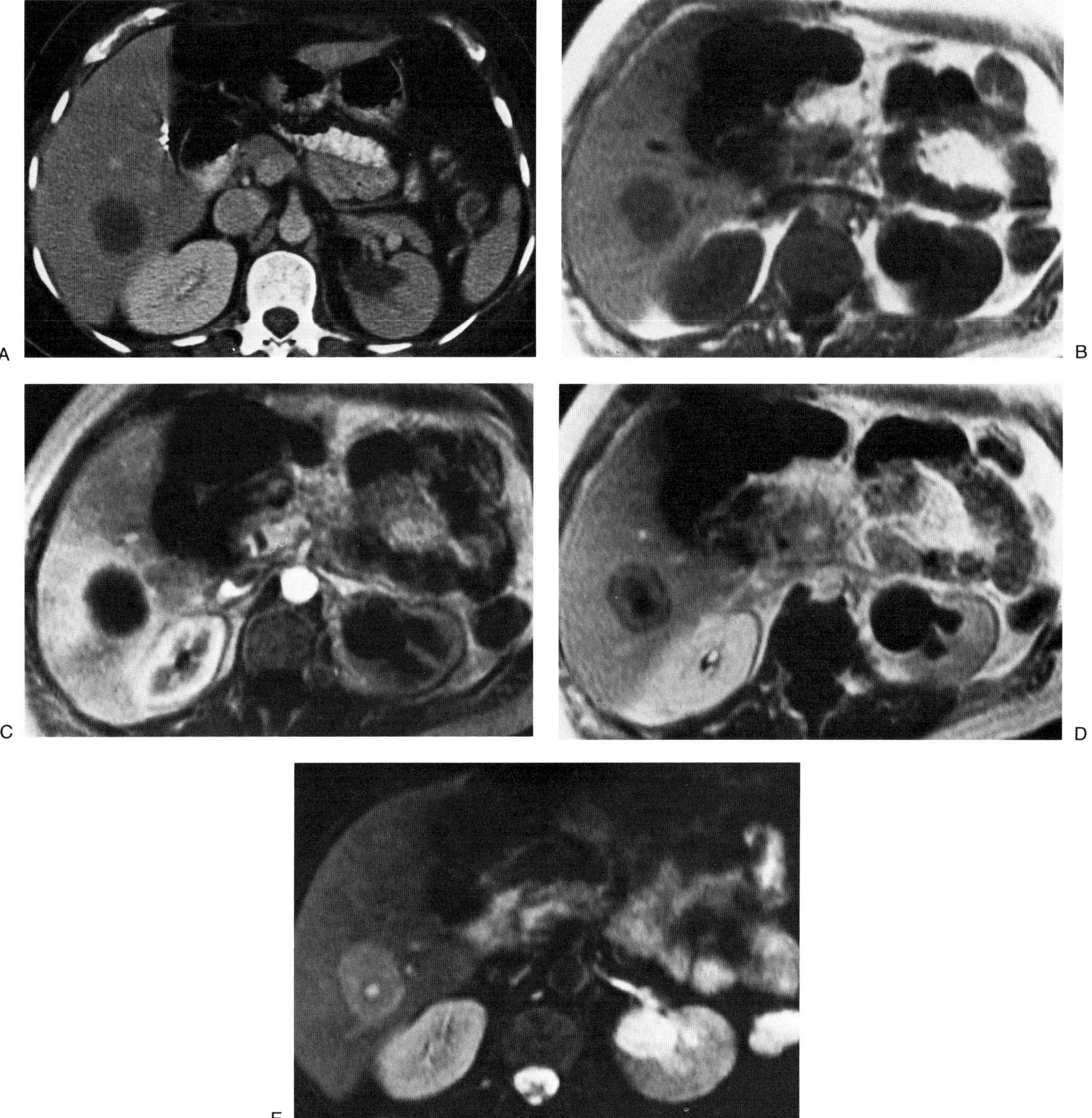

FIG. 30. Liver metastasis resembling an abscess. Contrast-enhanced CT (**A**), precontrast FLASH (**B**), 1-second (**C**) and 10-minute (**D**) postcontrast FLASH, and T2FS (**E**) images in a 44-year-old woman with colon cancer. The CT and precontrast FLASH images demonstrate a well-defined liver lesion. On the 1-second postcontrast FLASH image, substantial increased enhancement of the liver surrounding the lesion is compatible with an inflammatory reaction. On the 10-minute postcontrast image, the lesion is signal-void with a thick enhancing margin and a thin peripheral signal-void outer band are present. This target appearance, although present in this metastasis, is classic for an abscess; the target appearance is due to an enhancing capsule and perilesional edema. A similar concentric ring pattern.is apparent on the T2FS image, confirming that this lesion does not contain simple fluid.

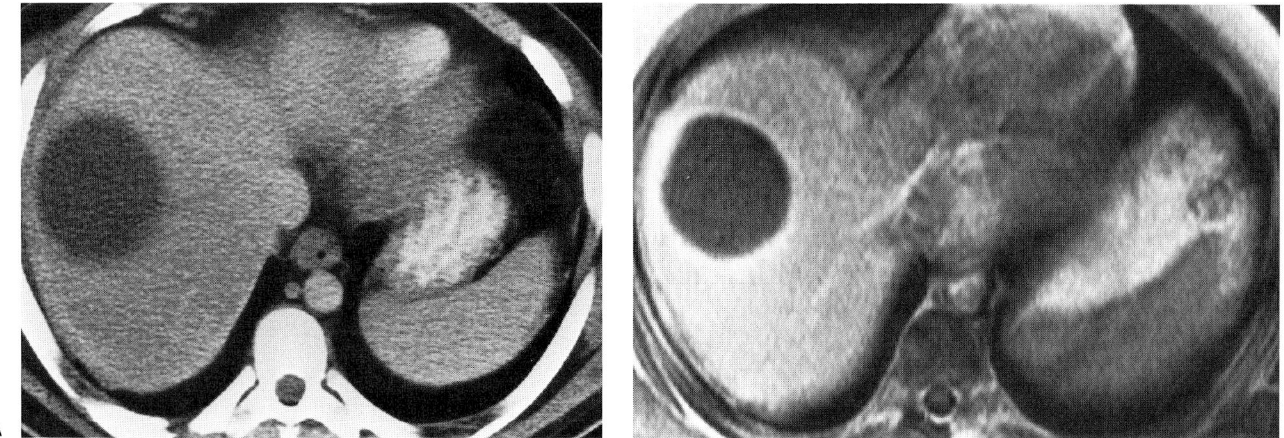

FIG. 31. Amebic abscess. Dynamic contrast-enhanced CT (**A**) and 45-second postcontrast FLASH (**B**) images of a 28-year-old man with an amebic abscess. The definition of the lesion is roughly comparable on the two images. Enhancement of the wall of the abscess is better shown on the MR image.

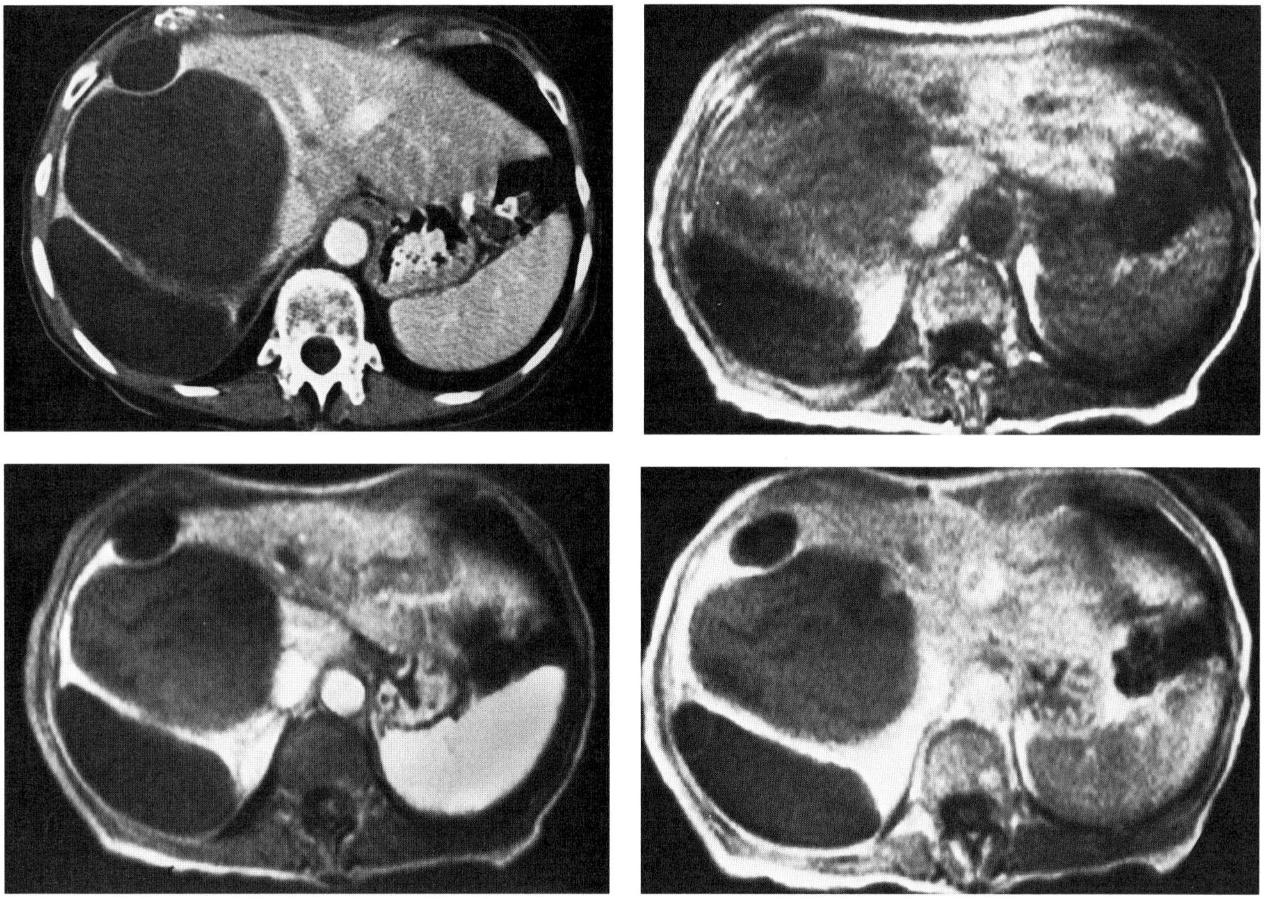

FIG. 32. Hydatid cysts with satellite cysts. CT (**A**), FLASH (**B**), 1-second (**C**) and 10-minute (**D**) postcontrast FLASH, and T2FS (**E**) images in a 77-year-old woman with a hepatic multilocular hydatid cyst. Internal calcified lesions are apparent in the main cyst on the CT images. On FLASH images the material in the main cyst is high in SI. No enhancement is present after contrast administration (C,D). These findings are compatible with proteinaceous and/or fibrinous debris. The T2FS image demonstrates the fibrous capsule and septations characteristic of this lesion. The main cyst is moderately low in SI and contains multiple high-SI septations. The low SI is compatible with proteinaceous and/or fibrinous material. The liver and spleen are low in SI on T2-weighted images, consistent with iron deposition in the RES. Note the high-SI uniform enhancement of the spleen on the 1-second postcontrast images. This is a nonspecific finding compatible with inflammatory or neoplastic disease (see Chapter 5).

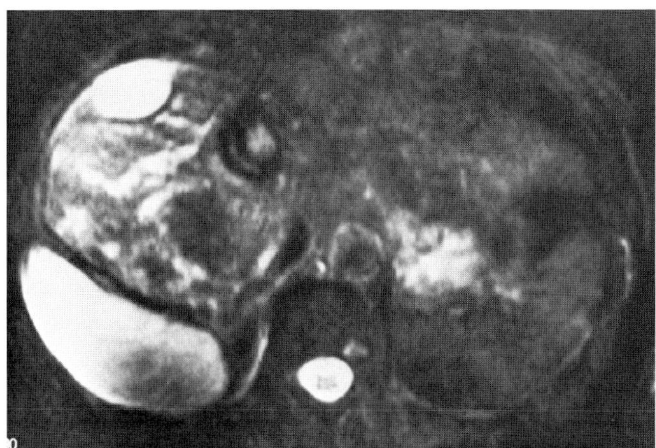

E

FIG. 32. *Continued.*

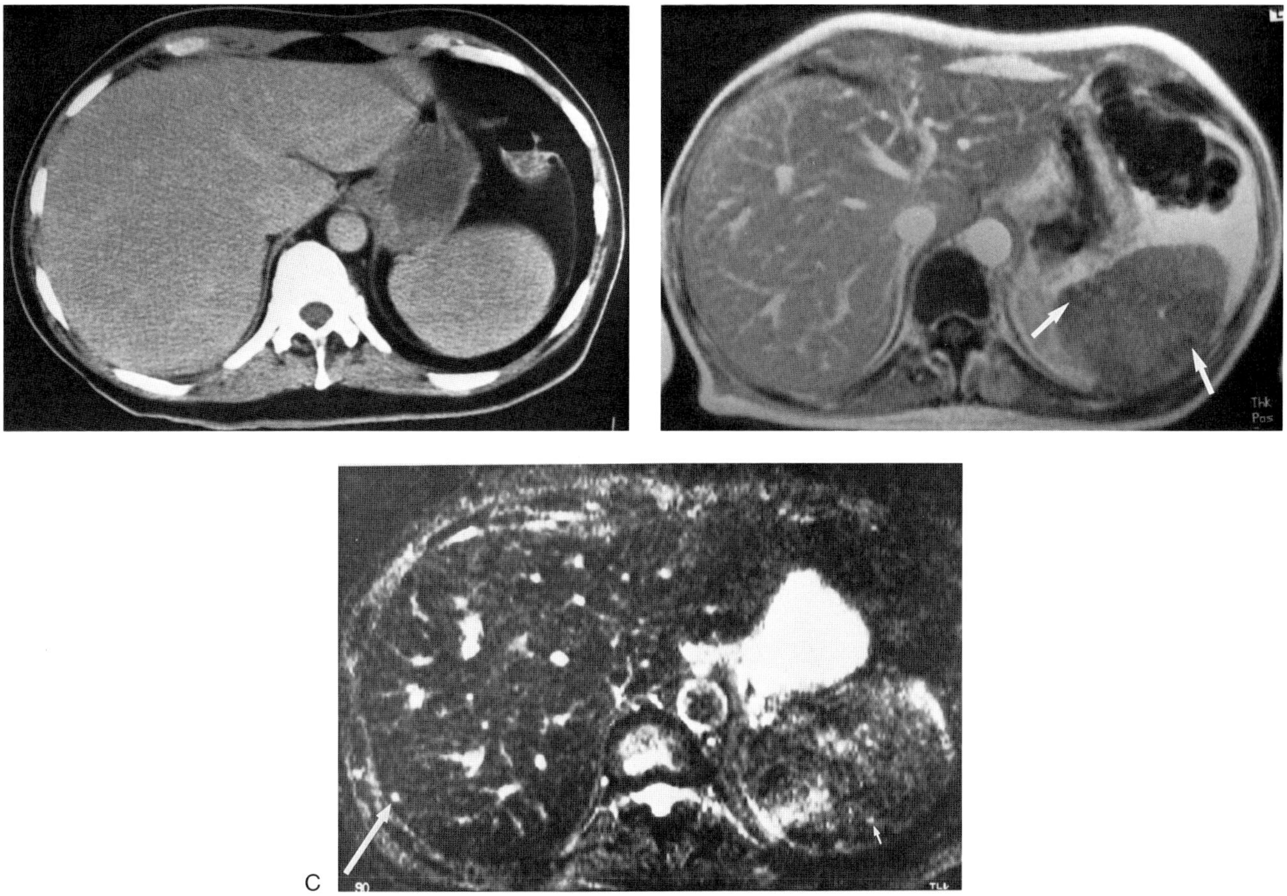

A

B

C

FIG. 33. Acute hepatosplenorenal candidiasis. Dynamic contrast-enhanced CT (**A**), 90-second postcontrast FLASH (130/4.5) (**B**), and T2FS (2300/80) (**C**), images in a 48-year-old man on consolidation chemotherapy for acute myelogenous leukemia with suspected hepatosplenic candidiasis. No lesions in the liver or spleen are apparent on the CT images (A). Gd-FLASH images did not demonstrate liver lesions but revealed numerous lesions (*white arrows*, B) in the spleen. The T2FS images (C) showed lesions smaller than 5 mm in the liver and spleen (C, *arrows*). The low SI of the liver and spleen is secondary to iron deposition. Reprinted with permission from ref. 63.

incidence of 16% for satellite cysts of hydatid cysts in a series of 185 patients (Fig. 32)(59). The fibrous capsule and internal septations are well shown on Gd-DTPA-enhanced T1-weighted and T2-weighted images (59). Calcification of the cyst wall and internal calcification are frequently identified on CT images; on MRI, however, calcification cannot be distinguished from the fibrous tissue of the capsule.

Fungal Infections

Fungal microabscesses are observed with increasing frequency as a complication of immunosuppression or an immunocompromised state (60–62). Patients on medical therapy for acute myelogenous leukemia (AML) are the group of patients most susceptible. The most common infecting organism is *Candida albicans*. Acute hepatosplenic candidiasis typically involves the liver and spleen, with other organs (such as the kidney) occasionally involved. Patient survival depends upon early diagnosis. Liver lesions are frequently <1 cm and subcapsular. The small size and peripheral nature of these lesions make them difficult to detect with standard spin echo sequences. Patients with AML undergo multiple blood transfusions, so the liver and spleen are usually low in SI in these patients (63). T2-weighted fat-suppressed spin echo may be of particular importance in detecting these lesions because of the high conspicuity of this sequence for small lesions and the absence of chemical shift artifact, which may mask small, peripheral lesions. MRI with T2-weighted fat suppression and dynamic Gd-DTPA-enhanced FLASH images is more sensitive for the detection of these lesions than is contrast-enhanced CT (64) (Fig. 33). MRI is also better able to detect lesions that have responded to antifungal therapy (64) (Fig. 34).

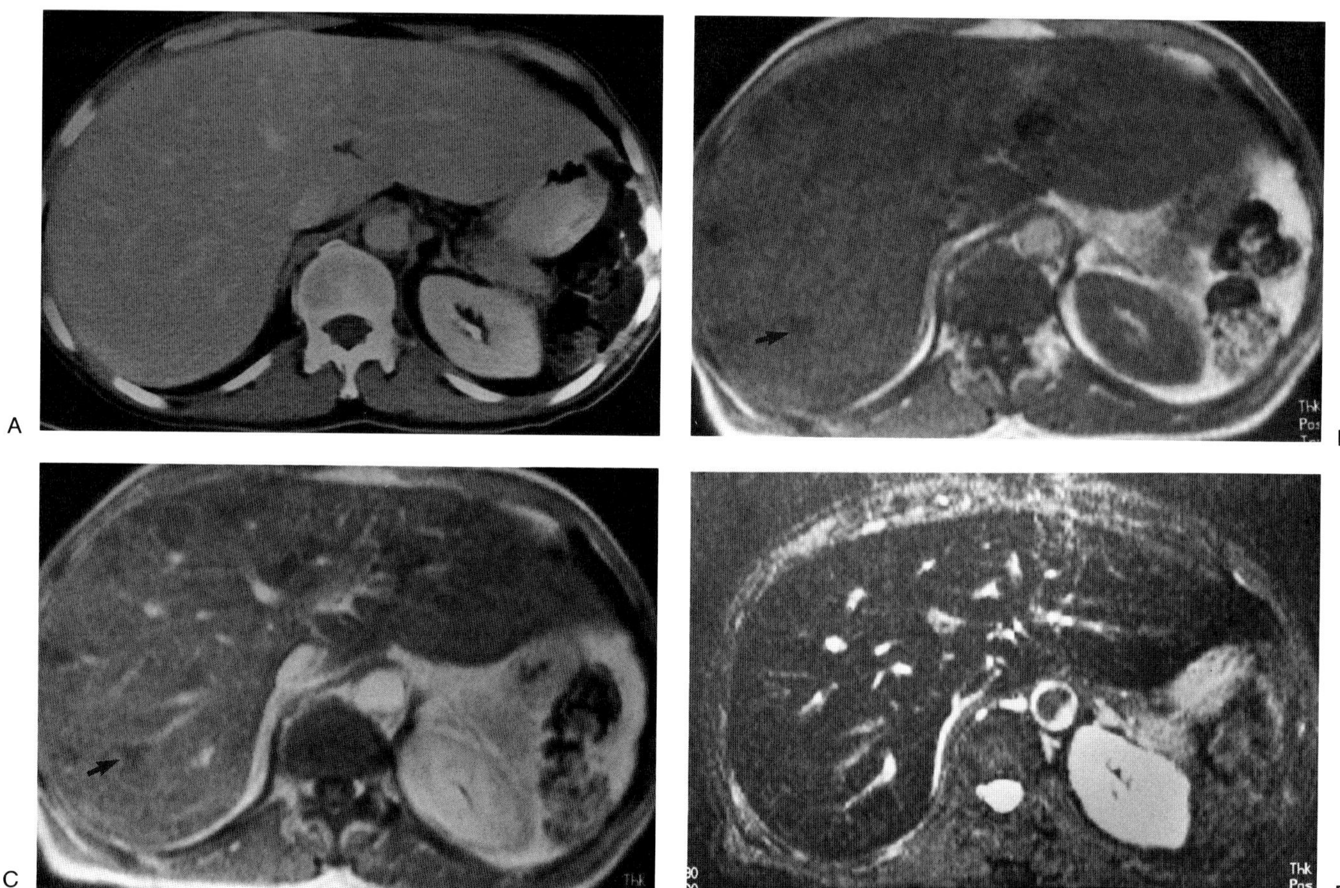

FIG. 34. Chronic treated hepatic candidiasis. Dynamic contrast-enhanced CT (**A**), FLASH (130/4.5) (**B**), 90-second postcontrast FLASH (130/4.5) (**C**), and T2FS (2300/80) (**D**) images of a 68-year-old man who had received 4 months of amphotericin B for hepatosplenic candidiasis. The spleen had been removed 1 year earlier. No lesions were identified on the CT studies. The Gd-FLASH images best defined multiple hepatic lesions that had irregular angular margins (C, *arrow*), with fewer lesions present on the precontrast FLASH image (B, *arrow*). The lesions were not identified on the T2FS image (C). The presence of large lesions with irregular margins on FLASH images with poor demonstration on T2FS images is consistent with treated lesions of candidiasis. Reprinted with permission from ref. 63.

LIVER TRANSPLANTS

MRI is suitable for the evaluation of liver transplants to assess the presence of complications including biloma, vascular thrombosis, vascular stenosis, and abscess (Fig. 35) (65,66). Preoperative evaluation of candidates for liver transplantation is particularly important for patients with malignant disease to exclude locally advanced or metastatic disease, which would preclude surgery.

NEW DIRECTIONS

Contrast Agents

Several types of contrast agents have been developed for use in liver studies, including positive contrast agents that undergo selective uptake by hepatocytes (manganese DPDP and gadolinium-EOB-DTPA) (67–70), a negative hepatobiliary agent (Fe-EHPG) (71), iron oxide particulate reticuloendothelial system (RES) agents (72–74), a positive hepatocyte/RES agent (liposomal Gd-DTPA) (75), and a negative hepatocyte receptor agent (AG-USPIO) (76,77). Combining contrast agents has also been investigated (78). The future clinical applications of these agents are yet to be determined. The largest human experience is with manganese DPDP and iron oxide particulate agents.

MR Imaging

Currently, fast T1-weighted sequences are robust and useful in MR studies (2–6). Modifications of T2-weighted sequences to acquire images during suspended respiration are under investigation. Many sequences use an echo train during one TR interval to generate fast T2-weighted images (79–83). Imaging times of some of these sequences are <1 second per image section [e.g., ultrafast low-angle RARE (U-FLARE)] (81). None of these sequences at present can generate images with an acceptable image quality for clinical examination except echo planar imaging. There seems to be a fairly unlimited capability of MRI to generate new sequences, some of which acquire new types of information such as magnetization transfer (84). It seems likely that the evolution of MR sequences is far from complete.

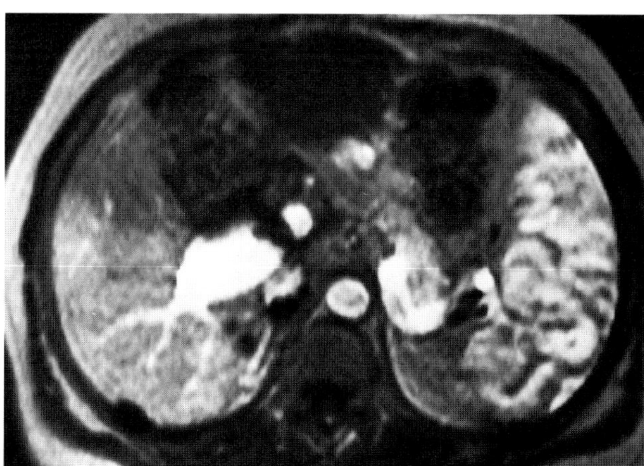

FIG. 35. Liver transplant. One-second postcontrast FLASH image in a 46-year-old woman with a liver transplant. The dilated right portal vein is appreciated as a fusiform Gd-DTPA-enhanced structure. Vascular stenosis is a common complication of liver transplantation.

REFERENCES

1. Gazelle GS, Haaga JR. Hepatic neoplasms: surgically relevant segmental anatomy and imaging techniques. *AJR* 1992;158: 1015–1018.
2. Semelka RC, Shoenut JP, Kroeker MA, Greenberg HM, Simm FC, Minuk GY, Kroeker R, Micflikier AB. Focal liver disease: comparison of dynamic contrast-enhanced CT and T2-weighted fat suppressed, FLASH, and dynamic gadolinium-enhanced MR imaging at 1.5T. *Radiology* 1992;184:687–694.
3. Semelka RC, Simm FC, Recht M, Deimling M, Lenz G, Laub GA. T1-weighted sequences of the liver—comparison of three techniques for single breath whole volume acquisition at 1.0 T and 1.5 T. *Radiology* 1991;180:629–635.
4. Taupitz M, Hamm B, Speidel A, Deimling M, Branding G, Wolf K-J. Multisection FLASH: method for breath-hold MR imaging of the entire liver. *Radiology* 1992;183:73–79.
5. Saini S, Li W, Wallner B, Hahn PF, Edelman RR. MR imaging of liver metastases at 1.5T: similar contrast discrimination with T1- and T2-weighted pulse sequences. *Radiology* 1991;181:449–453.
6. Edelman RR, Siegel JB, Singer A, Dupuis K, Longmaid HE. Dynamic MR imaging of the liver with Gd-DTPA: initial clinical results. *AJR* 1989;153:1213–1219.
7. Barnes PA, Thomas JL, Bernardino ME. Pitfalls in the diagnosis of hepatic cysts by computed tomography. *Radiology* 1981;141: 129–133.
8. Kadoya M, Matsui O, Nakanuma Y, et al. Ciliated hepatic foregut cyst: radiologic features. *Radiology* 1990;175:475–477.
9. Johnson CM, Sheedy PF, Stanson AW, Stephens DH, Hattery RR, Adson MA. Computed tomography and angiography of cavernous hemangiomas of the liver. *Radiology* 1981;138:115–121.
10. Li KC, Glazer GM, Quint LE, et al. Distinction of hepatic cavernous hemangioma from hepatic metastases with MR imaging. *Radiology* 1988;169:409–415.
11. Lombardo DM, Baker ME, Spritzer CE, Blinder R, Meyers W, Herfkens RJ. Hepatic hemangiomas vs metastases: MR differentiation at 1.5T. *AJR* 1990;155:55–59.
12. Schmiedl U, Kölbel G, Hess CF, Klose U, Kurtz B. Dynamic sequential MR imaging of focal liver lesions: initial experience in 22 patients at 1.5 T. *J Comput Assist Tomogr* 1990;14:600–607.
13. Hamm B, Fischer E, Taupitz M. Differentiation of hepatic hemangiomas from metastases by dynamic contrast-enhanced MR imaging. *J Comput Assist Tomogr* 1990;14:205–216.
14. Quinn SF, Benjamin GG. Hepatic cavernous hemangiomas: simple diagnostic sign with dynamic bolus CT. *Radiology* 1992;182:545–548.
15. Choi BI, Han MC, Park JH, Kim SH, Han MH, Kim C-W. Giant cavernous hemangioma of the liver: CT and MR imaging in 10 cases. *AJR* 1989;152:1221–1226.
16. Kerlin P, Davis GL, McGill DB, Weiland LH, Adson MA, Sheedy PR II. Hepatic adenoma and focal nodular hyperplasia: clinical, pathologic and radiologic features. *Gastroenterology* 1983;84: 994–1002.
17. Shortell CK, Schwartz SI. Hepatic adenoma and focal nodular hyperplasia. *Surg Gynecol Obstet* 1991;173:426–431.

18. Lee MJ, Saini S, Hamm B, et al. Focal nodular hyperplasia of the liver: MR findings in 35 proved cases. *AJR* 1991;156:317–320.
19. Mathieu D, Bruneton JN, Drouillard J, Pointreau CC, Vasile N. Hepatic adenomas and focal nodular hyperplasia: dynamic CT study. *Radiology* 1986;160:53–58.
20. Rogers JV, Mack LA, Freeny PC, Johnson ML, Sones PJ. Hepatic focal nodular hyperplasia: angiography, CT, sonography and scintigraphy. *AJR* 1981;137:983–990.
21. Mathieu D, Rahmouni A, Anglade M-C, et al. Focal nodular hyperplasia of the liver: assessment with contrast-enhanced Turbo-FLASH MR imaging. *Radiology* 1991;180:25–30.
22. Vilgrain V, Fléjou J-F, Arrivé L, et al. Focal nodular hyperplasia of the liver: MR imaging and pathological correlation in 37 patients. *Radiology* 1992;184:699–703.
23. Rummeny EJ, Wernecke K, Saini S, et al. Comparison between high-field-strength MR imaging and CT for screening of hepatic metastases: a receiver operating characteristic analysis. *Radiology* 1992;182:879–886.
24. Nelson RC, Chezmar JL, Sugarbaker PH, Murray DR, Bernardino ME. Preoperative localization of focal liver lesions to specific liver segments: utility of CT during arterial portography. *Radiology* 1990;176:89–94.
25. VanBeers B, Demeure R, Pringot J, et al. Dynamic spin-echo imaging with Gd-DTPA: value in the differentiation of hepatic tumors. *AJR* 1990;154:515–519.
26. Mirowitz SA, Lee JKT, Gutierrez E, Brown JJ, Heiken JP, Eilenberg SS. Dynamic gadolinium-enhanced rapid acquisition spin-echo MR imaging of the liver. *Radiology* 1991;179:371–376.
27. Adson MA, Van Heerden JA, Adson MH, Wagner JS, Ilstrup DM. Resection of hepatic metastases from colorectal cancer. *Arch Surg* 1984;119:647–651.
28. Morrow CE, Grage TB, Sutherland DER, Najarian JS. Hepatic resection for secondary neoplasms. *Surgery* 1982;92:610–614.
29. Wagner JS, Adson MA, Van Heerden JA, Adson MH, Ilstrup DM. The natural history of hepatic metastases from colorectal cancer: a comparison with resective treatment. *Ann Surg* 1984;197:502–508.
30. Sugarbaker PH, Kemeny N. Management of metastatic liver cancer. *Adv Surg* 1988;22:1–55.
31. Hughes KS, Rosenstein RB, Songhorabodi S, et al. Resection of the liver for colorectal carcinoma metastases: a multi-institutional study of long-term survivors. *Dis Colon Rectum* 1988;31:1–4.
32. Hughes KS, Simon R, Songhorabodi S, et al. Resection of the liver for colorectal carcinoma metastases: a multi-institutional study of indications for resection. *Surgery* 1988;103:278–288.
33. Doci R, Gennari L, Bignami P, Montalto F, Moralito A, Bozzetti F. One hundred patients with hepatic metastases from colorectal cancer treated by resection: analysis of prognostic determinants. *Br J Surg* 1991;78:797–801.
34. Stark DD, Wittenberg J, Butch RJ, Ferrucci JR Jr. Hepatic metastases: randomized, controlled comparison of detection with MR imaging and CT. *Radiology* 1987;165:399–406.
35. Zeman RK, Dritschillo A, Silverman PM, et al. Dynamic CT vs 0.5T MR imaging in the detection of surgically proven hepatic metastases. *J Comput Assist Tomogr* 1989;13:637–644.
36. Vassiliades VG, Foley WD, Alarcon J, et al. Hepatic metastases: CT versus MR imaging at 1.5T. *Gastrointest Radiol* 1991;16:159–163.
37. Jones EC, Chezmar JR, Nelson RC, Bernardino ME. The frequency and significance of small (<15mm) hepatic lesions detected by CT. *AJR* 1992;158:535–539.
38. Premkumar A, Sanders H, Marincola F, Feverstein I, Concepcion R, Schwartzentruber D. Visceral metastases from melanoma: findings on MR imaging. *AJR* 1992;158:293–298.
39. LaBerge JM, Laing FC, Federle MP, Jeffrey RB Jr, Lim RC Jr. Hepatocellular carcinoma: assessment of resectability by computed tomography and ultrasound. *Radiology* 1984;152:485–490.
40. Craig JR, Peters RL, Edmondson HA, Omata M. Fibrolamellar carcinoma of the liver: a tumor of adolescents and young adults with distinctive clinicopathologic features. *Cancer* 1980;46:372–379.
41. Berman MM, Libbey NP, Foster JH. Hepatocellular carcinoma: polygonal cell type with fibrous stroma—an atypical variant with a favorable prognosis. *Cancer* 1980;46:1448–1455.
42. Rummeny EJ, Weissleder R, Stark DD, et al. Primary liver tumors: diagnosis by MR imaging. *AJR* 1989;152:63–72.
43. Freeny PC, Baron RL, Teefey SA. Hepatocellular carcinoma: reduced frequency of typical findings with dynamic contrast-enhanced CT in a non-Asian population. *Radiology* 1992;182:143–148.
44. Kadoya M, Matsui O, Takashima T, Nonomura A. Hepatocellular carcinoma: correlation of MR imaging and histopathologic findings. *Radiology* 1992;183:819–825.
45. Ebara M, Watanabe S, Kita K, et al. MR imaging of small hepatocellular carcinoma: effect of intratumoral copper content on signal intensity. *Radiology* 1991;180:617–621.
46. Torres WE, Whitmire LF, Gedgaudas-McClees K, Bernardino ME. Computed tomography of hepatic morphologic changes in cirrhosis of the liver. *J Comput Assist Tomogr* 1986;10:47–50.
47. Stark DD, Hahn PF, Trey C, et al. MRI of the Budd-Chiari syndrome. *AJR* 1986;146:1141–1148.
48. Mathieu D, Vasile N, Menu Y, et al. Budd-Chiari syndrome: dynamic CT. Radiology 1987;165:409–413.
49. Gomori JM, Horev G, Tamary H, et al. Hepatic iron overload: quantitative MR imaging. *Radiology* 1991;179:367–369.
50. Siegelman ES, Mitchell DG, Rubin R, et al. Parenchymal versus reticuloendothelial iron overload in the liver: distinction with MR imaging. *Radiology* 1991;179:361–366.
51. Schertz LD, Lee JKT, Heiken JP, Molina PL, Totty WG. Proton spectroscopic imaging (Dixon method) of the liver: clinical utility. *Radiology* 1989;173:401–405.
52. Levenson H, Greensite F, Hoefs J, et al. Fatty infiltration of the liver: quantification with phase-contrast MR imaging at 1.5T vs biopsy. *AJR* 1991;156:307–312.
53. Halvorsen RA, Korobkin M, Ram RC, Thompson WM. CT appearance of focal fatty infiltration of the liver. *AJR* 1982;139:277–281.
54. Lewis E, Bernardino ME, Barnes PA, Parvey HR, SOO C-S, Chuang VP. The fatty liver: pitfalls in the CT and angiographic evaluation of metastatic disease. *J Comput Assist Tomogr* 1983;7:235–241.
55. Holley HC, Koslin DB, Berland LL, Stanley RJ. Inhomogeneous enhancement of liver parenchyma secondary to passive congestion: contrast-enhanced CT. *Radiology* 1989;170:795–800.
56. Bertel CK, Van Heerden JA, Sheedy PF. Treatment of pyogenic hepatic abscesses. *Arch Surg* 1986;121:554–558.
57. Ralls PW, Henley DS, Colletti PR, et al. Amebic liver abscess: MR imaging. *Radiology* 1987;165:801–804.
58. Landy MJ, Setiawan H, Hirsch G, Christensen EE, Conrad MR. Hepatic and thoracic amebiasis. *AJR* 1980;135:449–454.
59. Kalovidouris A, Voros D, Gouliamos A, Vlachos L, Papavasiliou C. Extracapsular (satellite) hydatid cysts. *Gastrointest Radiol* 1992;17:353–356.
60. Shirkhoda A, Lopez-Berestein G, Holbert JM, Lunga MA. Hepatosplenic fungal infection: CT and pathologic evaluation after treatment with liposomal amphotericin B. *Radiology* 1986;159:349–353.
61. Lewis JH, Patel HR, Zimmerman HJ. The spectrum of hepatic candidiasis. *Hepatology* 1982;2:479–487.
62. Myerowitz RL, Pazin GJ, Allen CM. Disseminated candidiasis: changes in incidence, underlying disease, and pathology. *Am J Clin Pathol* 1977;68:29–38.
63. Cho J-S, Kim EE, Varma DGK, Wallace S. MR imaging of hepatosplenic candidiasis superimposed on hemochromatosis. *J Comput Assist Tomogr* 1990;14:774–776.
64. Semelka RC, Shoenut PJ, Greenberg HM, Bow EJ. Detection of acute and treated lesions of hepatosplenic candidiasis: comparison of dynamic contrast enhanced CT and MR imaging. *JMRI* 1992;2:341–345.
65. Ledesma-Medina J, Dominguez R, Bowen A, Young LW, Bron KM. Pediatric liver transplantation (part 1). *Radiology* 1984;153:195–338.
66. Segel MC, Zajko AB, Bowen A, et al. Hepatic artery thrombosis after liver transplantation radiologic evaluation. *AJR* 1986;146:137–141.
67. Hamm B, Vogl TJ, Branding G, et al. Focal liver lesions: MR

imaging with Mn-DPDP—initial clinical results in 40 patients. *Radiology* 1992;182:167–174.
68. Lim KO, Stark DD, Leese PT, Pfefferbaum A, Rocklage SM, Quay SC. Hepatobiliary MR imaging: first human experience with Mn-DPDP. *Radiology* 1991;178:79–82.
69. Bernardino ME, Young SW, Lee JKT, Weinreb JC. Hepatic MR imaging with Mn-DPDP: safety, image quality, and sensitivity. *Radiology* 1992;183:53–58.
70. Schuhmann-Giampier G, Schmitt-Willich H, Press W-R, Negishi C, Weinmann H-J, Speck U. Preclinical evaluation of Gd-EOB-DTPA as a contrast agent in MR imaging of the hepato-biliary system. *Radiology* 1992;183:59–64.
71. Shtern F, Garrido L, Compton C, Swiniarski JK, Lauffer RB, Brady TJ. MR imaging of blood-borne liver metastases in mice: contrast enhancement with Fe-EHPG. *Radiology* 1991;178: 83–89.
72. Stark DD, Weissleder R, Elizondo G, et al. Superparamagnetic iron oxide: clinical application as a contrast agent for MR imaging of the liver. *Radiology* 1988;168:297–301.
73. Marchal G, Van Hecke P, Demaerel P, et al. Detection of liver metastases with superparamagnetic iron oxide in 15 patients: results of MR imaging at 1.5T. *AJR* 1989;152:771–775.
74. Fretz CJ, Stark DD, Metz CE, et al. Detection of hepatic metastases: comparison of contrast-enhanced CT, unenhanced MR imaging and iron oxide-enhanced MR imaging. *AJR* 1990; 155:763–770.
75. Unger EC, Winokur T, MacDougall P, et al. Hepatic metastases: liposomal Gd-DTPA-enhanced MR imaging. *Radiology* 1989;171:81–85.
76. Reimer P, Weissleder R, Lee AS, Wittenberg J, Brady TJ. Receptor imaging: application to MR imaging of liver cancer. *Radiology* 1990;177:729–734.
77. Weissleder R, Reimer P, Lee AS, Wittenberg J, Brady TJ. MR receptor imaging: ultrasmall iron oxide particles targeted to asialoglycoprotein receptors. *AJR* 1990;155:1161–1167.
78. Weissleder R, Saini S, Stark DD, Wittenberg J, Ferrucci JT. Dual-contrast MR imaging of liver cancer in rats. *AJR* 1988; 150:561–566.
79. Hennig J, Naureth A, Friedburg H. RARE imaging: a fast imaging method for clinical MR. *Magn Reson Med* 1986;3:823–833.
80. Jones RA, Rinck PA. Snapshot imaging using a FLARE sequence. *Magn Reson Med* 1991;21:282–287.
81. Norris DG. Ultrafast low-angle RARE: U-FLARE. *Magn Reson Med* 1991;17:539–542.
82. Feinberg DA, Oshio K. GRASE (gradient and spin-echo) MR imaging: a new fast clinical imaging technique. *Radiology* 1991;181:597–602.
83. Oshio K, Feinberg DA. GRASE (gradient- and spin-echo) imaging: a novel fast MRI technique. *Magn Reson Med* 1991;20:344–349.
84. Outwater E, Schnall MD, Braitman LE, Dinsmore BJ, Kressel HY. Magnetization transfer of hepatic lesions: evaluation of a novel contrast technique in the abdomen. *Radiology* 1992;182:535–540.

CHAPTER 4

The Gallbladder and the Biliary Tree

Richard C. Semelka, J. Patrick Shoenut, and Allan B. Micflikier

NORMAL ANATOMY

The gallbladder is an oval organ seated in the gallbladder fossa, which is located inferiorly between the right and left lobes of the liver. The anatomical components of the gallbladder are the fundus, body, neck, and cystic duct. The cystic duct joins the common hepatic duct to form the common bile duct. The normal gallbladder wall should not exceed 4 mm in thickness. The size and shape of the gallbladder can vary substantially, and its position can vary from deep in the interlobar fissure (intrahepatic gallbladder) to substantial inferior extension below the liver. The intrahepatic bile ducts are a component of the intrahepatic portal triad. The biliary tree is an arborized system. Subsegmental branches join to form segmental branches, which join to form right and left bile ducts, which join at the porta hepatis to form the common hepatic duct (CHD). The CHD joins with the cystic duct superior to the head of the pancreas to form the common bile duct (CBD). The CBD enters the head of the pancreas and in close approximation to the pancreatic duct enters the duodenum through the sphincter of Oddi. In patients younger than 60 years, the common hepatic duct should not exceed 6 mm in diameter. Beyond age 60, the normal CHD diameter may correspond to patient age in decades (e.g., 7 mm = 70 years old). The CHD and CBD are considered dilated if they measure >9 mm in diameter (1). Normal central intrahepatic ducts are frequently identified, and they should measure < 2 mm. Normal peripheral ducts are occasionally seen (2). The CBD should be visible along its entire length to the entry into the duodenum. The wall thickness of the biliary tree is 1 to 2 mm.

R. C. Semelka: Department of Radiology and Magnetic Resonance Services, University of North Carolina at Chapel Hill, Chapel Hill, North Carolina 27599.

J. P. Shoenut: University of Manitoba and Department of Medicine, Saint Boniface General Hospital, Winnipeg, Manitoba R2H 2A6.

A. B. Micflikier: Department of Medicine, University of Manitoba, Winnipeg, Manitoba R2H 2A6.

MR TECHNIQUE

The liver is the organ most affected by respiratory artifact and, as the intrahepatic bile ducts are small tubular structures within the liver, the biliary system is at a particular disadvantage for adequate demonstration. Phase artifact suppression is critical. Breath-hold FLASH is a useful sequence to study the biliary tree and should be acquired precontrast, immediately post-Gd-DTPA, and 10 minutes postcontrast (3). The precontrast and immediate postcontrast images are used mainly to image the hepatic parenchyma, as severe inflammatory enhancement of the bile duct wall is uncommon. The 10-minute postcontrast images permit ready distinction of enhanced hepatic vessels from nonenhanced bile ducts (Fig. 1). T1-weighted fat-suppressed spin echo, pre- and postcontrast, are recommended sequences. Gd-DTPA-enhanced fat suppression permits detection of abnormal extension of tumor or inflammatory periductal tissue into the liver (3). The addition of Gd-DTPA not infrequently results in increased ghosting artifact arising from respiratory motion of high-SI intrahepatic vessels containing Gd-DTPA. Multiple averaging alone has difficulty compensating for this ghosting artifact, and respiratory-ordered phase encoding may be desirable. The gallbladder is well examined with fat suppression. The combined Gd-DTPA-enhanced fat-suppressed sequence is successful for imaging inflammatory disease.

BENIGN DISEASES OF THE BILIARY TREE

Calculous Disease

The most common disease of the biliary tree is stone formation. Five hundred thousand cholecystectomies

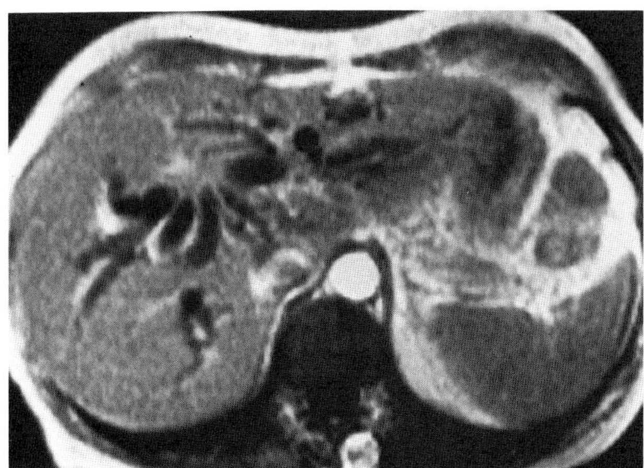

FIG. 1. Dilatation of the intrahepatic bile ducts. A 10-minute postcontrast FLASH image in a 64-year-old woman with gallbladder cancer demonstrates high-grade dilatation of the intrahepatic bile ducts, which are signal void. Intrahepatic vessels are high in SI at 10 minutes postcontrast, so distinction between ducts and vessels is readily apparent.

are performed each year in the United States, representing a billion dollar industry. In recent years, laparoscopic cholecystectomy has offered a minimally invasive alternative to open cholecystectomy (4). The two principal types of calculi are the cholesterol stone and the pigment stone. The cholesterol stone contains 70% to 90% cholesterol. The pigment stone contains a wide variety of organic and inorganic substances, with calcium bilirubinate being a major component (40% to 50% of dry weight). Approximately 80% of calculi in North America and Europe are cholesterol stones. Pigment stones develop most frequently in Asians and in patients with cirrhosis or chronic hemolytic anemia.

Presentation is most frequent in the fifth and sixth decades, although both cholesterol and pigment calculi have been reported in childhood. In women younger than 30 years, gallstones are associated with pregnancy. American Indians have the highest known prevalence of cholesterol gallstones. Low-calorie dieting may predispose obese subjects to gallstone formation by decreasing the nucleating time of cholesterol crystals in the gallbladder (5). The time lag between stone formation and clinical symptoms has been estimated at 12 years. Bile composition includes bile salts (65% to 90%), phospholipid (2% to 25%), and cholesterol (5%).

Pigment stones are frequently apparent on CT images because of the high calcium content, whereas cholesterol stones are more difficult to identify because they frequently are of soft tissue density (6). All calculi on MR images are signal void. This is because stones lack mobile protons and cannot generate a signal in response to excitation. The signal intensity of bile is very high on T2-weighted images but varies from dark (water intensity) to bright (fat intensity) on T1-weighted images, presumably because of variations in bile content of various lipids and bile salt (Fig. 2). Calculi are well shown on MR images in which bile is high in SI (Fig. 3). Small calculi are routinely identified (Fig. 4).

Cholecystitis

Acute Cholecystitis

Acute cholecystitis is caused by obstruction of the cystic duct by a calculus in 95% of patients. The acute inflammation of the gallbladder wall secondary to obstruction is caused by the toxic effects of bile salts. Lipids may also penetrate the Rokitansky-Aschoff sinus and cause an irritant reaction. Acalculous cholecystitis may develop in patients secondary to previous surgery, recent trauma, or sepsis (7). Findings in acute cholecystitis include gallbladder enlargement, gallbladder wall thickening, and pericholecystic fluid (8). Clinically, patients present with right upper quadrant pain (Murphy's sign). Serious complications of acute cholecystitis include gangrene, abscess, and rupture.

The high sensitivity of the Gd-DTPA-enhanced fat-suppressed MR sequence to inflammatory changes makes this an optimal MR technique to assess patients in whom a diagnosis of acute cholecystitis is entertained but findings of traditional imaging techniques such as sonography are equivocal (Fig. 5). Intrahepatic periportal high SI on T2-weighted images is observed in a variety of liver, biliary, and pancreatic diseases, including acute cholecystitis (9). Other acute gallbladder diseases include gallbladder wall hemorrhage (hemobilia) and gallbladder abscess (10).

Chronic Cholecystitis

Chronic cholecystitis results from chronic inflammation of the gallbladder secondary to calculous disease. This is the most common form of clinical gallbladder disease. Etiological factors include all those related to gallstones. Morphologically, the gallbladder wall is thickened, as seen in acute cholecystitis. Histologically, the mucosa is congested with lymphocytic infiltration, occasionally with the complete destruction of the mucosa. The gallbladder is usually reduced in size and is irregular in shape.

On MR the Gd-DTPA-enhanced fat-suppressed images frequently demonstrate a small, irregularly shaped gallbladder with a thickened, mildly enhancing wall. A distinguishing feature between acute and chronic cholecystitis on MR images is the degree of mural enhancement (Fig. 6).

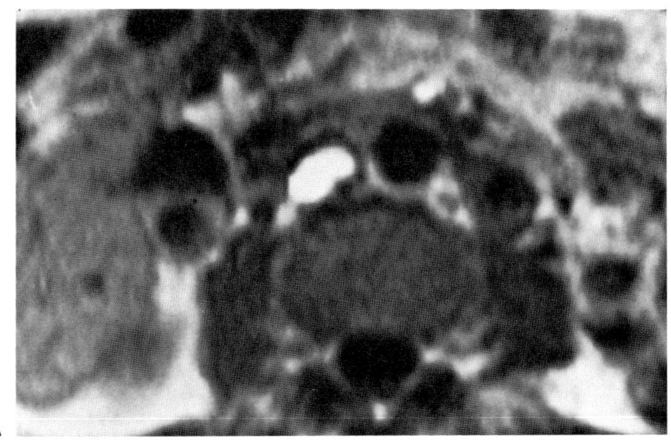

A

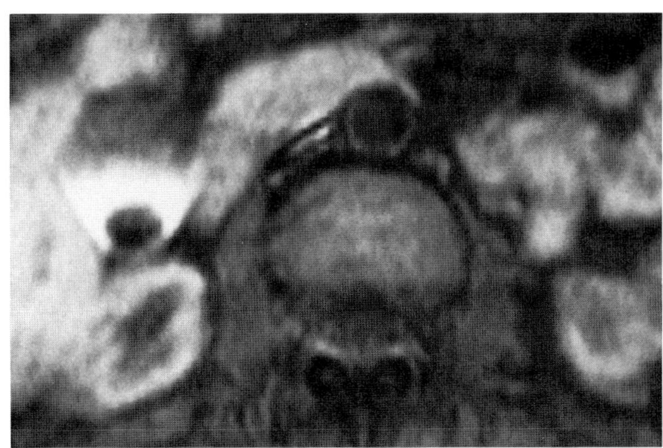

B

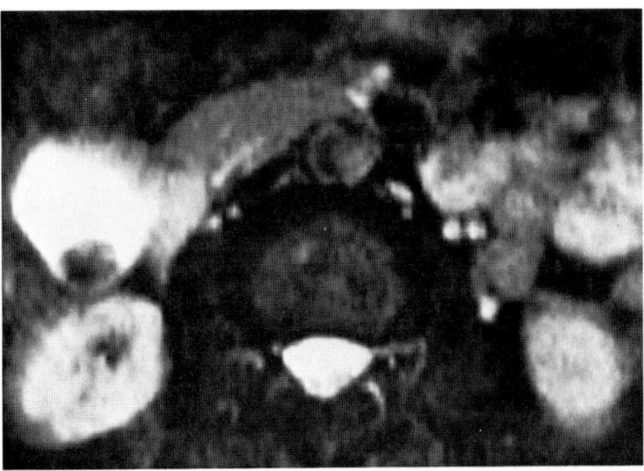

C

FIG. 2. Gallstones. Precontrast FLASH (**A**), T1FS (**B**), and T2FS (**C**) images in a 43-year-old woman with cholelithiasis. The signal-void calculus is well shown on all images. Layering of low-SI bile on top of high-SI bile is apparent on the T1-weighted images. Bile may be either high or low SI on T1-weighted images because of variations in bile composition.

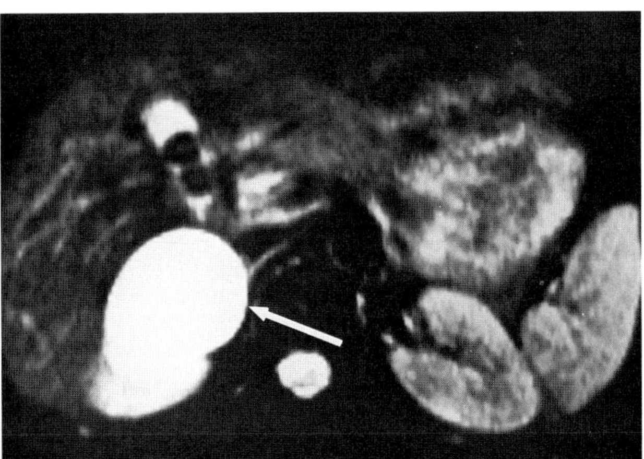

FIG. 3. Gallstones. T2-weighted fat-suppressed spin echo image in a 32-year-old woman demonstrates signal-void gallstones in a background of high-SI bile, rendering excellent conspicuity. Incidental note is made of a large cyst arising from the upper pole of the right kidney (*arrow*).

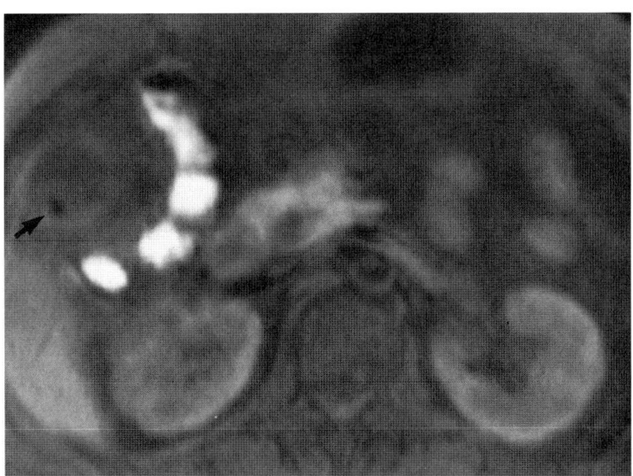

FIG. 4. Small gallstone. T1-weighted fat-suppressed spin echo image in a 38-year-old woman demonstrates a 2-mm calculus in the gallbladder (*black arrow*).

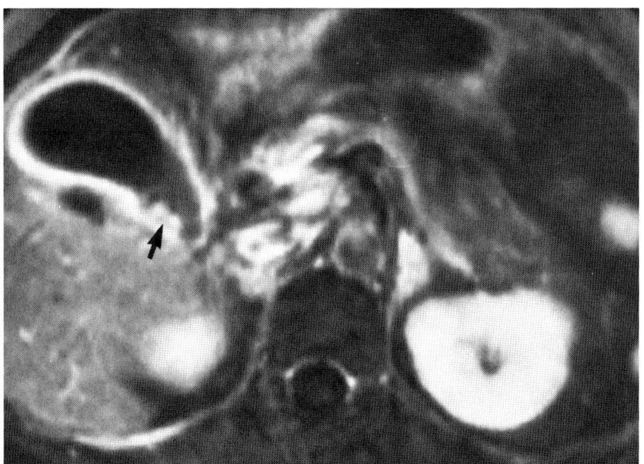

FIG. 5. Acute cholecystitis. Gd-DTPA-enhanced T1FS image in a 71-year-old women with acute cholecystitis. The gallbladder measures 5 mm in thickness and demonstrates substantial enhancement consistent with acute cholecystitis. Note is also made of two small enhancing polyps in the gallbladder (*arrow*).

Ampullary Stenosis

Ampullary stenosis most frequently occurs in the context of choledocholithiasis as a sequela of stone passage. The degree of dilatation of the biliary tree is usually moderate but can be severe. The absence of substantial dilatation of the pancreatic duct and the inability to demonstrate a duodenal or pancreatic tumor usually permit distinction from malignant disease on tomographic studies (Fig. 7). A small periampullary cancer is difficult to exclude, and endoscopic retrograde cholangiopancreatography (ERCP) is often necessary to make the diagnosis.

Choledocholithiasis

The diagnosis of choledocholithiasis can be difficult from CT images because of the tomographic nature of the technique and the frequent soft tissue attenuation of cholesterol stones (11). MRI may be superior to CT at detecting common duct stones, since T2-weighted images have higher contrast between a signal-void calculus and high-SI bile. Intrahepatic biliary dilatation may not be present despite extrahepatic biliary obstruction (12,13). ERCP is the technique of choice, since diagnosis and treatment can be performed during the same procedure.

Sclerosing Cholangitis

Primary sclerosing cholangitis (PSC) may occur in isolation, but 70% of the patients have inflammatory bowel disease, usually ulcerative colitis (14). PSC is also associated with other autoimmune conditions such as retroperitoneal fibrosis. Destruction of the intra- and extrahepatic biliary tree occurs from an inflammatory reaction that results in fibrosis. The etiology is unknown; possible mechanisms include immunological disorders, bile and biliary mucosal abnormalities, and infection (15). Male patients are twice as likely to be affected, usually between the ages of 25 and 45. No specific medical treatment exists. Secondary sclerosing cholangitis is seen in the context of preexisting biliary disease such as prior surgery, biliary stones, or prior infection.

Sclerosing cholangitis is characterized by dilated segments of the biliary tree interspersed with narrowed segments, resulting in a beaded and stenotic appearance (16–18). Bile duct walls are also thickened, usually to 3

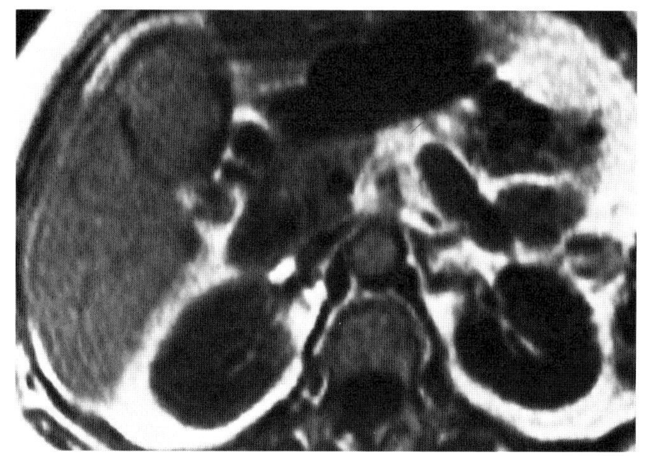

A

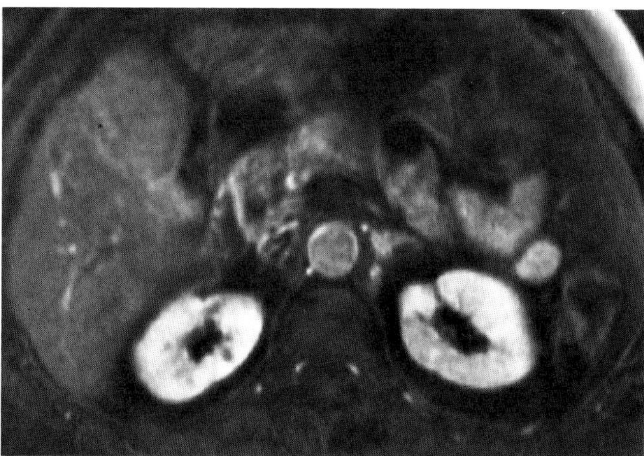

B

FIG. 6. Chronic cholecystitis. Precontrast FLASH (**A**) and Gd-DTPA-enhanced T1FS (**B**) in a 70-year-old woman with chronic cholecystitis. Gallbladder wall thickening is apparent on the FLASH and Gd-DTPA-enhanced T1FS images. Minimal enhancement is present, confirming that active inflammation is not present.

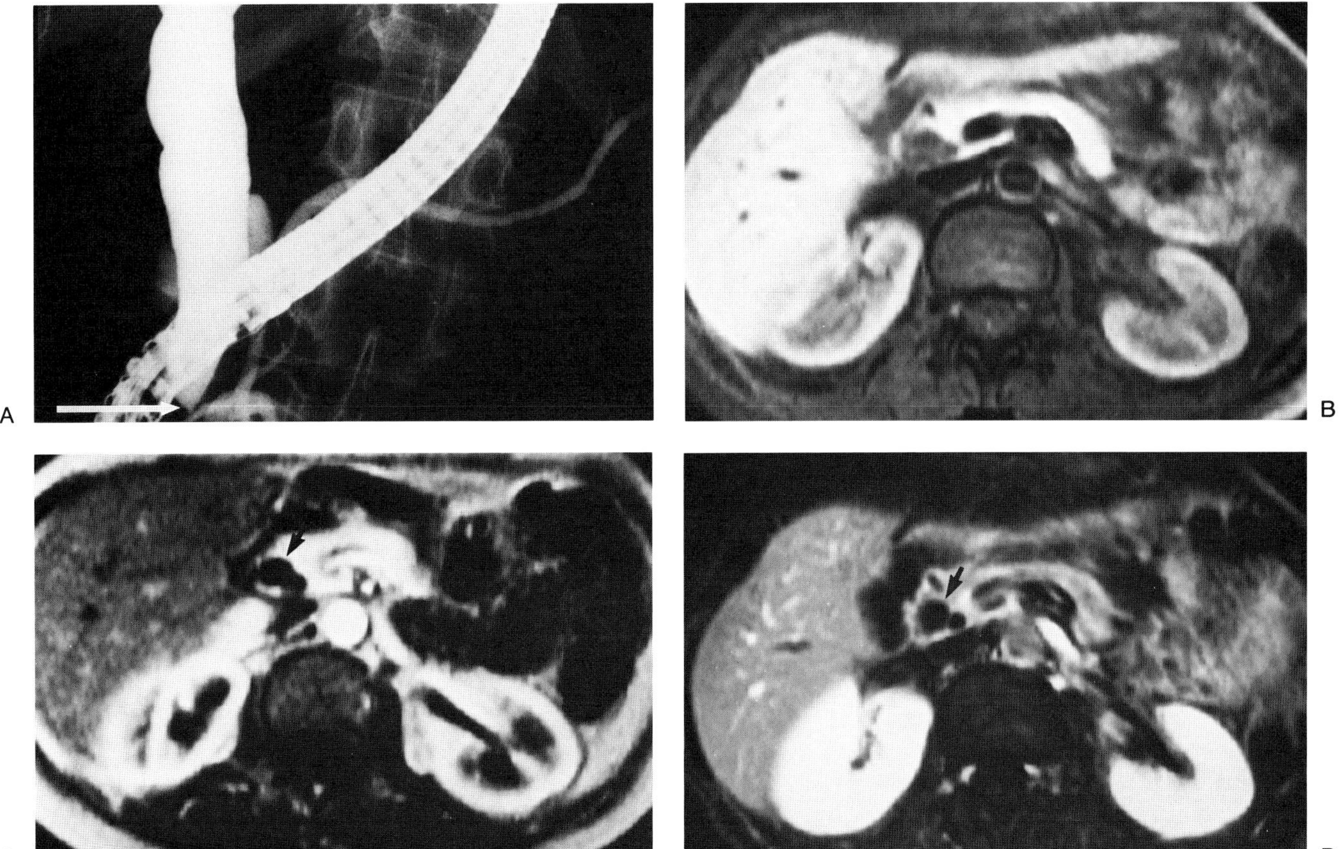

FIG. 7. Ampullary stenosis. Endoscopic retrograde cholangiopancreatography (**A**), fat-suppressed spin echo MR (**B**), immediate postcontrast FLASH (**C**), and Gd-DTPA-enhanced fat-suppressed spin echo MR (**D**) images in a 49-year-old woman with ampullary stenosis. On the ERCP image (A), the typical smoothly tapered narrowing of the CBD at the level of the ampulla of Vater is characteristic of ampullary stenosis (*arrow*). On the MR images, normal high-SI pancreatic tissue surrounds the dilated CBD on the fat-suppressed image (B) and the duct narrows in a smoothly tapered fashion into the duodenum. The Gd-DTPA-enhanced FLASH (C) fat-suppressed MR image (D) shows high contrast between pancreatic tissue and the signal-void CBD (*arrow*). Note the high contrast enhancement of normal pancreatic tissue on the FLASH image, which is a consistent finding on immediate postcontrast images. Reprinted with permission from ref. 3.

to 4 mm (18,19). The major differential diagnosis is cholangiocarcinoma. Bile duct wall thickening and dilatation are also features of cholangiocarcinoma. These entities can be distinguished on the basis of the degree of dilatation of the biliary tree; it is severe in malignant disease and moderate to mild in benign disease (20). The wall thickness in benign disease usually does not exceed 5 mm; in malignant disease, however, the wall thickness frequently exceeds 5 mm (19). Gd-DTPA-enhanced fat-suppressed spin echo images are somewhat successful in demonstrating the bile duct wall in sclerosing cholangitis. As the inflammatory process is mild, substantial enhancement is not present (3). On tomographic images mild duct wall thickening, beading, and segments of narrowing and dilatation are observed (Fig. 8). Diagnosis is usually made on the basis of ERCP findings.

Mirrizzi's Syndrome

Compression of the CHD by a calculus in the cystic duct is termed *Mirrizzi's syndrome* (21). This syndrome can occur with the gallbladder in place or after cholecystectomy. The recognition of this entity is important because CBD exploration alone would not demonstrate the cause of obstruction.

Cystic Diseases of the Biliary Tree

Choledochal cyst, choledochocele, and Caroli's disease are conditions that result from dilatation of various parts of the biliary tree. Caroli's disease is the dilatation of distal intrahepatic bile ducts, which follow a segmen-

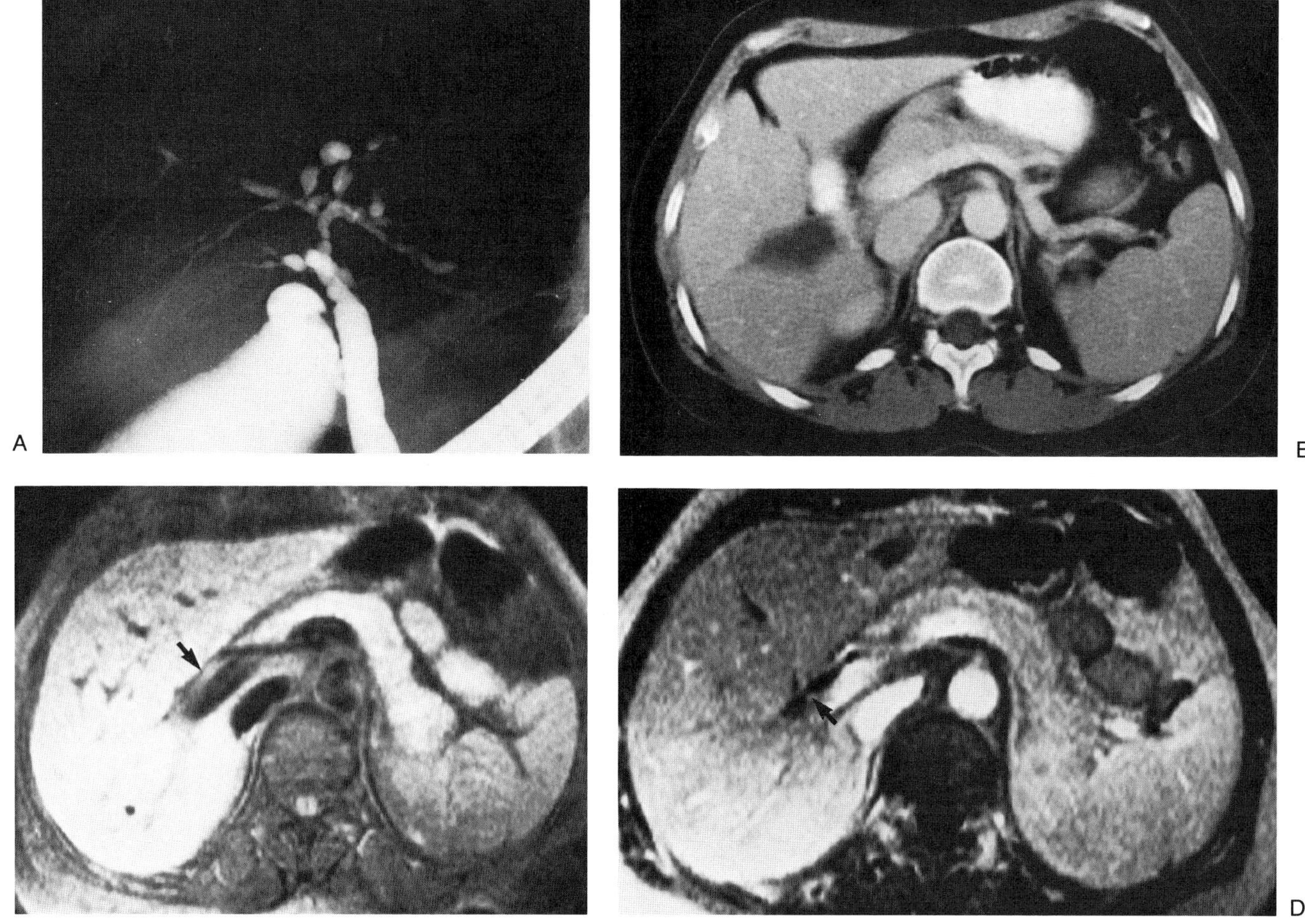

FIG. 8. Primary sclerosing cholangitis with minimal ductal dilatation. Endoscopic retrograde cholangiopancreatography (**A**), contrast-enhanced CT (**B**), fat-suppressed MR (**C**), and 10-minute postcontrast FLASH (**D**) images in a 41-year-old woman with PSC. The ERCP image (A) shows multiple smoothly tapered narrowings in the biliary system, diagnostic of PSC. Multiple beaded narrowings are present throughout the biliary tree. The lack of areas of substantial dilatation makes detection of ductal abnormalities difficult. Mild thickening of the CHD wall is identified on the T1FS image (*arrow,* C). A smooth narrowing of the common hepatic duct can be appreciated on the 10-minute postcontrast FLASH image (*arrow*). Reprinted with permission from ref. 3.

tal distribution. Choledochal cysts may have a variety of locations and appearances, but most typically appear as a uniform dilatation of the intrahepatic bile duct. An increased incidence of biliary tree malignant neoplasms is associated with this condition (22,23). A choledochocele is a termination of the distal CBD into the duodenum, forming a cystic structure (24).

Oriental Cholangiohepatitis

Oriental cholangiohepatitis is endemic in Southeast Asia. Infection by *Escherichia coli* and *Ascaris lumbricoides* is often demonstrated. Biliary dilatation and multiple calculi are imaging features (25).

Infective Cholangitis

Infective cholangitis results from infection of the biliary tree secondary to gastrointestinal organisms. Duct wall thickening and ductal dilatation are imaging features.

MALIGNANT DISEASES

Gallbladder Cancer

Gallbladder cancer is a rare neoplasm more commonly seen in female than male patients. Tumors occur in elderly patients (older than 60 years). There is a strong association with calculous disease, in that approximately 75% of patients have gallstones. The 5-year survival is poor. The most common cell type is adenocarcinoma, which may be papillary. Squamous cell and scirrhous forms have also been reported. Gallbladder cancer is characterized on imaging studies by a mass filling or replacing the gallbladder or by a mass protruding into the gallbladder lumen (26–30). Tumor invasion of adjacent liver, duodenum, and pancreas is a frequent occurrence (Fig. 9). Focal or diffuse thickening of the gallbladder wall of >1 cm is highly suggestive of the diagnosis (Fig. 10).

Cholangiocarcinomas

Cholangiocarcinoma is a primary malignant neoplasm of bile ducts which has different disease associations than has gallbladder cancer. Long-term survival for patients with cholangiocarcinoma is better than that for patients with gallbladder cancer even when the disease is advanced. In North America, cholangiocarcinoma is associated most commonly with ulcerative colitis, often with preexisting sclerosing cholangitis (31). Other associations include aniline dye exposure, liver fluke infestation, and choledochal cyst. Tumors occur in older patients (>60 years). The tumor histology is usually

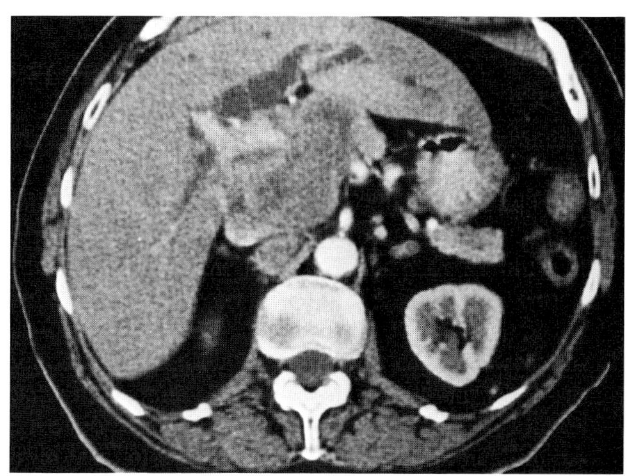

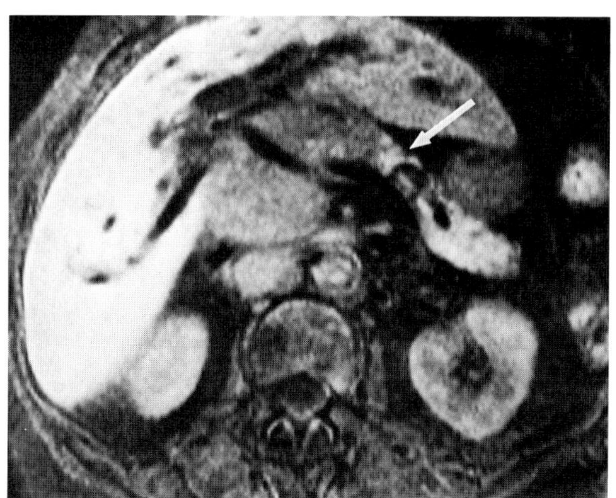

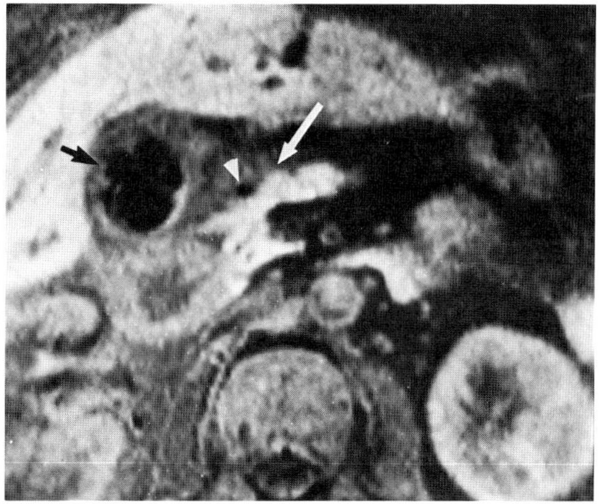

FIG. 9. Gallbladder cancer. Contrast-enhanced CT (**A**) and T1FS MR (**B,C**) images in a 74-year-old woman with gallbladder cancer. Computed tomography (**A**) and MR (**B**) images from a comparable tomographic level show a large tumor mass in the region of the porta hepatis causing high-grade obstruction of intrahepatic bile ducts. The higher contrast resolution on the fat-suppressed MR image (**B**) permits better distinction of high-SI normal pancreas (*arrow*) from the tumor mass. On more inferior sections, calculi are demonstrated on CT (not shown) and MR images (*arrow,* C) within the tumor mass, consistent with gallbladder cancer. A scalloped margin well demonstrated between the tumor and the high-SI head of the pancreas (*white arrow*,C) is compatible with invasion. Invasion of the duodenal wall and encasement of the gastroduodenal artery (*arrowhead*, C) are also shown. Reprinted with permission from ref. 3.

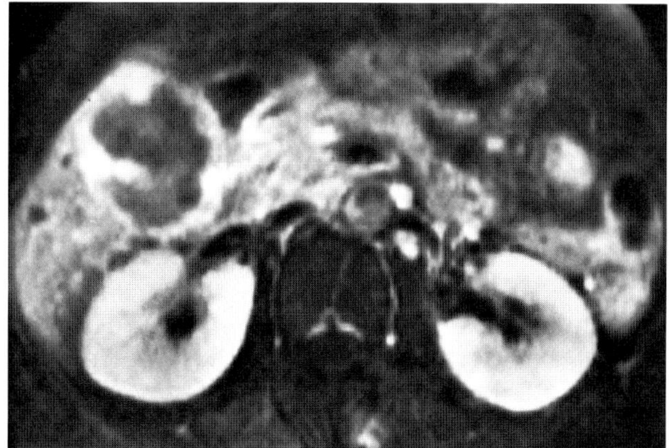

FIG. 10. Gallbladder cancer. Gd-DTPA-enhanced T1FS image in a 62-year-old woman with gallbladder cancer. Irregular thickening associated with increased enhancement is indicative of the gallbladder cancer.

consistent with mucus-secreting adenocarcinoma. The presenting features are jaundice and weight loss in over 75% of patients. Tumors are classified as central or peripheral in location. Central tumors are lesions arising from the main hepatic ducts, the CHD, or the CBD, and peripheral tumors arise from peripheral intrahepatic branches (32–39). Cholangiocarcinoma occurs most frequently (about 50% of cases) at the junction of the right and left hepatic ducts; these are termed Klatskin tumors (34). Tumors at the CHD and CBD are next in frequency, followed by intrahepatic peripheral tumors. Peripheral tumors do not cause significant impairment in overall liver function, so these tumors tend to present later as a large mass lesion (33,37,39) (Fig. 11). Determination of the proximal extent of tumor is critical for patient management to determine resectability and patient prognosis (40,41).

The presence of high-grade obstruction of the biliary tree and a wall thickness of >5 mm are findings on CT images consistent with cholangiocarcinoma (19). These features have also been observed on MR images (3). On Gd-DTPA-enhanced fat-suppressed MR images, cholangiocarcinoma enhances to a moderate extent. The enhancement of the tumor permits better delineation of intrahepatic tumor extension than on CT images (Fig. 12). Ductal tumors that arise in the intrapancreatic portion of the CBD are well delineated on fat-suppressed images as low-SI masses set in the high-SI of the head of the pancreas (Fig. 13).

Periampullary Carcinomas

Tumors that arise in the region of the ampulla are termed *periampullary carcinomas.* Patients present with obstruction of both the CBD and the pancreatic ducts. The presentation is similar to that of pancreatic ductal adenocarcinoma. The prognosis of periampullary carcinoma, however, is much better than that of pancreatic cancer, with an 85% 5-year survival after Whipple surgery for localized lesions and a 10% to 25% 5-year survival for more infiltrative tumors (42). Patients with ulcerative colitis and Gardner's syndrome are at increased risk of developing the neoplasm. *Ascaris* infection carries a significant predisposition. Periampullary tumors can range in size from millimeters to larger than 10 centimeters. Symptoms will depend on the proximity of the origin of the tumor to the ampulla. The closer the tumor origin is to the ampulla, the sooner the patient presents with signs of obstruction. The tumor can occasionally be

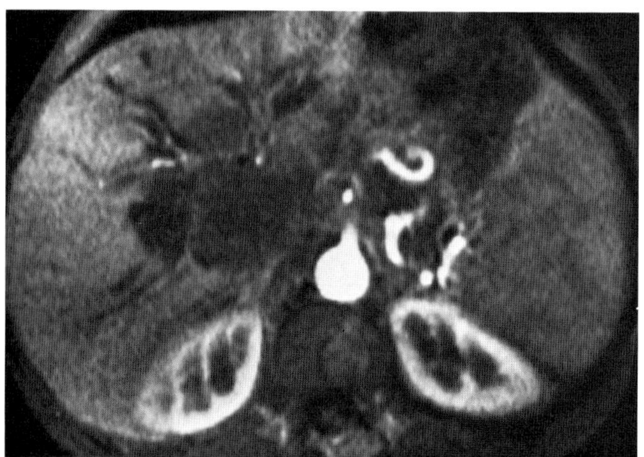

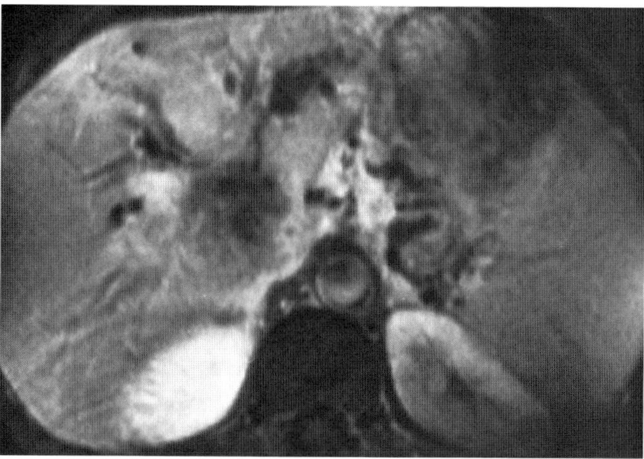

FIG. 11. Intrahepatic (peripheral) cholangiocarcinoma. One-second postcontrast FLASH (**A**) and Gd-DTPA-enhanced T1FS (**B**) images in a 47-year-old man with intrahepatic cholangiocarcinoma. A large intrahepatic mass is present, which encases the celiac axis (A). The Gd-DTPA-enhanced T1FS image shows low SI centrally within the tumor (B), consistent with a hypovascular lesion. Dilatation of intrahepatic signal-void bile ducts is identified.

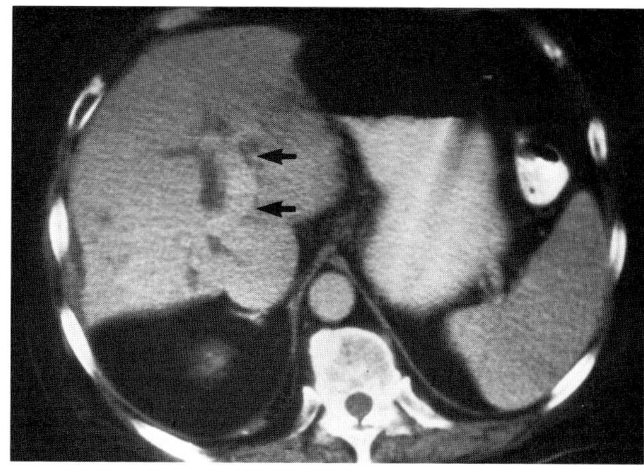

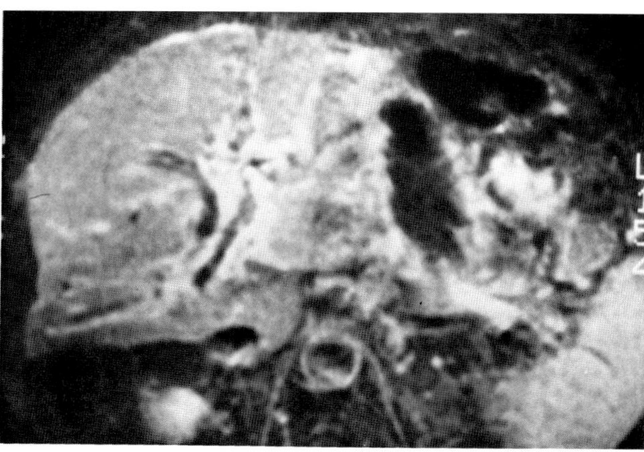

FIG. 12. Cholangiocarcinoma with proximal extension into liver. Contrast-enhanced CT (**A**) and Gd-DTPA-enhanced fat-suppressed spin echo (**B**) in a 75-year-old man with cholangiocarcincma. Dilated intrahepatic ducts are shown on the CT image; however, the intrahepatic portion of the tumor cannot be visualized because of diminished contrast resolution. On the MR image, enhancing periportal tissue can be appreciated extending into the liver. Surgical biopsies confirmed that this tissue was cholangiocarcinoma. The slightly high-attenuation tube-shaped structure on the CT image is the left portal vein (*arrow*). Reprinted with permission from ref. 3.

visualized on fat-suppressed spin echo as a low-SI mass in the region of the ampulla (Fig. 14). Diminished heterogeneous enhancement occurs after intravenous Gd-DTPA administration.

Biliary Cystadenomas/Cystadenocarcinomas

These rare tumors form a heterogeneous group. Tumors typically are quite large and have a multilocular appearance (43–45).

NEW DIRECTIONS

New lipophilic contrast agents that undergo uptake and excretion by hepatocytes provide enhancement of the biliary system (46,47). The application to biliary disease has not been ascertained as yet.

A gradient echo technique termed PSIF has been used in two-dimensional (2D) and 3D acquisition to acquire images of the biliary tree. With these techniques, the biliary tree is high in SI, which facilitates 3D image reconstruction (48).

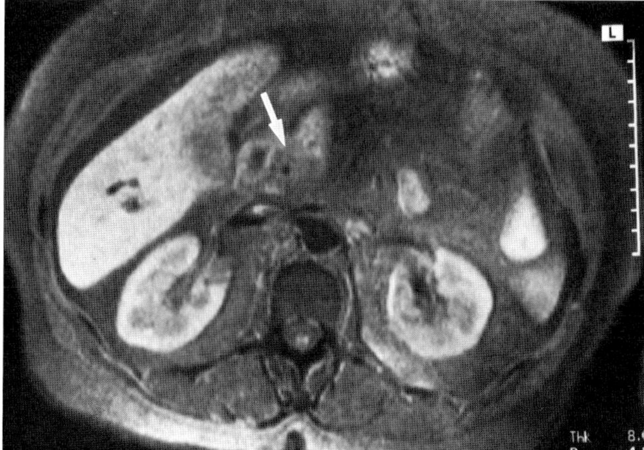

FIG. 13. Cholangiocarcinoma of the intrapancreatic portion of the CBD. T1-weighted fat-suppressed spin echo image in a 68-year-old woman with cholangiocarcinoma. An irregular low-SI circumferential mass is noted surrounding the CBD in the head of the pancreas (*arrow*).

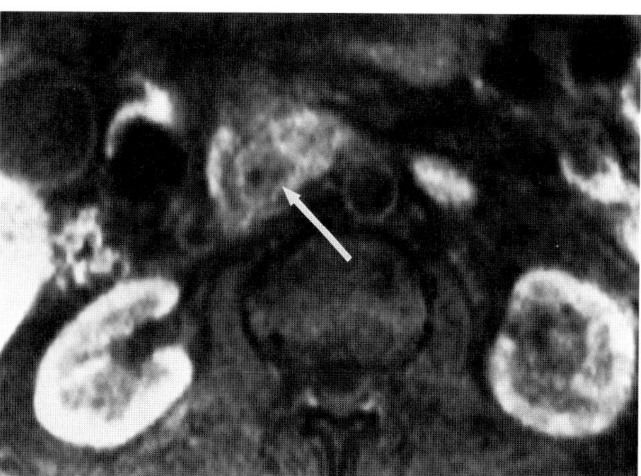

FIG. 14. Periampullary carcinoma. T1-weighted fat-suppressed spin echo image in 67-year-old man with a periampullary carcinoma. Low-SI tumor tissue (*white arrow*) is well demonstrated in a background of higher-SI pancreatic tissue at the level of the ampulla of Vater.

REFERENCES

1. Baron RL, Stanley RJ, Lee JKT, et al. A prospective comparison of the evaluation of biliary obstruction using computed tomography and ultrasonography. *Radiology* 1982;145:91–98.
2. Liddell RM, Baron RL, Ekstrom JE, Varnell RM, Shuman WP. Normal intrahepatic bile ducts: CT depiction. *Radiology* 1990;176:633–635.
3. Semelka RC, Shoenut JP, Kroeker MA, Hricak H, Minuk GY, Yaffe CS, Micflikier AB. Bile duct disease: prospective comparison of ERCP, CT, and fat suppression MRI. *Gastrointest Radiol* 1992;17:347–352.
4. Olsen DO. Laparoscopic cholecystectomy. *Am J Surg* 1991; 161:339–344.
5. Marks JW, Bonorris GG, Albers G, Schoenfield LJ. The sequence of biliary events preceding the formation of gallstones in humans. *Gastroenterology* 1992;103:566–570.
6. Berk RN, Ferrucci JT, Fordtran JS, Cooperberg PL, Weissmann HS. The radiological diagnosis of gallbladder disease. *Radiology* 1981;141:49–56.
7. Glenn F. Acute acalculous cholecystitis. *Ann Surg* 1979;189:458.
8. Kane RA, Costello P, Duszlack E. Computed tomography in acute cholecystitis: new observations. *AJR* 1983;141:697–701.
9. Matsui O, Kadoya M, Takashima T, Kamayam T, Yoshikawa J, Tamura S. Intrahepatic periportal abnormal intensity on MR images: an indication of various hepatobiliary diseases. *Radiology* 1989;171:335–338.
10. Terrier F, Becker CD, Stoller C, Triller JK. Computed tomography in complicated cholecystitis. *J Comput Assist Tomogr* 1984;8:58–62.
11. Baron RL. Common bile duct stones: reassessment of criteria for CT diagnosis. *Radiology* 1987;162:419–424.
12. Shanser JD, Korobkin M, Goldberg HI, Rohlfing BM. Computed tomographic diagnosis of obstructive jaundice in the absence of intrahepatic ductal dilatation. *AJR* 1978;1341: 389–392.
13. Pedrosa CS, Casanova R, Lezana AH, Fernandex MC. Computed tomography in obstructive jaundice: part II. The cause of obstruction. *Radiology* 1981;139:635–645.
14. LaRusso NF, Wiesner RH, Ludwig J, MacCarty RL. Current concepts: primary sclerosing cholangitis. *N Engl J Med* 1984;310:899–903.
15. Lindor KD, Wiesner RH, MacCarty RL, et al. Advances in primary sclerosing cholangitis. *Am J Med* 1990;89:73–80.
16. Rahn NH III, Koehler RE, Weyman PJ, Truss CD, Sagel SS, Stanley RJ. CT appearance of sclerosing cholangitis. *AJR* 1983;141:549–552.
17. Majoie CBLM, Reeders JWAJ, Sanders JB, Huibregtse K, Jansen PLM. Primary sclerosing cholangitis: a modified classification of cholangiographic findings. *AJR* 1991;157:495–497.
18. Teefey SA, Baron RL, Rohrmann CA, Shuman WP, Freeny PC. Sclerosing cholangitis: CT findings. *Radiology* 1988;169:635–639.
19. Schulte SJ, Baron RL, Teffey SA, Rohrmann CA Jr, Freeny PC, Shuman WP, Foster MA. CT of the extrahepatic bile ducts: wall thickness and contrast enhancement in normal and abnormal ducts. *AJR* 1990;154:79–85.
20. Baron RL, Stanley RJ, Lee JKT, Koehler RE, Levitt RG. Computed tomographic features of biliary obstruction. *AJR* 1983;140:1173–1178.
21. Htoo MM. Surgical implications of stone impaction in the gallbladder neck with compression of the common bile duct (Mirrizzi's syndrome). *Clin Radiol* 1983;3:651–655.
22. Rattner DW, Schapiro RH, Warshaw AL. Abnormalities of the pancreatic and biliary ducts in adult patients with choledochal cysts. *Arch Surg* 1983;118:1068–1073.
23. Sorensen KW, Glazer GM, Francis IR. Diagnosis of cystic ectasia of intrahepatic bile ducts by computed tomography. *J Comput Assist Tomogr* 1982;6:486–489.
24. Pollack M, Shirkhoda A, Charnsangavej C. Computed tomography of choledochocele. *J Comput Assist Tomogr* 1985;9:360–362.
25. Van Sonnenberg E, Casola G, Cubberley DA, et al. Oriental cholangiohepatitis: diagnostic imaging and interventional management. *AJR* 1986;146:327–331.
26. Itai Y, Araki T, Yoshikawa K, Furui S, Yashiro N, Tasaka A. Computed tomography of gallbladder carcinoma. *Radiology* 1980;137:713–718.
27. Smathers R, Lee JKT, Heiken JP. Differentiation of complicated cholecystitis from gallbladder carcinoma by computed tomography. *AJR* 1984;143:255–259.
28. Weiner SN, Koenigsberg M, Morehouse H, Hoffman J. Sonography and computed tomography in the diagnosis of carcinoma of the gallbladder. *AJR* 1984;142:735–739.
29. Yeh H-C. Ultrasonography and computed tomography of carcinoma of the gallbladder. *Radiology* 1979;159:167–173.
30. Sagoh T, Itoh K, Togashi K, et al. Gallbladder carcinoma: evaluation with MR imaging. *Radiology* 1990;174:131–136.
31. MacCarty RL, LaRusso NF, May GR, et al. Cholangiocarcinoma complicating primary sclerosing cholangitis: cholangiographic appearances. *Radiology* 1985;156:43–46.
32. Itai Y, Araki T, Furui S, Yashiro N, Ohtomo K, Lio M. Computed tomography of primary intrahepatic biliary malignancy. *Radiology* 1983;147:485–490.
33. Choi BI, Park JH, Kim YI, et al. Peripheral cholangiocarcinoma and clonorchiasis: CT findings. *Radiology* 1988;169:149–153.
34. Carr DH, Hadjis NS, Banks LM, Hemingway AP, Blumgart LH. Computed tomography of hilar cholangiocarcinoma: a new sign. *AJR* 1985;145:53–56.
35. Thorsen MK, Quiroz F, Lawson TL, Smith DF, Foley DW, Stewart ET. Primary biliary carcinoma: CT evaluation. *Radiology* 1984;152:479–483.
36. Engels JT, Balfe DM, Lee JKT. Biliary carcinoma: CT evaluation of extrahepatic spread. *Radiology* 1989;172:35–40.
37. Itai Y, Araki T, Furui S, Yashiro N, Ohtomo K, Lio M. Computed tomography of primary intrahepatic biliary malignancy. *Radiology* 1983;147:485–490.
38. Dooms GC, Kerlan RK Jr, Hricak H, Wall SD, Margulis AR. Cholangiocarcinoma: imaging by MR. *Radiology* 159:89–94, 1986.
39. Hamrick-Turner J, Abbitt PL, Ros PR. Intrahepatic cholangiocarcinoma: MR appearance. *AJR* 1992;158:77–79.
40. Ham JM, Mackenzie DC. Primary carcinoma of the extrahepatic bile ducts. *Surg Gynecol Obstet* 1964;118:977–983.
41. Adson MA, Farrell MB. Hepatobiliary cancer: Surgical considerations. *Mayo Clin Proc* 1981;56:686–699.
42. Yamaguchi K, Enjoji M. Carcinoma of the ampulla of Vater: a clinico-pathologic study and pathologic staging of 109 cases of carcinoma and 5 cases of adenoma. *Cancer* 1987;59:506–515.
43. Stanley J, Vujic I, Schabel SI, Gobien RP, Reines HD. Evaluation of biliary cystadenoma and cystadenocarcinoma. *Gastrointest Radiol* 1983;8:245–248.
44. Choi BI, Lim JH, Han MC, et al. Biliary cystadenoma and cystadenocarcinoma: CT and sonographic findings. *Radiology* 1989; 171:57–61.
45. Kokubo T, Itai Y, Ohtomo K, Itoh K, Kawauchi N, Minami M. Mucin-hypersecreting intrahepatic biliary neoplasms. *Radiology* 1988;168:609–614.
46. Lim KO, Stark DD, Leese PT, Pfefferbaum A, Rocklage SM, Quay SC. Hepatobiliary MR imaging: first human experience with Mn-DPDP. *Radiology* 1991;178:79–82.
47. Schuhmann-Giampier G, Schmitt-Willich, Press W-R, Negishi C, Weinmann H-J, Speck U. Preclinical evaluation of Gd-EOB-DTPA as a contrast agent in MR imaging of the hepato-biliary system. *Radiology* 1992;183:59–64.
48. Wallner BK, Schumacher KA, Weidenmaier W, Friedrich JM. Dilated biliary tract: evaluation with MR cholangiography with T2-weighted contrast-enhanced fast sequence. *Radiology* 1991;181:805–808.

CHAPTER 5

The Spleen

Richard C. Semelka and J. Patrick Shoenut

NORMAL ANATOMY

The spleen is situated posteriorly in the left upper quadrant of the abdomen. The spleen is typically crescent-shaped, with the lateral border convex, conforming to the abdominal wall and left hemidiaphragm, and the medial border concave, conforming to the stomach and left kidney. The splenic hilum is directed anteromedially, and the splenic artery and vein enter the spleen at this location. The splenic vein follows a relatively straight course along the posterior surface of the body and tail of the pancreas. The splenic artery is slightly superior to the vein and is often tortuous. The spleen is suspended by diaphragmatic attachments and by the splenorenal and splenocolic ligaments. The short gastric veins travel in the splenolenal ligament. These commonly dilate in the presence of portal hypertension. Isolated dilatation of these vessels is seen in splenic vein thrombosis.

The splenic index is the most accurate method for judging splenic size on tomographic images. The splenic index is a product of the length, width, and thickness of the spleen (in centimeters). Splenic length is derived from the number of contiguous transverse sections in which the spleen is identified. The width is the longest dimension of the spleen on any tomographic image. The thickness is the radial measurement of the spleen diameter at the splenic hilum. Normal spleen size corresponds to an index of 120 to 480 cm^3 (1).

The spleen is composed of white and red pulp. The red pulp is further divided into two components based on blood circulation or pathways. One pathway involves the passage of blood cells through a filtration process in the splenic chords, which is termed the *open circulation* and is functionally slow. The other pathway is direct passage through capillaries in the splenic sinuses to the splenic vein, which is termed the *closed circulation* and is functionally rapid (2).

R. C. Semelka: Department of Radiology and Magnetic Resonance Services, University of North Carolina at Chapel Hill, Chapel Hill, North Carolina 27599.

J. P. Shoenut: University of Manitoba and Department of Medicine, Saint Boniface General Hospital, Winnipeg, Manitoba R2H 2A6.

MR TECHNIQUE

The most important technique to evaluate the spleen is a dynamic breath-hold sequence acquired immediately after intravenous Gd-DTPA administration (3,4). This sequence assesses the compartments of the normal spleen and the presence of focal mass lesions.

NORMAL VARIANTS AND CONGENITAL ANOMALIES

The normal spleen may be variable in shape and location. Clefts and lobulations are particularly common. A cleft may be difficult to distinguish from a laceration; however, a cleft should have smooth, tapered margins and there should be no sign of adjacent soft tissue changes (e.g., free blood or fluid).

Accessory spleens are frequently observed on tomographic images. Usually, the presence of accessory spleens is not important except to distinguish them from other mass lesions. It is important to detect accessory spleens in patients who are scheduled for splenectomy for hypersplenism. If accessory spleens are not identified and removed, they can hypertrophy and hypersplenism can recur (5,6).

Asplenia/polysplenia syndromes are associated with congenital cardiac anomalies and situs abnormalities. Asplenia is associated with bilateral right-sided pulmonary anatomy and usually presents early with severe cardiac malformation (7). Polysplenia is associated with bilateral left-sided pulmonary anatomy and tends to be associated with less severe forms of congenital cardiac disease (8).

SPLENIC ENHANCEMENT

Fundamental to the detection of splenic abnormalities is the appreciation that the normal spleen enhances in an arciform fashion on immediate postcontrast images and then shows uniform high SI at 40 to 60 seconds (3,4,9–13). An advantage of MRI over most CT scanning is that the entire spleen can be examined in one phase of contrast enhancement. A previous study examined the splenic enhancement pattern in a nonselected group of 137 patients (3). One hundred eight patients (79%) had an arciform enhancement pattern, which was considered normal. This included all patients with no disease demonstrated, patients with splenomegaly on the basis of portal hypertension or as an isolated finding, and many patients with inflammatory and malignant disease. Twenty-two patients (16%) had uniformly high SI, and these included patients with inflammatory and neoplastic disease and those with focal fatty infiltration of the liver and liver enzyme abnormalities. Importantly, no normal individuals had uniform enhancement. Seven patients (5%) had uniformly low-SI spleens, and all of those patients had undergone recent multiple blood transfusions. Iron deposition in the reticuloendothelial systems of the spleen increased T2 relaxation (14), which outweighed the T1-shortening effect of Gd-DTPA. Figure 1 illustrates examples of the three patterns of dynamic splenic contrast enhancement. All three enhancement patterns can be observed in the presence of mass lesions. A fourth category, irregular enhancement, is seen in the context of diffuse splenic invasion by tumor, usually lymphoma (Fig. 2).

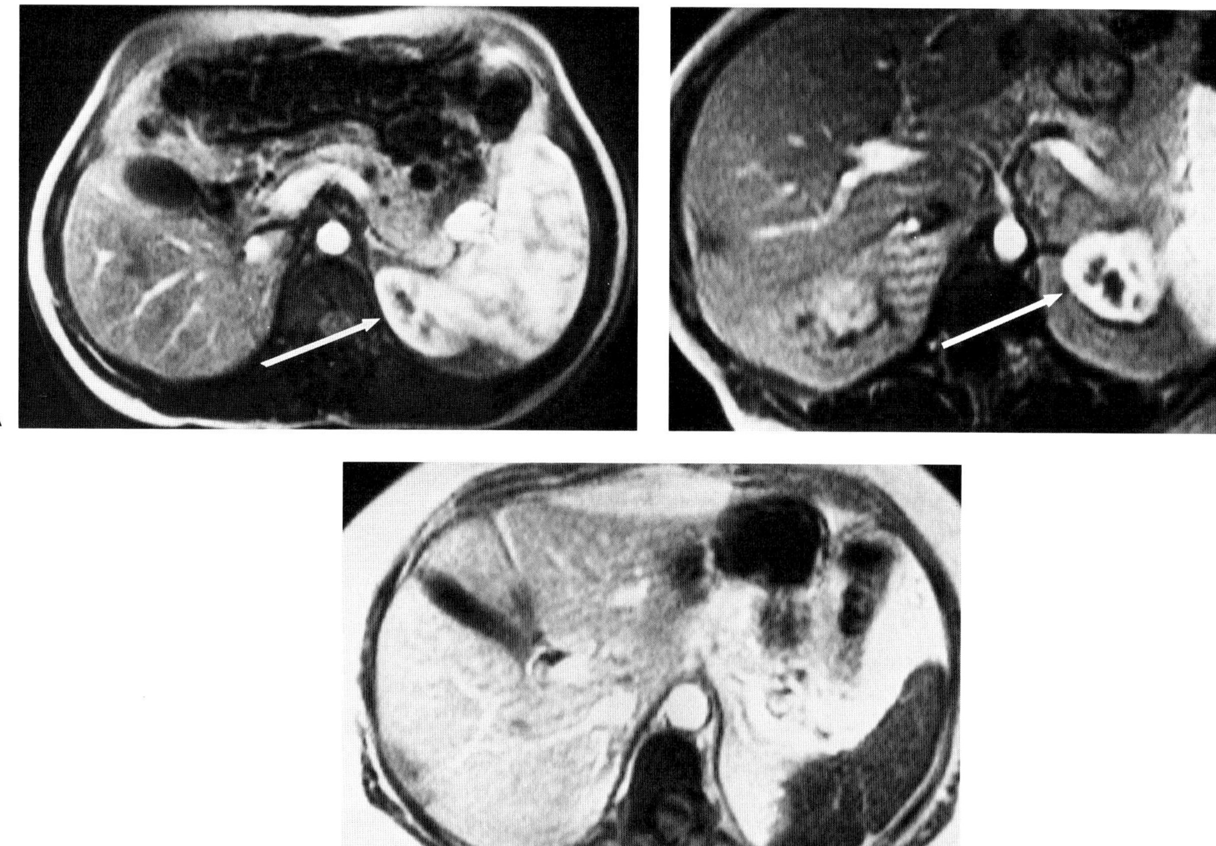

FIG. 1. Dynamic splenic enhancement patterns. Arciform (**A**), uniform high-SI (**B**), and uniform low-SI (**C**) enhancement patterns. The arciform enhancement pattern occurred in a 41-year-old woman with a polygonal gammopathy and isolated splenomegaly (A); the uniform high-SI pattern occurred in a 68-year-old man with liver metastases from colon cancer which were responding to treatment with 5-fluorouracil (B); and the uniform low-SI pattern occurred in a 57-year-old woman with treated acute myelogenous leukemia who had undergone multiple blood transfusions within the last year (C). A and B include the upper pole of the left kidney (*white arrow*). The appearance of intense renal cortical enhancement and high corticomedullary difference confirms that the images were acquired in the dynamic phase. Reprinted with permission from ref. 3.

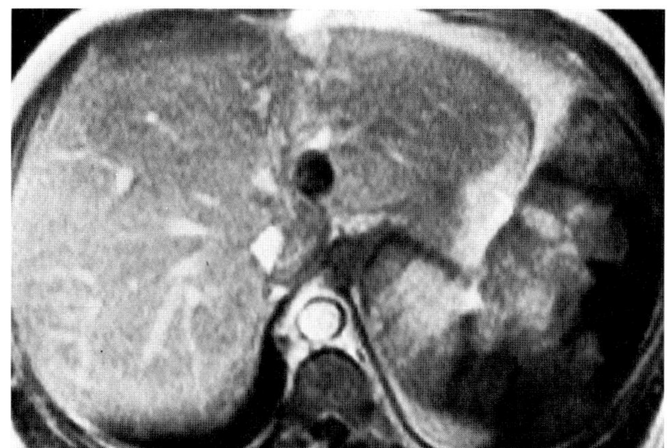

FIG. 2. Splenic infiltration with non-Hodgkin's lymphoma. One-second post-Gd-DTPA FLASH image in a 44-year-old man with non-Hodgkin's lymphoma. Irregular patchy enhancement is present in the spleen, which indicates diffuse splenic infiltration by tumor.

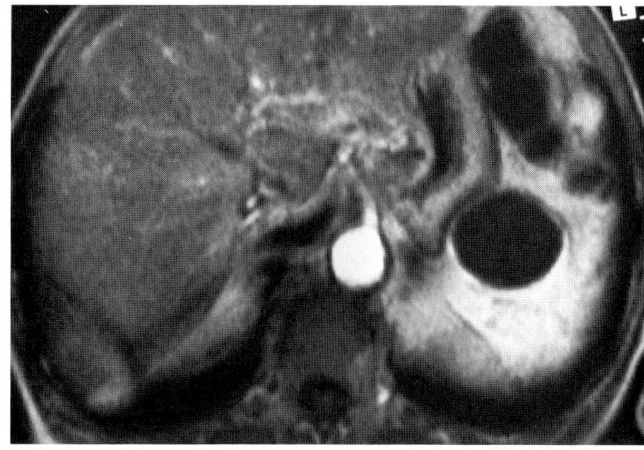

FIG. 3. Splenic pseudocyst. This 1-second post-Gd-DTPA FLASH image in a 70-year-old man demonstrates a well-defined signal-void lesion consistent with a splenic pseudocyst.

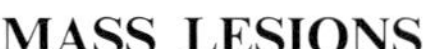

MASS LESIONS

Benign Lesions

The two most frequent benign lesions in the spleen are cysts and hemangiomas. The three most common forms of cysts are posttraumatic pseudocysts and epidermoid and hydatid cysts (15). Posttraumatic pseudocyst is the most common form of cyst, accounting for approximately 80% of cysts (Fig. 3). The diagnosis of a cyst is best made on postcontrast images, as cysts do not enhance.

Hemangiomas of the spleen are rare, but they represent the most common form of benign splenic tumor (16–18). Splenic hemangiomas typically have a different enhancement pattern from that of hepatic hemangiomas. These lesions usually remain lower in SI than adjacent spleen (Fig. 4).

Hamartomas are rare benign lesions. These lesions are noteworthy because they can have a large, aggressive appearance simulating a malignant tumor (Fig. 5).

Malignant Tumors

Lymphoma and Other Hematopoietic Malignant Neoplasms

The most common malignant neoplasm to involve the spleen is lymphoma, both Hodgkin's and non-Hodg-

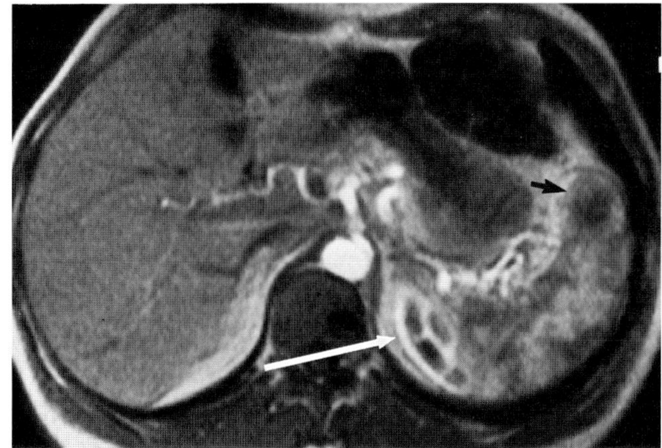

A

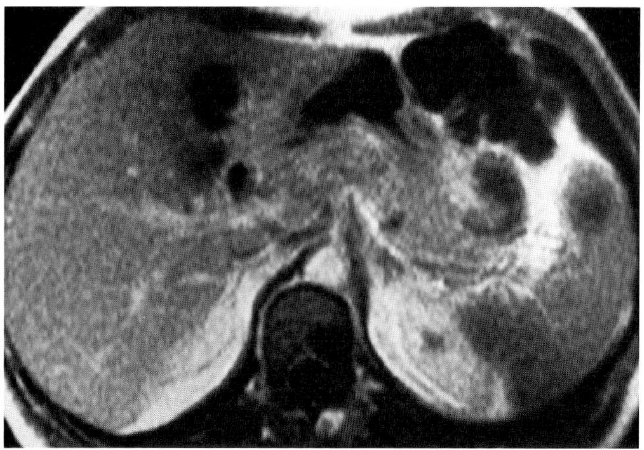

B

FIG. 4. Hemangioma. One-second (**A**) and 10-minute (**B**) post-Gd-DTPA FLASH images in a 52-year-old man with an incidental splenic mass. The high corticomedullary difference of the kidney (*white arrow*) confirms the dynamic nature of the study on the 1-second post-Gd-DTPA images (**A**). The splenic lesion is apparent on the 1-second post-Gd-DTPA image (*black arrow,* A) and remains well shown 10 minutes post-Gd-DTPA (B). Benign lesions frequently do not become isointense with splenic parenchyma on later post-Gd-DTPA images, unlike malignant lesions. Reprinted with permission from ref. 3.

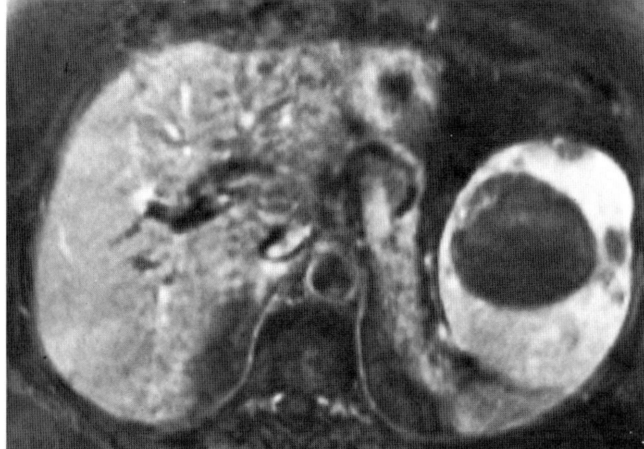

FIG. 5. Hamartoma. Gd-DTPA-enhanced T1FS image in an 80-year-old woman with a splenic hamartoma. A large mass lesion is present within the spleen, which contains central, well-defined cystic spaces.

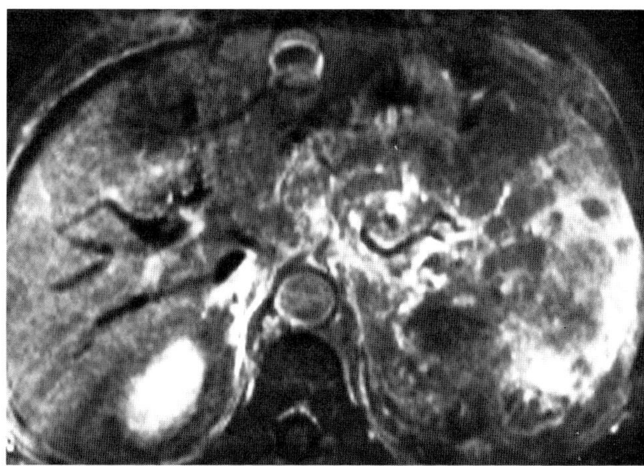

FIG. 7. Non-Hodgkin's lymphoma. Gd-DTPA-enhanced T1FS image in a 75-year-old man with non-Hodgkin's lymphoma. A large tumor mass in the left upper abdomen involves spleen, stomach, left adrenal gland, and retroperitoneal adenopathy. Invasion of spleen and contiguous upper abdominal organs is a finding suggestive of lymphoma.

kin's types (18,19). Acute and chronic leukemia and malignant histiocytosis also involve the spleen. Dynamic postcontrast images are critical to obtain in patients with lymphoma as the presence of arciform enhancement excludes tumor involvement. Diffuse lymphomatous involvement of the spleen results in an irregular enhancement pattern with large irregular patches of low- and high-SI tissue (Fig. 6). Large tumor masses in the left upper quadrant that invade local organs such as stomach, pancreas, adrenal gland, and spleen are most frequently lymphomas (Fig. 7). Focal mass lesions can be distinguished from the normal arciform enhancement of the spleen (Fig. 8). Lymphomatous involvement of the spleen occurs as focal mass lesions or as diffuse involvement.

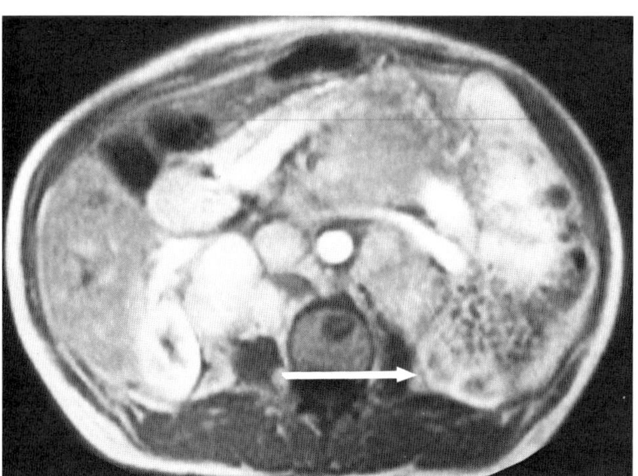

FIG. 6. Splenic infiltration with non-Hodgkin's lymphoma. One-second post-Gd-DTPA FLASH image in a 62-year-old woman with non-Hodgkin's lymphoma. Irregular patchy contrast enhancement is identified. The superior pole of the left kidney is present on this image, and the presence of a high corticomedullary difference confirms that this image was acquired in the perfusion phase. Note that irregular enhancement has a variety of appearances (see Fig. 2). Reprinted with permission from ref. 3.

Malignant mass lesions have a greater tendency than benign lesions to become isointense with splenic parenchyma after contrast enhancement. This equilibration can occur in as short a time as 1 minute after contrast administration (Fig. 8).

Metastases

Metastatic disease to the spleen is usually a late occurrence in patients with diffuse metastatic disease to other organs (20,21). Metastases appear as discrete nodules or as aggregate tumor masses that disrupt the splenic architecture (Fig. 9). The tumors that most frequently metastasize to the spleen are melanoma and breast and lung cancer. The infrequent demonstration of metastases on CT images is due in part to rapid equilibration between tumor and splenic parenchyma after contrast enhancement. Mirowitz et al. observed that at 2 minutes post Gd-DTPA, splenic metastases may become isointense with spleen (4). On conventional spin echo images metastases tend to be low in SI on T1-weighted images and high in SI on T2-weighted images (22). The SI of lesions tends to parallel that of splenic tissue rendering noncontrast images of limited value.

Infectious Lesions

Histoplasmosis, tuberculosis, and echinococcosis are the three nonviral infections that most frequently affect the spleen in the host with normal immune status. Viral infection frequently results in splenomegaly. Epstein-

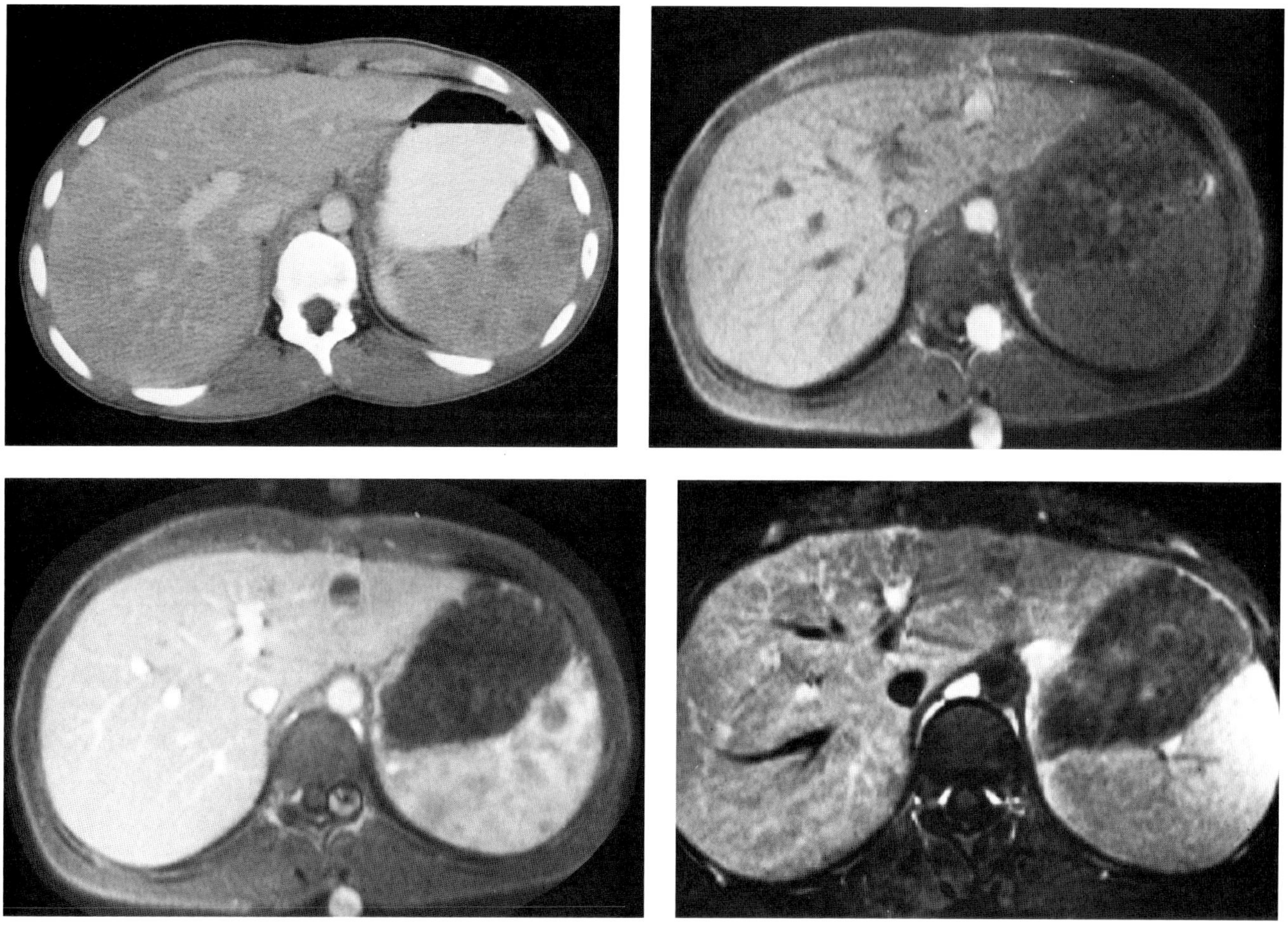

FIG. 8. Focal splenic lesions. Contrast-enhanced CT (**A**), pre-Gd-DTPA FLASH (**B**), 1-second post-Gd-DTPA FLASH (**C**), and Gd-DTPA-enhanced T1FS (**D**) images in a 16-year-old boy with Hodgkin's disease. Multiple focal lesions identified on the CT images (A) were not apparent on pre-Gd-DTPA MR images (B) but were identified on the dynamic Gd-DTPA-enhanced MR images (C). Distinction could be made between focal rounded lesions and the background tubular arciform pattern. Subsequent post-Gd-DTPA MR images (D) showed loss of contrast between spleen and focal lesions. Reprinted with permission from ref. 3.

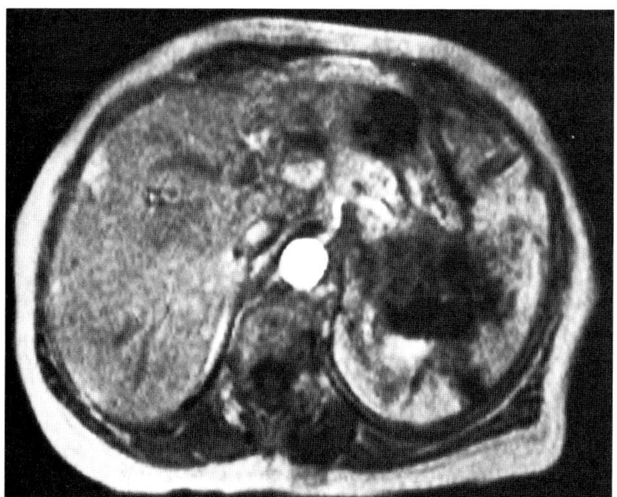

FIG. 9. Splenic metastases. One-second postcontrast FLASH Gd-DTPA-enhanced T1FS image in an 80-year-old woman with macrocystic cystadenocarcinoma of the pancreas demonstrates multiple low-SI metastatic lesions in the spleen.

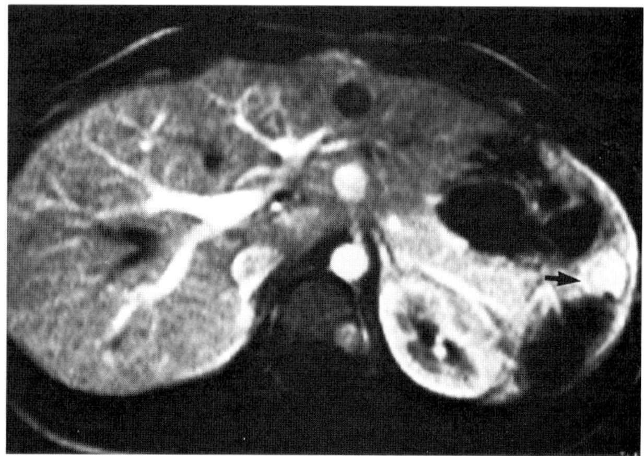

FIG. 10. Splenic trauma. One-second post-Gd-DTPA FLASH image in a 36-year-old man 3 months after abdominal trauma. A small anterior portion of the spleen is seen to enhance (*black arrow*) while the larger posterior portion of the spleen is signal void, consistent with devascularization.

Barr, varicella, and cytomegalovirus are the three most common viral agents.

In the immunocompromised host *Candida albicans* is a common infection (23,24). Fungal microabscesses are identified as high-SI foci on T2-weighted images (25) and do not enhance with Gd-DTPA (see Chapter 3, Figs. 33 and 34).

TRAUMA

The spleen is the abdominal organ most frequently ruptured in trauma. Before CT, splenic laceration usually necessitated splenectomy. Current practice is to reevaluate an injured spleen serially with tomographic imaging (26,27). A rare sequela of splenic rupture is seeding of the peritoneal cavity with splenic tissue, which may result in splenosis. Traumatic injury of the spleen is well shown on postcontrast CT and MR images. Devascularization is particularly well seen on postcontrast MR images because of the high sensitivity of MR for Gd-DTPA (Fig. 10).

NEW DIRECTIONS

Iron oxide particulate contrast is particularly well suited for studying the spleen as it is selectively taken up by the reticuloendothelial system. This agent may be useful in demonstrating diffuse lymphomatous infiltration of the spleen (28,29).

REFERENCES

1. Strijk SP, Wagener DJT, Bogman MJJT, de Pauw BE, Wobbes T. The spleen in Hodgkin disease: diagnostic value of CT. *Radiology* 1986;154:753–757.
2. Weiss L. The red pulp of the spleen: structural basis of blood flow. *Clin Haematol* 1983;12:375–393.
3. Semelka RC, Shoenut JP, Lawrence PH, Greenberg HM, Madden TP, Kroeker MA: Spleen: dynamic enhancement patterns using Gd-DTPA enhanced gradient echo MR images. *Radiology* 1992;185:479–482.
4. Mirowitz SA, Brown JJ, Lee JKT, Heiken JP. Dynamic gadolinium-enhanced MR imaging of the spleen: normal enhancement patterns and evaluation of splenic lesions. *Radiology* 1991;179:681–686.
5. Ambriz P, Munoz R, Quintanar E, Sigler L, Aviles A, Pizzuto J. Accessory spleen compromising response to splenectomy for idiopathic thrombocytopenic purpura. *Radiology* 1985;155:793–796.
6. Beahrs JR, Stephens DH. Enlarged accessory spleens: CT appearance in postsplenectomy patients. *AJR Am J Roentgenol* 1981;141:483–486.
7. Rao BK, Shore RM, Lieberman LM, Polcyn RE. Dual radiopharmaceutical imaging in congenital asplenia syndrome. *Radiology* 1982;145:805–810.
8. DeMaeyer P, Wilms G, Baert AL. Polysplenia. *J Comput Assist Tomogr* 1981;5:104–105.
9. Glazer GM, Axel L, Goldberg HI, Moss AA. Dynamic CT of the normal spleen. *AJR Am J Roentgenol* 1981;137:343–346.
10. Mirowitz SA, Gutierrez E, Lee JKT, Brown JJ, Heiken JP. Normal abdominal enhancement patterns with dynamic gadolinium-enhanced MR imaging. *Radiology* 1991;180:637–640.
11. Hamed MM, Hamm B, Ibrahim ME, Taupitz M, Mahfouz AE. Dynamic MR imaging of the abdomen with gadopentatate dimeglumine: normal enhancement patterns of the liver, spleen, stomach, and pancreas. *AJR Am J Roentgenol* 1992;158:303–307.
12. Semelka RC, Hricak H, Tomei E, Floth A, Stoller M. Obstructive nephropathy: evaluation with dynamic Gd-DTPA-enhanced MR imaging. *Radiology* 1990;175:797–803.
13. Taylor AJ, Dodds WJ, Erickson SJ, Stewart ET. CT of acquired abnormalities of the spleen. *AJR Am J Roentgenol* 1991;157:1213–1219.
14. Siegelman ES, Mitchell DG, Rubin R, et al. Parenchymal versus reticuloendothelial iron overload in the liver: distinction with MR imaging. *Radiology* 1991;179:361–366.
15. Dachman AH, Ros PR, Murari PJ, Olmsted WW, Lichtenstein JE. Nonparasitic splenic cysts: a report of 52 cases with radiologic-pathologic correlation. *AJR Am J Roentgenol* 1986;147:537–542.
16. Ros PR, Moser RP Jr, Dachman AH, Murari PJ, Olmsted WW. Hemangioma of the spleen: radiologic-pathologic correlation in ten cases. *Radiology* 1987;162:73–77.
17. Disler DG, Chew FS. Splenic hemangioma. *AJR Am J Roentgenol* 1991;157:44.
18. Bragg DG, Colby TV, Ward JH. New concepts in the non-Hodgkin lymphoma: radiologic implications. *Radiology* 1986;159:289–304.
19. Castellino RA. Hodgkin disease: practical concepts for the diagnostic radiologist. *Radiology* 1986;159:305–310.
20. Freeman MH, Tonkin AK. Focal splenic defects. *Radiology* 1976;121:689–692.
21. Piekarski J, Federle MP, Moss AA, London SS. CT of the spleen. *Radiology* 1980;135:683–689.
22. Hahn PF, Weissleder R, Stark DD, Saini S, Elizondo G, Ferrucci JT. MR imaging of focal splenic tumors. *AJR Am J Roentgenol* 1988;150:823–827.
23. Shirkhoda A, Lopez-Berestein G, Holbert JM, Luna MA. Hepatosplenic fungal infection: CT and pathologic evaluation after treatment with liposomal amphotericin B. *Radiology* 1986;159:349–353.
24. Berlow ME, Spirt BA, Weil L. CT follow-up of hepatic and splenic fungal microabscesses. *J Comput Assist Tomogr* 1984;8:42–45.
25. Semelka RC, Shoenut JP, Greenberg HM, Bow EJ. Detection of acute and treated lesions of hepatosplenic candidiasis: Comparison of dynamic contrast-enhanced CT and MR imaging. *J Magn Reson Imag* 1992;2:341–345.
26. Berger PE, Kuhn JP. CT of blunt abdominal trauma in childhood. *AJR Am J Roentgenol* 1981;136:105–110.
27. Federle MP, Goldberg HI, Kaiser JA, Moss AA, Jeffrey RB, Mall JC. Evaluation of abdominal trauma by computed tomography. *Radiology* 1981;138:637–744.
28. Weissleder R, Hahn PF, Stark DD, et al. Superparamagnetic iron oxide: enhanced detection of focal splenic tumors with MR imaging. *Radiology* 1988;169:399–403.
29. Weissleder R, Elizonda G, Stark DD, et al. The diagnosis of splenic lymphoma by MR imaging: value of superparamagnetic iron oxide. *AJR Am J Roentgenol* 1989;152:175–180.

CHAPTER 6

The Pancreas

Richard C. Semelka, J. Patrick Shoenut, Mervyn A. Kroeker, and Allan B. Micflikier

NORMAL ANATOMY

The anatomical divisions of the pancreas include the head, neck, uncinate process, body, and tail. The usual shape of the pancreas resembles a field hockey stick. The tail is located in the region of the splenic hilum, and the body is oriented in an oblique fashion extending to the right of midline. The neck of the pancreas passes anterior to the portal vein and curves posteriorly and inferiorly to form the head of the pancreas. The uncinate process is a medial triangle-shaped extension of the head of the pancreas. The uncinate process lies posterior to the superior mesenteric vein.

The anatomical relationship of the head of the pancreas includes the second portion of the duodenum laterally, the gastroduodenal artery anteriorly, the inferior vena cava posterolaterally, the third portion of the duodenum posteroinferiorly, and the superior mesenteric vessels medially. Considerable variation in the size of the head of the pancreas occurs.

The splenic vein lies on the dorsal surface of the body and tail of the pancreas. This constant relationship is an important landmark for the identification of the pancreatic body. The left adrenal gland is seated posterior to the splenic vein. The tail of the pancreas frequently drapes over the left kidney and terminates in the splenic hilum. The stomach lies anterior to the pancreas and is separated from it by parietal peritoneum and the lesser sac. The transverse mesocolon forms the inferior boundary of the lesser sac and is formed by the fusion of parietal peritoneal leaves, which cover the anterior surface of the pancreas. The lesser sac and transverse mesocolon are important, as they represent common pathways for fluid tracking and accumulation in acute pancreatitis.

The outer surface of the pancreas may vary in appearance from smooth to lobulated. In elderly patients fatty replacement of the pancreas occurs frequently as a normal degenerative process and results in a feathery, lobulated appearance.

The pancreatic duct is frequently identified on fat-suppressed spin echo and immediate dynamic Gd-DTPA-enhanced FLASH images. The duct should not exceed 1 to 2 mm in diameter in normal subjects. The normal pancreatic head should measure 2 to 2.5 cm in diameter, with the remainder of the gland approximately 1 to 2 cm thick. The main pancreatic duct continues from the body of the pancreas through the head and empties through the sphincter of Oddi into the second part of the duodenum. This main duct is termed the *duct of Wirsung*. A smaller accessory duct or duct of Santorini extends from the duct of the body of the pancreas through the neck and enters separately into the duodenum in a more proximal location.

The pancreas performs two distinct functions involving two specific cell types: exocrine function performed by acinar cells and endocrine function performed by islet cells. The major hormones released by the pancreas are insulin and glucagon.

MR TECHNIQUE

The most important sequence for imaging the pancreas is fat-suppressed T1-weighted spin echo (1–3). The

R. C. Semelka: Department of Radiology and Magnetic Resonance Services, University of North Carolina at Chapel Hill, Chapel Hill, North Carolina 27599.

J. P. Shoenut: University of Manitoba and Department of Medicine, Saint Boniface General Hospital, Winnipeg, Manitoba R2H 2A6.

M. A. Kroeker: Department of Radiology, University of Manitoba, Winnipeg, Manitoba R2H 2A6.

A. B. Micflikier: Department of Medicine, University of Manitoba, Winnipeg, Manitoba R2H 2A6.

high aqueous protein content of normal pancreatic tissue results in a relatively high SI on fat-suppressed images. Pancreatic tumors do not contain aqueous protein and therefore appear as low-SI focal masses (2). Chronic pancreatitis also has diminished SI and appears as diffuse low-SI changes in the pancreas (2).

Immediate post-Gd-DTPA-enhanced images are a useful adjunct to fat-suppressed images in that they demonstrate the capillary phase of enhancement of the pancreas. Dynamic imaging is particularly important in the investigation of islet cell tumors, which may be very vascular. Other applications include the investigation of pancreatic ductal cancer and pancreatitis. Non-fat suppressed T1-weighted images are most useful to demonstrate inflammatory peripancreatic changes in acute pancreatitis. The normal appearance of the pancreas on pre- and post-Gd-DTPA-enhanced images is illustrated in Fig. 1.

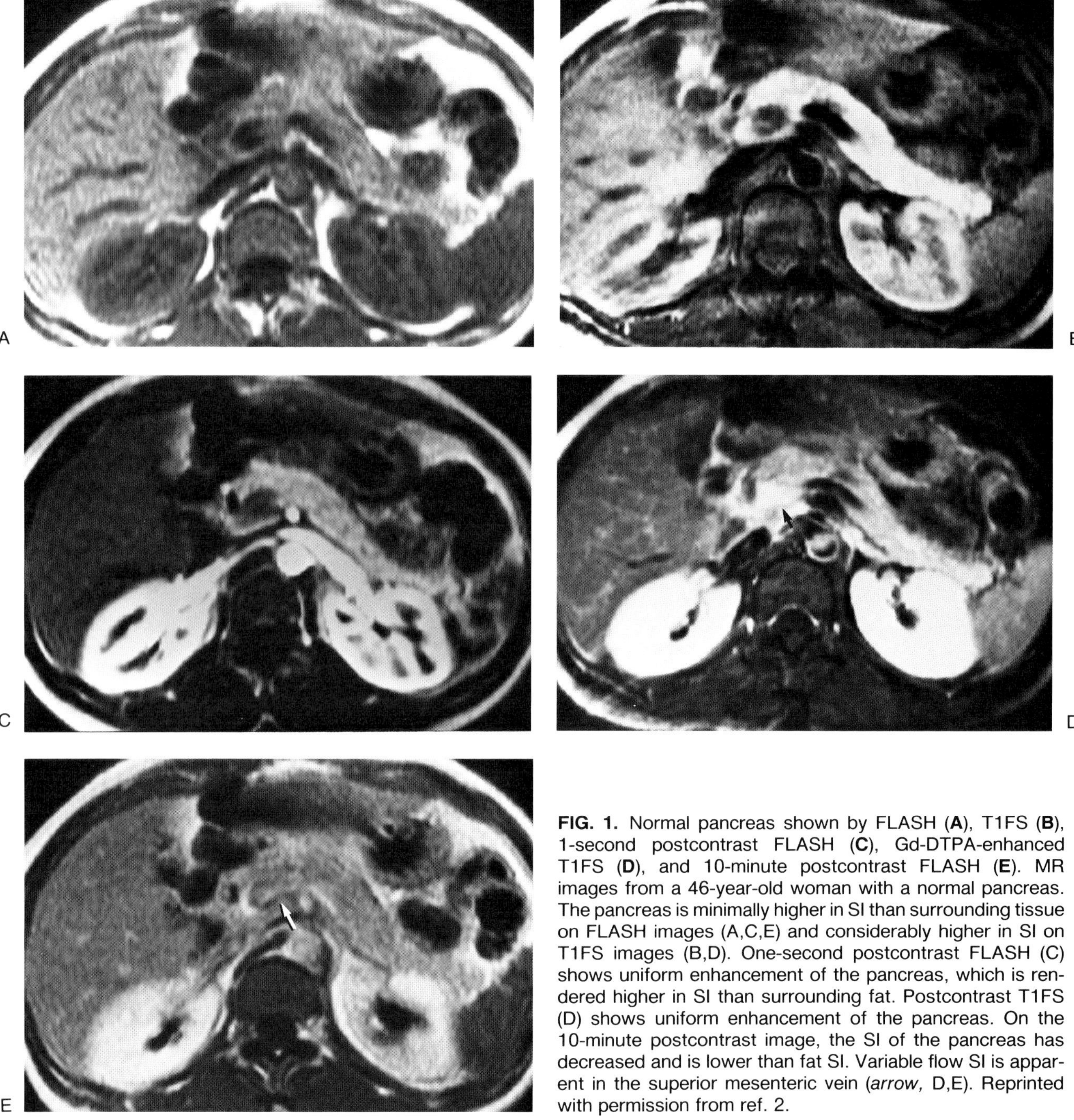

FIG. 1. Normal pancreas shown by FLASH (**A**), T1FS (**B**), 1-second postcontrast FLASH (**C**), Gd-DTPA-enhanced T1FS (**D**), and 10-minute postcontrast FLASH (**E**). MR images from a 46-year-old woman with a normal pancreas. The pancreas is minimally higher in SI than surrounding tissue on FLASH images (A,C,E) and considerably higher in SI on T1FS images (B,D). One-second postcontrast FLASH (C) shows uniform enhancement of the pancreas, which is rendered higher in SI than surrounding fat. Postcontrast T1FS (D) shows uniform enhancement of the pancreas. On the 10-minute postcontrast image, the SI of the pancreas has decreased and is lower than fat SI. Variable flow SI is apparent in the superior mesenteric vein (*arrow,* D,E). Reprinted with permission from ref. 2.

DEVELOPMENTAL ANOMALIES

Pancreas divisum is the most clinically important and common major anatomical variant. This results from the failure of embryological fusion of the head and body of the pancreas. These portions of the pancreas have separate ductal systems; the head is drained by the duct of Wirsung and the body by the duct of Santorini. The incidence of this anomaly varies from 1.3% to 6.7% of the population (4). The definitive diagnostic procedure is endoscopic retrograde cholangiopancreatography with injection of both pancreatic ducts. On tomographic images separate entry of both ducts with no communication between them can occasionally be demonstrated (Fig. 2).

Pancreatic divisum on occasion results in recurrent acute pancreatitis. It is believed that there is a partial obstruction to the passage of pancreatic exocrine secretions from the dorsal pancreas through the narrow orifice at the duodenum, which may result in a leak of secretions into the pancreatic tissue, causing pancreatitis.

MASS LESIONS

Adenocarcinomas

Pancreatic ductal adenocarcinoma accounts for 95% of the malignant tumors of the pancreas. Pancreatic adenocarcinoma is the fourth most common cause of cancer death in the United States (5). The lesion is more common in males and blacks (6). The age range for tumor occurrence is the fourth through eighth decades, with tumor incidence peaking in the eighth decade (7). The tumor carries a poor prognosis, with a 5-year survival of 5% (6). Approximately 60% of pancreatic adenocarcinomas occur in the head, 15% in the body, 5% in the tail,

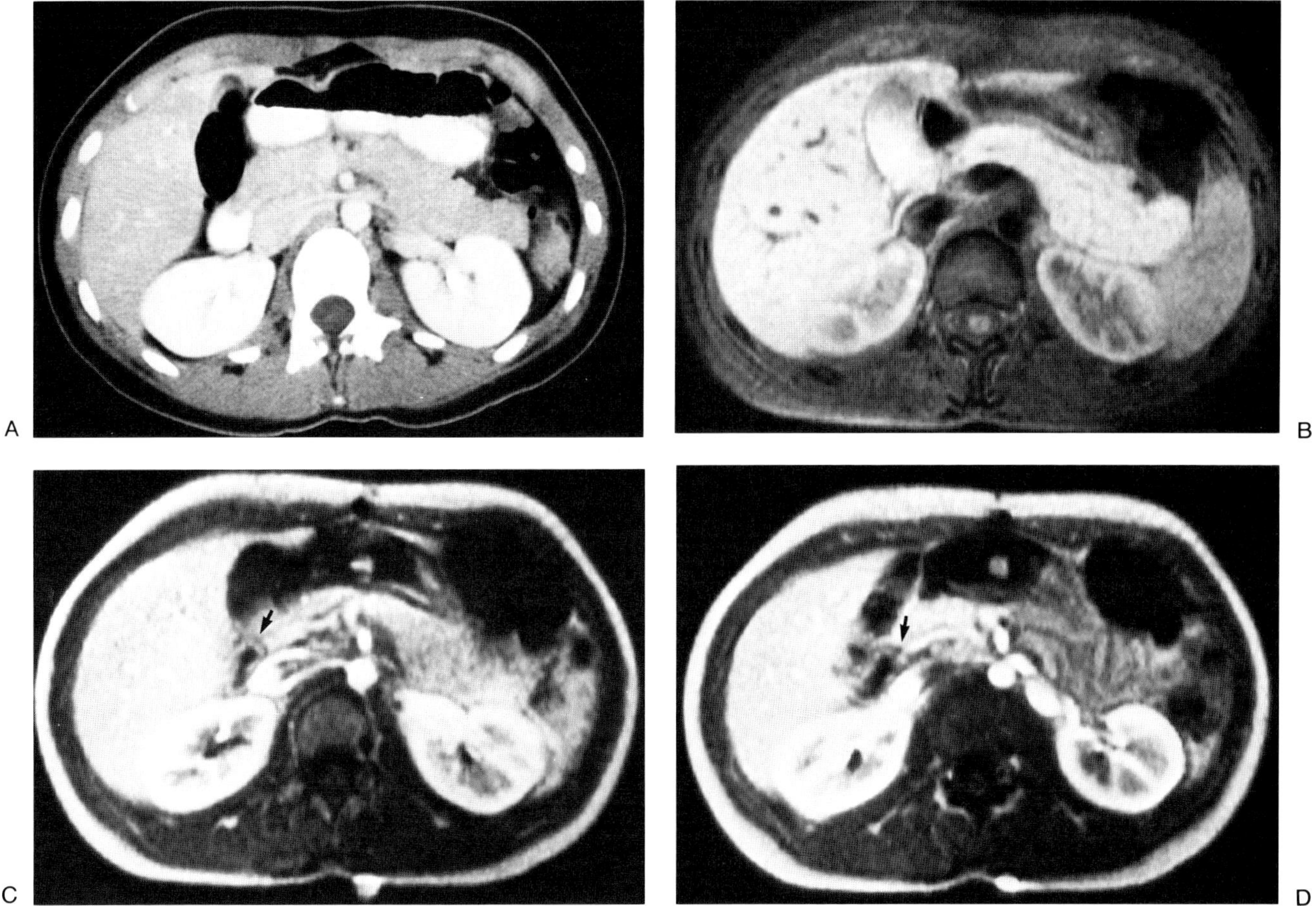

FIG. 2. Pancreas divisum. Contrast-enhanced CT (**A**), precontrast T1FS (**B**), and 1-second postcontrast FLASH (**C,D**) images in a 24-year-old woman with surgically proven pancreas divisum. No pancreatic calcifications are present in the CT study (A). The precontrast T1FS image shows a normal high-SI pancreas (B). Gd-DTPA-enhanced FLASH images show normal pancreatic enhancement (C,D). Separate entry into the duodenum of the ducts of Santorini (*arrow,* C) and Wirsung (*arrow,* D) can be identified with no continuity between the ducts. Reprinted with permission from ref. 49.

and 20% diffusely (8). Since tumors in the head of the pancreas are in intimate relation to the common bile duct, they tend to present when smaller than tumors in the body or tail, as they cause obstruction of the CBD and jaundice. Painless jaundice is the classic presenting feature of pancreatic cancer.

Pancreatic cancer tends to present late, when the disease is advanced. At initial investigation 65% of patients have advanced local disease or distant metastases, 21% have localized disease with spread to regional lymph nodes, and only 14% have tumor confined to the pancreas (9). The most common sites of metastases, in order of decreasing frequency, are liver, regional lymph nodes, peritoneum, and lungs (8). The rich lymphatic supply and lack of a capsule account for the early spread of cancer to regional lymph nodes, which include peripancreatic, periaortic, pericaval, periportal, and celiac. Calcification rarely occurs in pancreatic cancer, although the tumor can occur in a pancreas containing calcification.

Pancreatic cancer of the head of the pancreas causes abrupt obstruction of the CBD and the pancreatic duct (10). This appearance on ERCP studies has been termed the "double duct sign." This phenomenon can also be seen in patients with focal pancreatitis. Other secondary features of pancreatic cancer include the presence of lymphadenopathy, liver metastases, and encasement of the celiac axis or superior mesenteric artery (8,11). On tomographic images vascular encasement is observed as a loss of the fat plane around vessels (12). Only liver metastases are an absolute indication of malignancy, as lymphadenopathy and vascular encasement may occur, although rarely, in inflammatory disease.

The presence of a mass in the head of the pancreas causing dilatation of the CBD and pancreatic duct and atrophy of the body and tail of the pancreas is a common tomographic appearance of pancreatic cancer. This appearance can be seen in focal pancreatitis of the pancreatic head. Secondary features are important assessments to increase confidence in the diagnosis of pancreatic cancer. A small percentage of cases will remain indeterminate, and CT-guided biopsy will be necessary to make the diagnosis. False-negative biopsies do occur, and imaging follow-up is frequently necessary in the presence of negative biopsies.

Pancreatic cancers enhance to a lesser extent than does normal pancreatic tissue because of their desmoplastic, fibrotic composition (13). It is therefore critical in contrast-enhanced studies to exploit this difference in vascularity by imaging in the dynamic capillary phase of enhancement. Thin image section thickness is also helpful. Conventional spin echo images have been limited in the evaluation of pancreatic cancer (14). Fat-suppressed MR images have inherently superior contrast resolution to CT for imaging of the pancreas and may be superior in detecting small non-organ deforming tumors (Fig. 3).

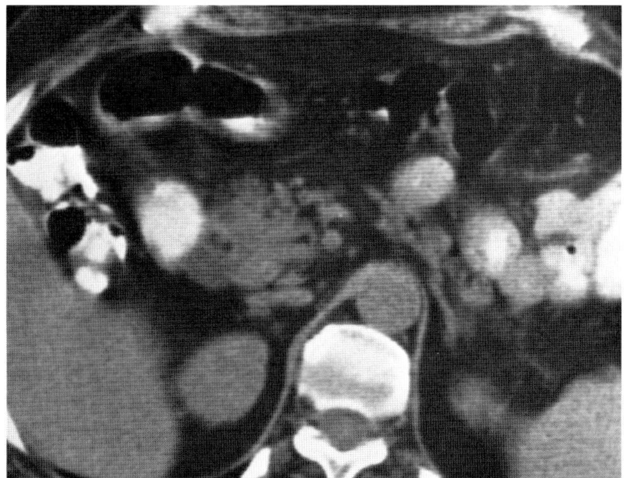
A

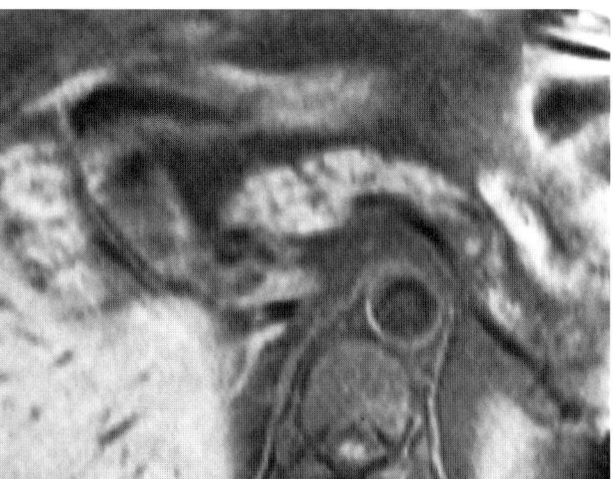
B

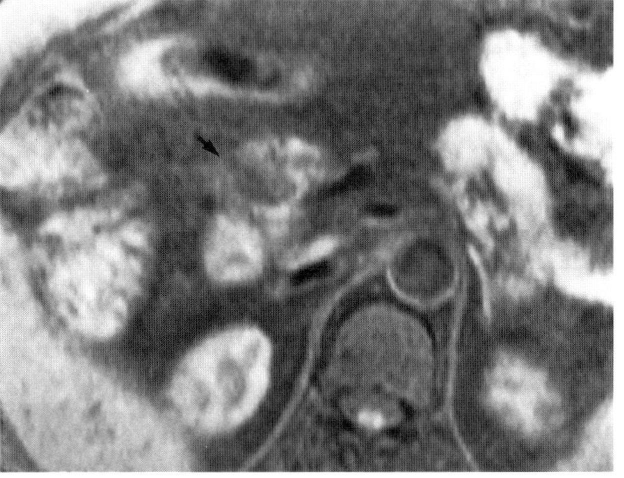
C

FIG. 3. Pancreatic cancer. Noncontrast 5-mm CT (**A**) and T1FS (**B,C**) images in a 62-year-old woman with pancreatic cancer. The CT image does not demonstrate the non-contour deforming pancreatic cancer. The MR image of the body of the pancreas is unremarkable (B), while a low-SI non-contour deforming lesion (*arrow,* C) is present in the neck of the pancreas, which was subsequently found to be a pancreatic cancer at surgery.

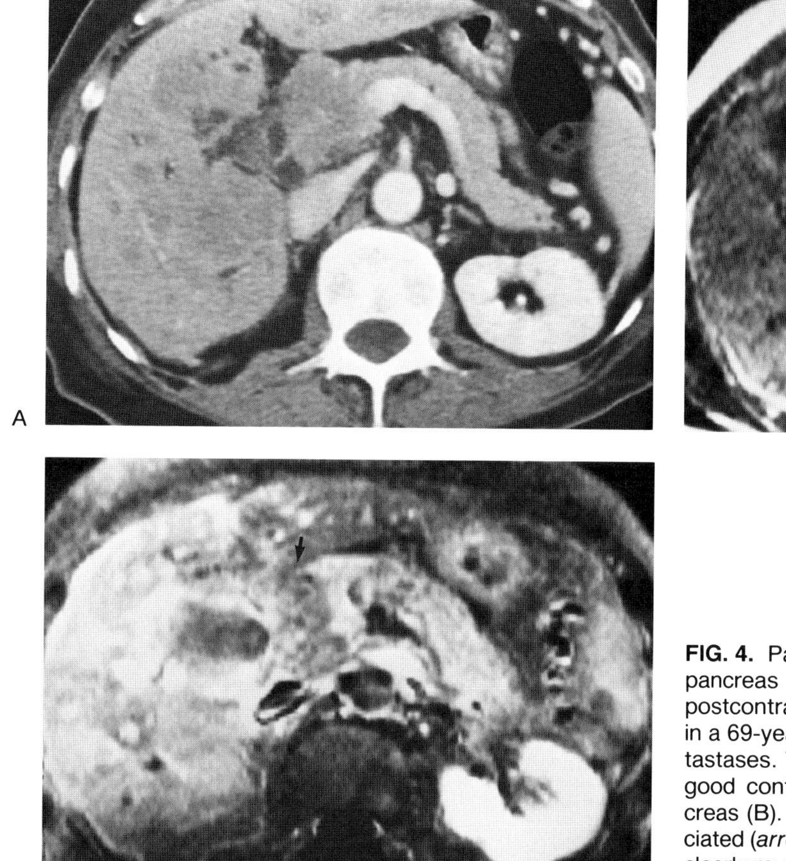

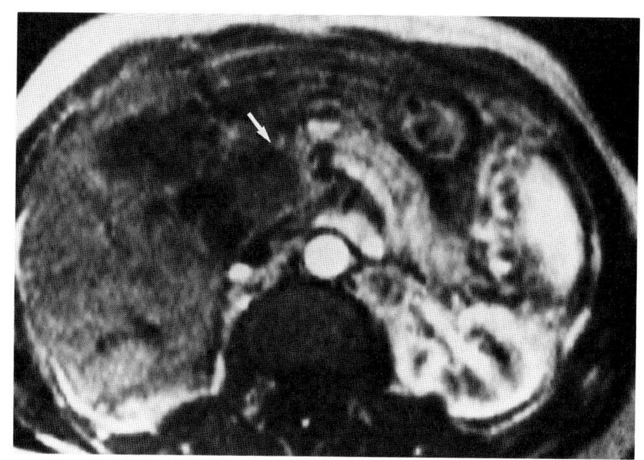

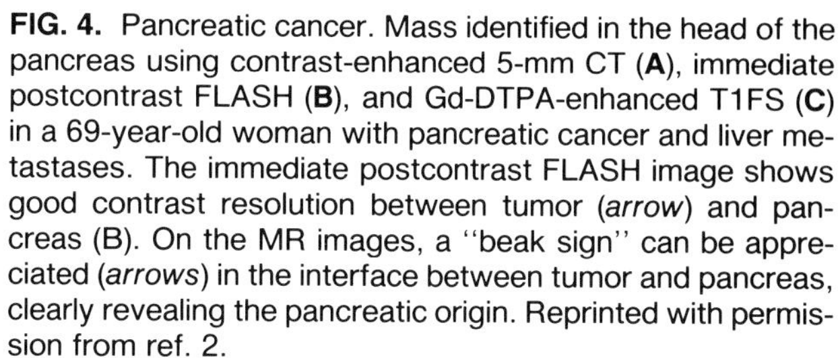

FIG. 4. Pancreatic cancer. Mass identified in the head of the pancreas using contrast-enhanced 5-mm CT (**A**), immediate postcontrast FLASH (**B**), and Gd-DTPA-enhanced T1FS (**C**) in a 69-year-old woman with pancreatic cancer and liver metastases. The immediate postcontrast FLASH image shows good contrast resolution between tumor (*arrow*) and pancreas (B). On the MR images, a "beak sign" can be appreciated (*arrows*) in the interface between tumor and pancreas, clearly revealing the pancreatic origin. Reprinted with permission from ref. 2.

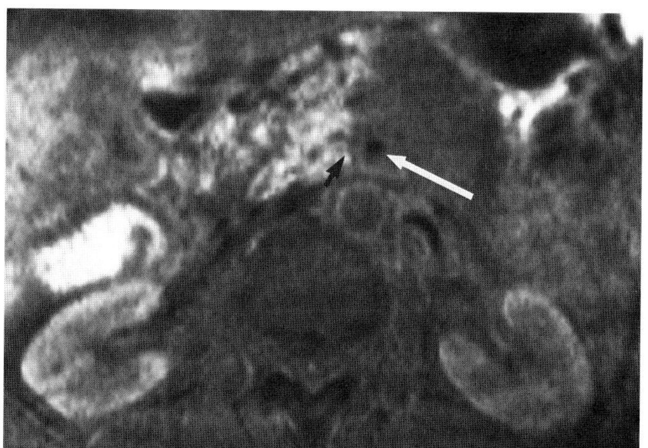

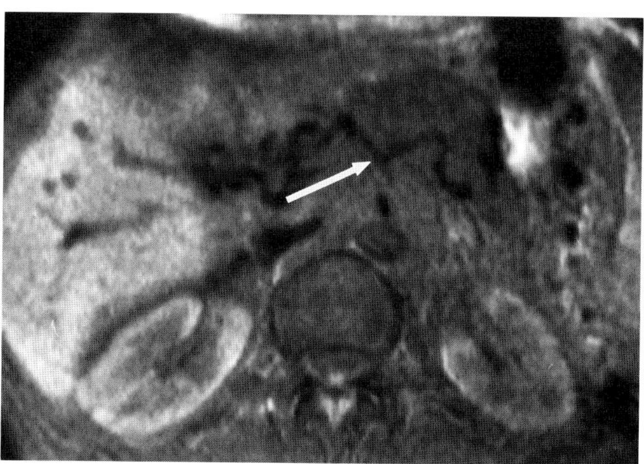

FIG. 5. Pancreatic cancer arising from the body of the pancreas. T1FS images in a 64-year-old woman with pancreatic cancer. A large, low-SI mass involves the body and tail of the pancreas, with encasement of the SMA (*white arrow,* **A**) and, on a higher section, encasement of the celiac axis (**B**). Extensive retroperitoneal adenopathy is also present (A,B). A transition from normal high-SI pancreas to pancreatic cancer is well shown (*black arrow,* A). Tumors of the body and tail of the pancreas tend to present when the tumor is advanced and large.

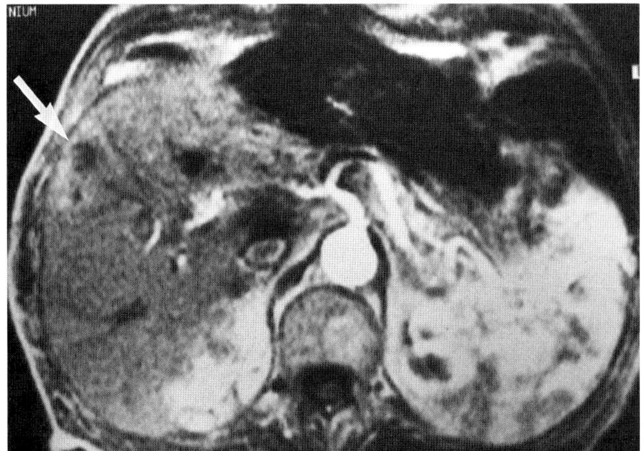

FIG. 6. Liver metastases from pancreatic cancer. One-second postcontrast FLASH image in a 71-year-old man with liver metastases from pancreatic cancer. Metastases demonstrate irregular peripheral enhancement with low-SI centers (*arrow*) on immediate postcontrast images. The central low SI reflects the desmoplastic character of the primary tumor.

Normal pancreatic tissue is well delineated from tumor, and tumor margins are well shown on MR images in the head (Fig. 4), body (Fig. 5), and tail regions. Pancreatic cancers appear as low-SI masses on T1FS images with good contrast resolution from normal pancreatic tissue, which is high in SI. Pancreatic tissue distal to pancreatic cancer may on occasion be lower in SI than is normal pancreatic tissue, which presumably reflects the decrease of proteinaceous fluid content secondary to obstruction of the pancreatic duct. In these cases Gd-DTPA in combination with fat suppression aids in delineating the tumor (see Fig. 4).

Focal, heterogeneously enhancing mass lesions with low-SI centers are characteristic of liver metastases from pancreatic cancer on immediate postcontrast FLASH images (Fig. 6). The low-SI centers of metastatic lesions presumably reflect the desmoplastic nature of the primary tumor. Lymphadenopathy is equally well shown on MR and CT images. Vellet et al. described better demonstration of vascular encasement on regular T1-weighted spin echo images when compared with CT images (15).

There may be a future role for the routine use of fat-suppressed MRI in the evaluation of pancreatic cancer because of the superior ability of MR to detect non-organ-deforming tumors compared to CT. Since surgery remains the main therapy of patients with pancreatic cancer (6), earlier detection of potentially curable disease may result in improved patient survival.

Islet Cell Tumors

Islet cell tumors are of neuroendocrine origin, and the great majority arise from the pancreas. These tumors are rare, with a reported incidence of <1 per 100,000 (16). These tumors have been classified as hormonally functional or nonfunctional (16). The histology of islet cell tumors, in decreasing order of frequency, includes insulinoma, gastrinoma, glucagonoma, vipoma, and somatostatinoma. The last two tumors are extremely rare.

Hormonally functional tumors tend to present when the lesions are small; symptoms related to the hormones secreted by the tumors are the presenting indicators (Fig. 7). Nonfunctional tumors account for approximately 15% of islet cell tumors and tend to present with symptoms due to large tumor mass (17,18).

Insulinomas

Insulinomas are the most frequent islet cell tumors and are frequently functional. These tumors are usually

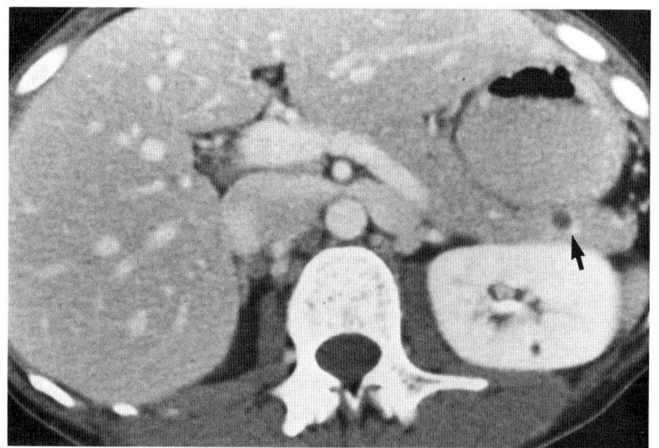

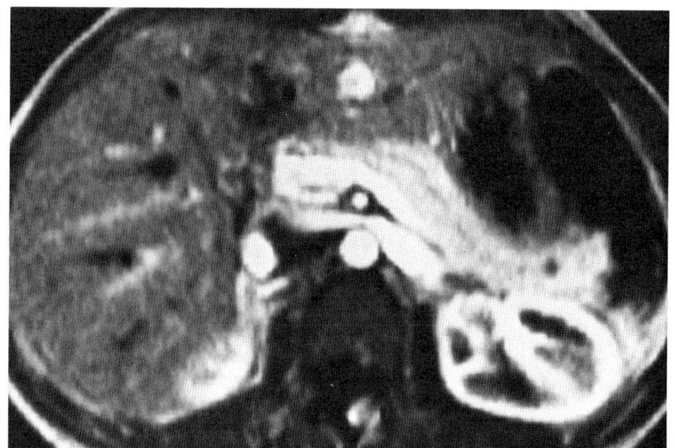

FIG. 7. Small functional islet cell tumor. Dynamic contrast-enhanced CT (**A**) and 1-second postcontrast FLASH (**B**) images in a 42-year-old woman with multiple endocrine neoplasia (MEN) Type I syndrome and elevated serum gastrin. CT and MR images demonstrate a 7-mm low-density/SI lesion in the tail of the pancreas. On the CT image a partial enhancing rim (*arrow,* A) is apparent. Rim enhancement on CT and MR images is characteristic of islet cell tumors.

very vascular. Angiography has been reported as superior to CT in detecting these tumors because of their small size and increased vascularity (19). The high sensitivity of MRI to Gd-DTPA enhancement results in high conspicuity of vascular insulinomas (20) (Fig. 8). Comparative sensitivity to other techniques is uncertain at present. Liver metastases from insulinomas have a typical peripheral ring-like enhancement. This pattern can also be observed in the primary pancreatic lesion, particularly when it is large. This feature distinguishes islet cell tumors from ductal adenocarcinomas. Other features include lack of vascular encasement and absence of central necrosis in large tumors.

Gastrinomas

Gastrinomas secrete gastrin, causing elevated acid production by the gastric mucosa, which results in peptic ulcer disease. This clinical picture is called the Zollinger-Ellison syndrome. Ulcers located in the postbulbar region of the duodenum or in the jejunum, particularly if multiple, should suggest the diagnosis of a gastrinoma. Esophagitis is often observed in these patients.

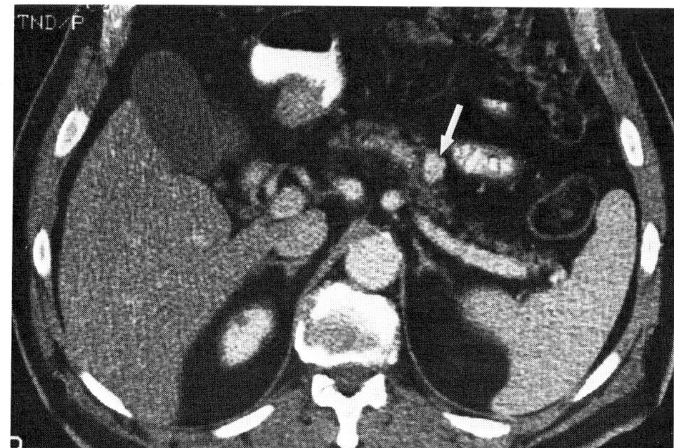

A

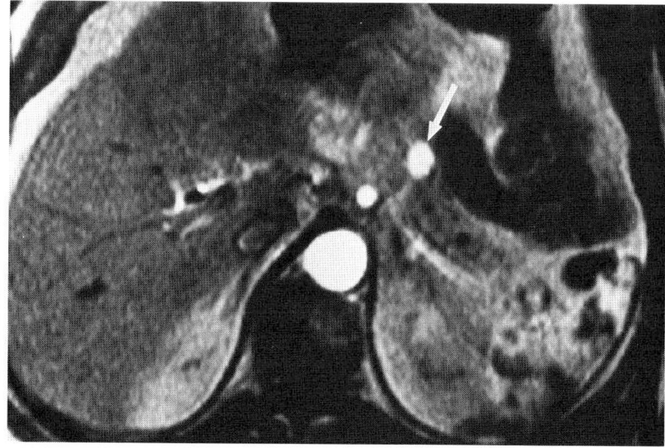
B

FIG. 8. Dynamic contrast-enhanced CT (**A**) and 1-second post-Gd-DTPA FLASH MR (**B**) images in a 78-year-old man with insulinoma. Good conspicuity of the 1.5-cm enhancing tumor arising from the body of the pancreas is apparent on both CT and MR images (*white arrow*). More intense enhancement is present on the MR image. Reprinted with permission from ref. 20.

Gastrinomas are not as frequently hypervascular as are insulinomas. The superior detection of gastrinomas compared with insulinomas is primarily due to the larger size of these tumors at presentation, which is approximately 4 cm, compared with 2 cm for insulinomas. CT is able to detect gastrinomas reliably when the tumor is larger than 3 cm but performs less well in the detection of smaller tumors (21). Conventional MRI has been limited in the detection of gastrinomas (22).

On fat-suppressed MR images, gastrinomas are low in SI and are separable from normal high-SI pancreatic tissue (Fig. 9). Gastrinomas occur most frequently in the region of the head of the pancreas, including the pancreatic head, duodenum, stomach, and lymph nodes in a territory termed the *gastrinoma triangle* (16). The anatomical boundaries of the triangle are the porta hepatis as the superior point of the triangle and the second and third parts of the duodenum as the base. Gastrinomas have a peripheral ring-like enhancement observed both in the primary lesion and in hepatic metastases (Fig. 10). The enhancing ring of the primary tumor is often difficult to appreciate because of similar enhancement of the surrounding pancreatic parenchyma, which also enhances.

Hepatic metastases are best shown on T2-weighted images. Islet cell tumor metastases to the liver in general are well shown on MR images. Typically, lesions are very high in SI and have well-defined margins. This appearance may be confused with hemangiomas, which have a similar appearance. Islet cell liver metastases are differentiated from hemangiomas by the relatively uniform ring-like enhancement pattern, which fades with time (20). This appearance is better shown on MR than CT images because of the higher sensitivity of MR to contrast enhancement, MR's faster intravenous contrast injection, and its greater imaging temporal resolution (Fig. 11). The ring can be thin (see Chapter 3, Fig. 13) or thick (Fig. 12), presumably because of differences in vascularity.

Glucagonomas

Glucagonomas are considerably rarer than insulinomas or gastrinomas. These tumors are frequently malignant, with liver metastases present at the time of diagnosis (16). The MR appearance of the primary tumor and of liver metastases is similar to that of gastrinomas (Fig. 13).

Cystic Neoplasms

Two forms of cystic neoplasm are described: microcystic adenoma (formerly serous cystadenoma) and macrocystic adenoma (formerly mucinous cystadenoma).

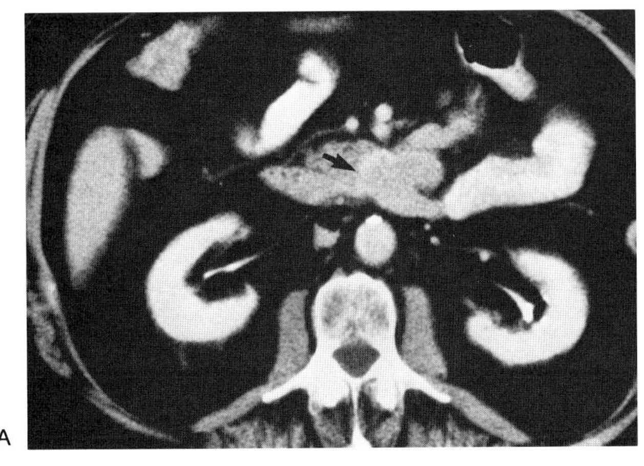

A

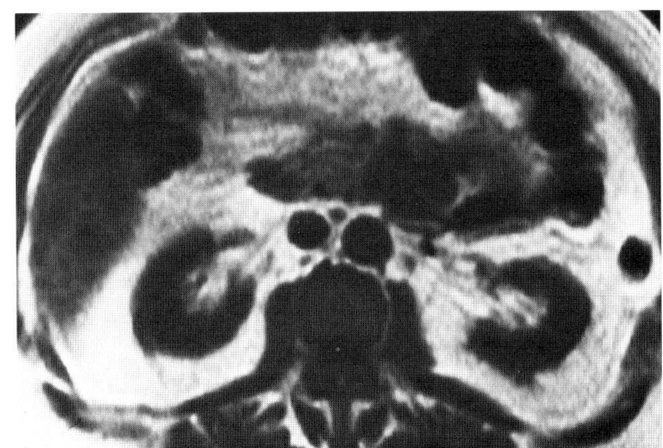

B

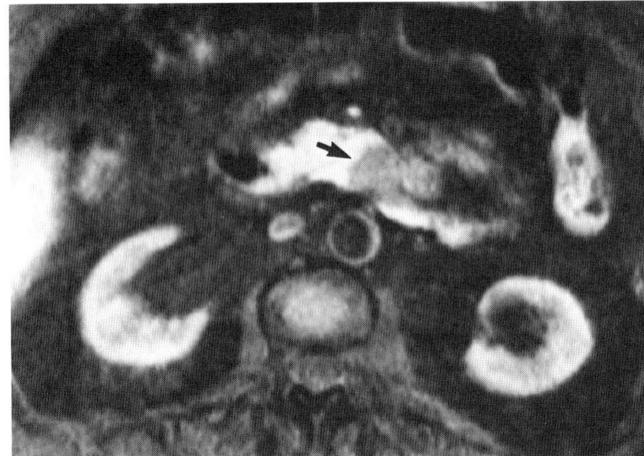

C

FIG. 9. Dynamic contrast-enhanced CT (**A**), FLASH (**B**), and fat-suppressed spin echo MR (**C**) images in a 78-year-old man with a gastrinoma. There is higher conspicuity of the 2-cm tumor arising from the uncinate process of the pancreas on the T1FS image (*arrow,* C) than on either the CT or the FLASH image. This tumor was initially missed on the CT study. An enhancing rim is apparent on the CT image (*arrow,* A). Reprinted with permission from ref. 20.

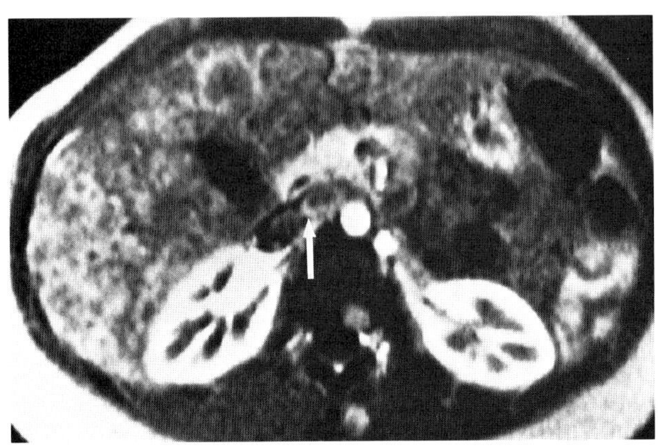

FIG. 10. One-second post-Gd-DTPA FLASH MR image in a 35-year-old woman with a gastrinoma. Distinct ring enhancement is appreciated in the primary tumor posterior to the head of the pancreas (*arrow*) and in the multiple hepatic metastases. Reprinted with permission from ref. 20.

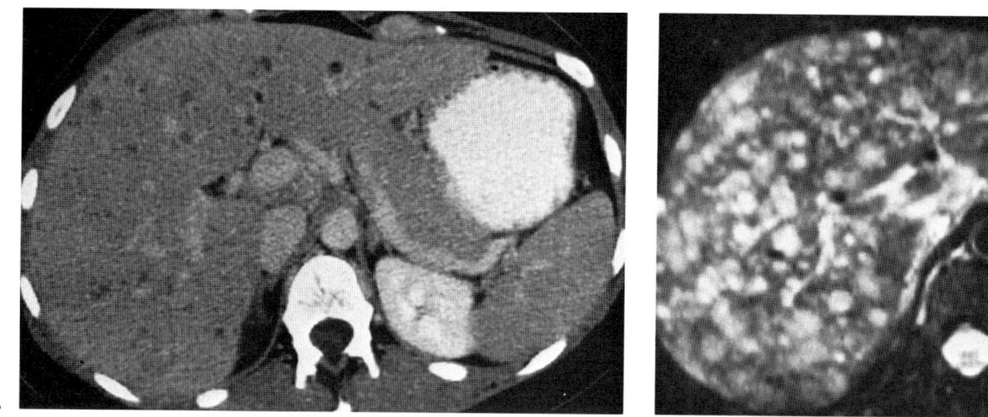

FIG. 11. Dynamic contrast-enhanced CT (**A**) and T2FS (2300/80) MR (**B**) images in a 35-year-old woman with a gastrinoma (same patient as in Fig. 10). A greater number of liver metastases are identified on the T2FS images. Reprinted with permission from ref. 20.

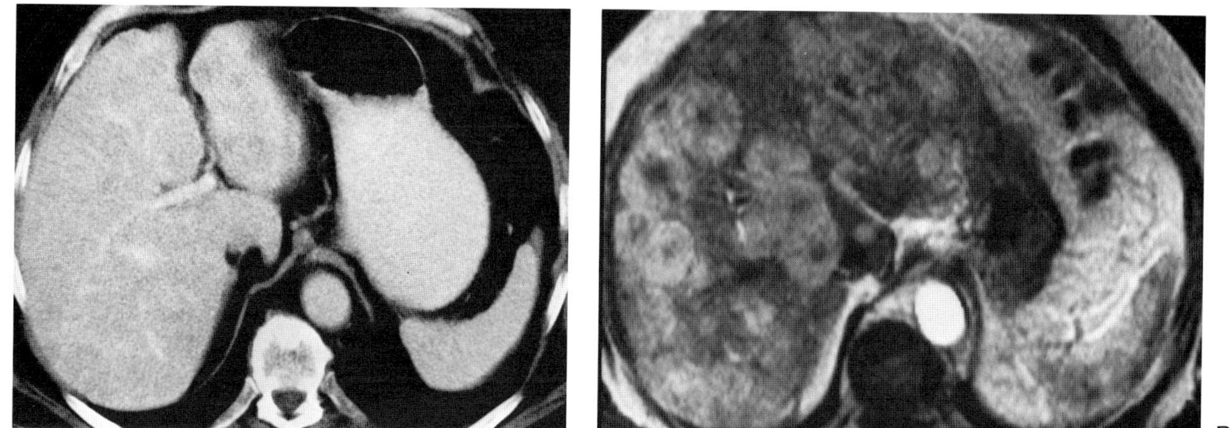

FIG. 12. Dynamic contrast-enhanced CT (**A**) and 1-second post-Gd-DTPA FLASH MR (**B**) images in a 78-year-old man with a gastrinoma (same patient as in Fig. 9). Ring-like enhancement of multiple hepatic metastases is better shown on the enhanced MR image. Reprinted with permission from ref. 20.

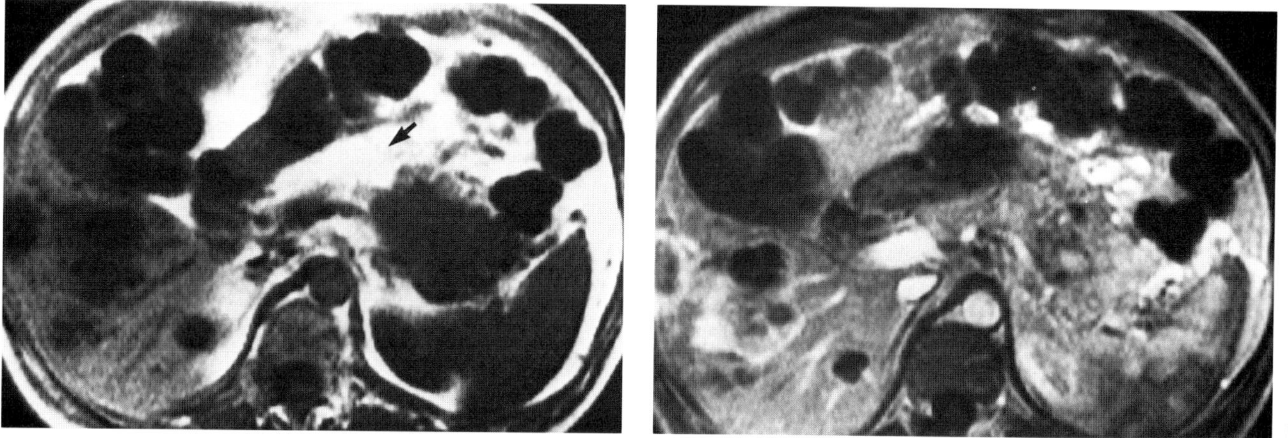

FIG. 13. Glucagonoma. FLASH (**A**) and 1-second postcontrast FLASH (**B**) images in a 43-year-old man with a glucagonoma and liver metastases. A 5-cm tumor arises from the tail of the pancreas. Extensive fatty replacement of the remainder of the pancreas is shown by high SI identical to that of subcutaneous fat (*arrow,* A). Multiple liver lesions are also identified and demonstrate peripheral rim enhancement immediately after Gd-DTPA injection. This appearance is typical for liver metastases from neuroendocrine tumors.

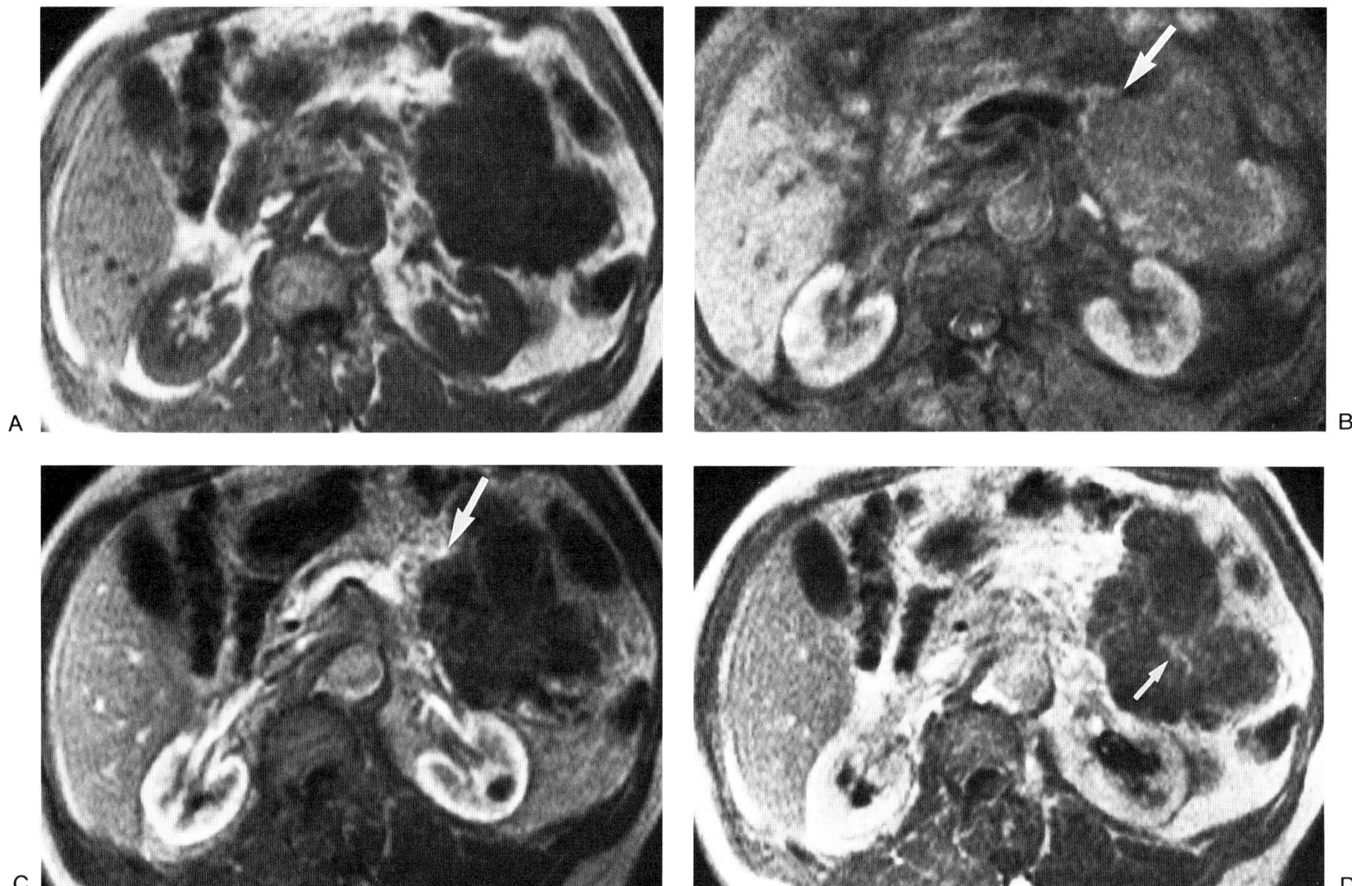

FIG. 14. Microcystic cystadenoma. FLASH (**A**), T1FS (**B**), 1-second (**C**), and 10-minute (**D**) postcontrast FLASH MR images in a 68-year-old man with a 12-cm microcystic cystadenoma. A low-SI mass arising from the tail of the pancreas is apparent on the FLASH and T1FS images. The mass shows minimal enhancement with Gd-DTPA. A high-SI irregular linear density is identified in the center of the mass on the 10-minute postcontrast FLASH image, consistent with a central scar (*arrow,* D). The tumor is clearly shown to arise from the tail of the pancreas by the demonstration of a "beak sign" (B,C).

Microcystic adenoma is a benign neoplasm characterized by multiple tiny cysts (22,23). This tumor frequently occurs in older patients and has an increased association with von Hippel-Lindau disease (24). The tumor occasionally contains a central scar. Tumors range in size from 1 to 12 cm, with an average diameter at presentation of 5 cm. The lesion has either a smooth or a nodular contour. On MR images the tumors are well defined and do not demonstrate invasion of fat or adjacent organs (Fig. 14) (25).

Macrocystic adenoma/adenocarcinoma are mucin-containing tumors that are malignant or have malignant potential (17,19). These tumors occur more frequently in female patients (6:1), and approximately one-half occur in patients between the ages of 40 and 60 years (26). These tumors usually are located in the body and tail of the pancreas. These tumors are large (mean diameter, 10 cm), multiloculated, and encapsulated (27). Large, irregular cystic spaces are separated by thick septa (Fig. 15). The mucin produced by these tumors may result in primary tumors and metastases that are high in SI on T1- and T2-weighted images (Fig. 16).

FIG. 16. Macrocystic cyst adenocarcinoma liver metastases. FLASH (**A**), T1FS (**B**), 1-second postcontrast FLASH (**C**), and T2FS (**D**) images in a 57-year-old woman with macrocystic cystadenocarcinoma of the pancreas and liver metastases. Metastases are high in SI on FLASH (A), T1FS (B), and T2FS (C) images, consistent with the SI of mucin. Layering of proteinaceous material is observed in some metastases on the T2FS (D) images. Irregular peripheral enhancement is present on dynamic Gd-DTPA-enhanced images (*arrow,* C), consistent with metastatic disease.

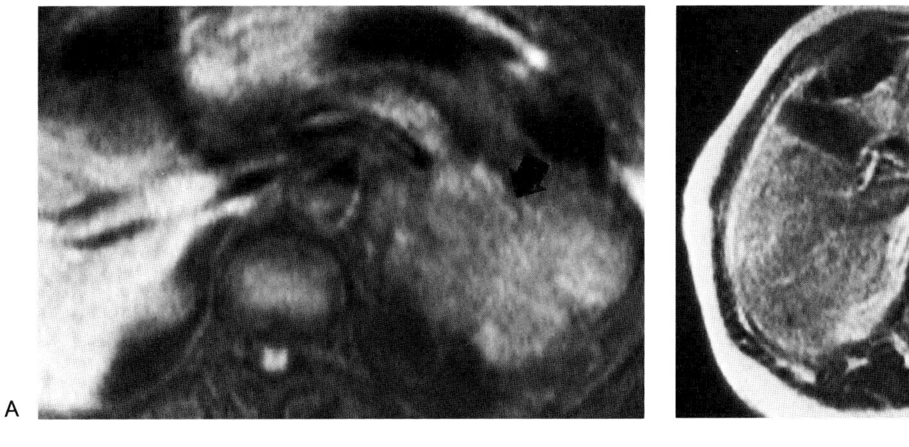

A

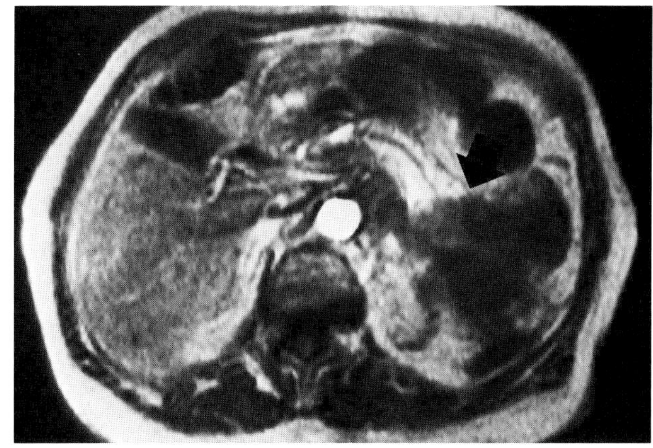

B

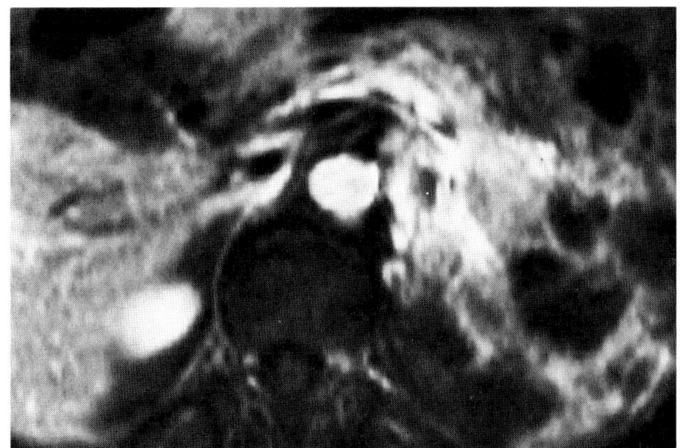

C

FIG. 15. Macrocystic cystadenocarcinoma. T1FS (**A**), 1-second postcontrast FLASH (**B**), and Gd-DTPA-enhanced T1FS (**C**) images in a 74-year-old woman with macrocystic cystadenocarcinoma. A large, low-SI tumor mass is identified on the T1FS image arising from the tail of the pancreas (*large black arrow*). After Gd-DTPA administration multiple large irregular signal-void defects are noted in the mass, consistent with cysts. Invasion of the spleen and multiple liver metastases are also present, confirming the malignant nature of this tumor.

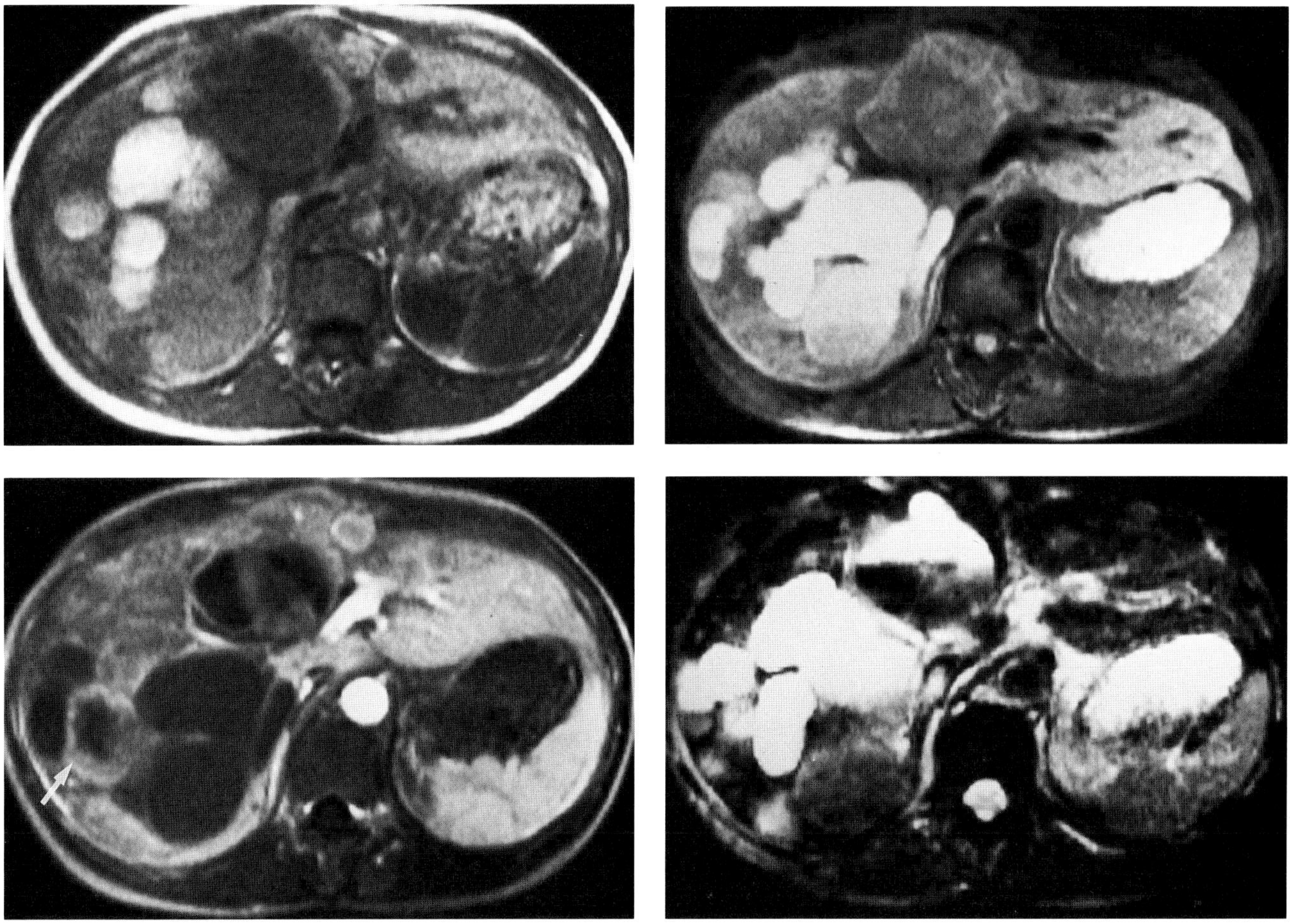

A

B

C

D

Rare Pancreatic Neoplasms

Papillary epithelial neoplasm is a rare, low-grade malignant lesion that most frequently occurs in women between 20 and 30 years of age (28). Pleomorphic carcinoma is a rare malignant cancer that follows an aggressive course and has a poor prognosis, with metastases to multiple organs (29).

Metastases and Lymphoma

Metastases and lymphoma can involve lymph nodes in the region of the pancreas or can directly invade the pancreas (30) (Fig. 17). Primary malignant neoplasms that involve peripancreatic nodes include gastrointestinal, kidney, breast, lung, prostate, and melanoma. Nodal masses in the region of the head of the pancreas can simulate pancreatic ductal cancer.

INFLAMMATORY DISEASE

Acute Pancreatitis

Pancreatitis occurs secondarily to chronic alcoholism, gallstones, hypercalcemia, hyperlipoproteinemia, blunt abdominal trauma, penetrating peptic ulcer diseases, viral infections (most frequently Epstein-Barr), and certain drugs (31). A predisposition can also be inherited as an autosomal dominant trait (32).

Acute pancreatitis most frequently results from excessive alcohol intake or gallstone disease (33). Alcohol-related acute pancreatitis usually results in acute recurrent pancreatitis. Gallstone-related pancreatitis more typically results in a single attack of pancreatitis. The passage of biliary sludge has recently been implicated in cases of acute pancreatitis (34). At least 95% of patients with acute pancreatitis experience severe midepigastric pain that radiates to the back. Nausea and vomiting occur in 75% to 85% of patients, and fever occurs in approximately 50%.

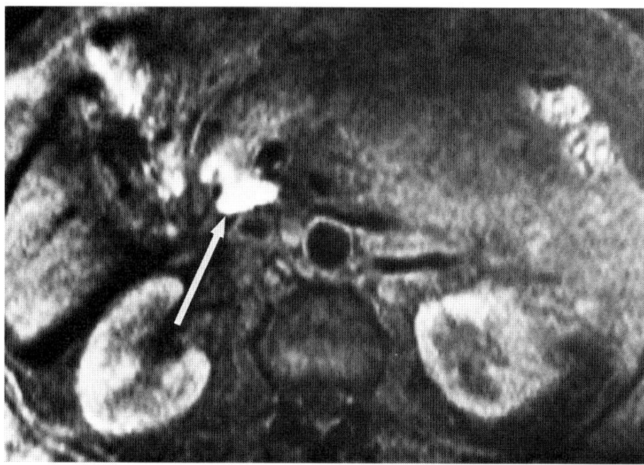

FIG. 17. Lymphoma. T1FS image in a 68-year-old man with a large lymphomatous mass in the left upper abdomen. Extensive lymphomatous involvement of the pancreas is present, causing diffuse SI loss of the pancreas. Sparing of the head and uncinate process is present, demonstrated by retention of the normal high SI of pancreatic tissue (*white arrow*). Paraaortic and paracaval adenopathy is also apparent.

Acute pancreatitis results from the exudation of fluid containing activated proteolytic enzymes into the interstitium of the pancreas and leakage of this fluid into surrounding tissue (35,36). Trypsin is suspected to be the primary enzyme involved in the coagulative necrosis.

MR is limited in the investigation of pancreatitis for two reasons. The first is that, in mild cases, physical examination and biochemistry are sufficient to establish the diagnosis and no imaging procedures are necessary. The second reason is that, in fulminant cases of pancreatitis, patients are generally too sick to warrant an MR study, with the further difficulty of managing life support systems in an MR facility. MR is useful, however, in detecting changes of pancreatitis and distinguishing acute from chronic forms. The acutely inflamed pancreas has normal SI on fat-suppressed spin echo images and normal parenchymal enhancement. Noncontrast T1-weighted images demonstrate a dusky or hazy appearance of peripancreatic fat, consistent with inflammatory changes. CT shows a normal-appearing gland in about one-third of cases of acute pancreatitis. MRI may be more sensitive than CT in detecting more subtle changes of acute pancreatitis (Fig. 18). In patients with acute or chronic pancreatitis or alcoholism, the serum amylase may be normal. In these cases either CT or MRI may be helpful to detect inflammatory changes.

Early in the course of acute pancreatitis, the pancreas enlarges, adopting a swollen appearance, and there is blurring of the pancreatic margins (37,38). In more severe cases fluid dissects into the anterior perirenal space. Free fluid collections can accumulate in peripancreatic tissue and in the lesser sac. These free fluid collections do not constitute pseudocysts, as it takes approximately 3 to 6 weeks for a capsule to develop to form a pseudocyst. These fluid collections are also more transient than pseudocysts and can resolve or progress at a more rapid rate.

In severe acute pancreatitis, fluid dissects from the peripancreatic tissue along the gastrohepatic, gastrosplenic, and gastrocolic ligaments; the transverse mesocolon; and the root of the mesentery (35,36). There is a good correlation between the extent of pancreatic fluid accumulation and mortality (39–41); however, the correlation between imaging findings and clinical outcome is not exact.

Recent CT reports suggest that pancreatic necrosis, as determined by lack of enhancement of pancreatic parenchyma on dynamic contrast-enhanced CT, has important prognostic implications. Dynamic Gd-DTPA-enhanced MR images may be more accurate than

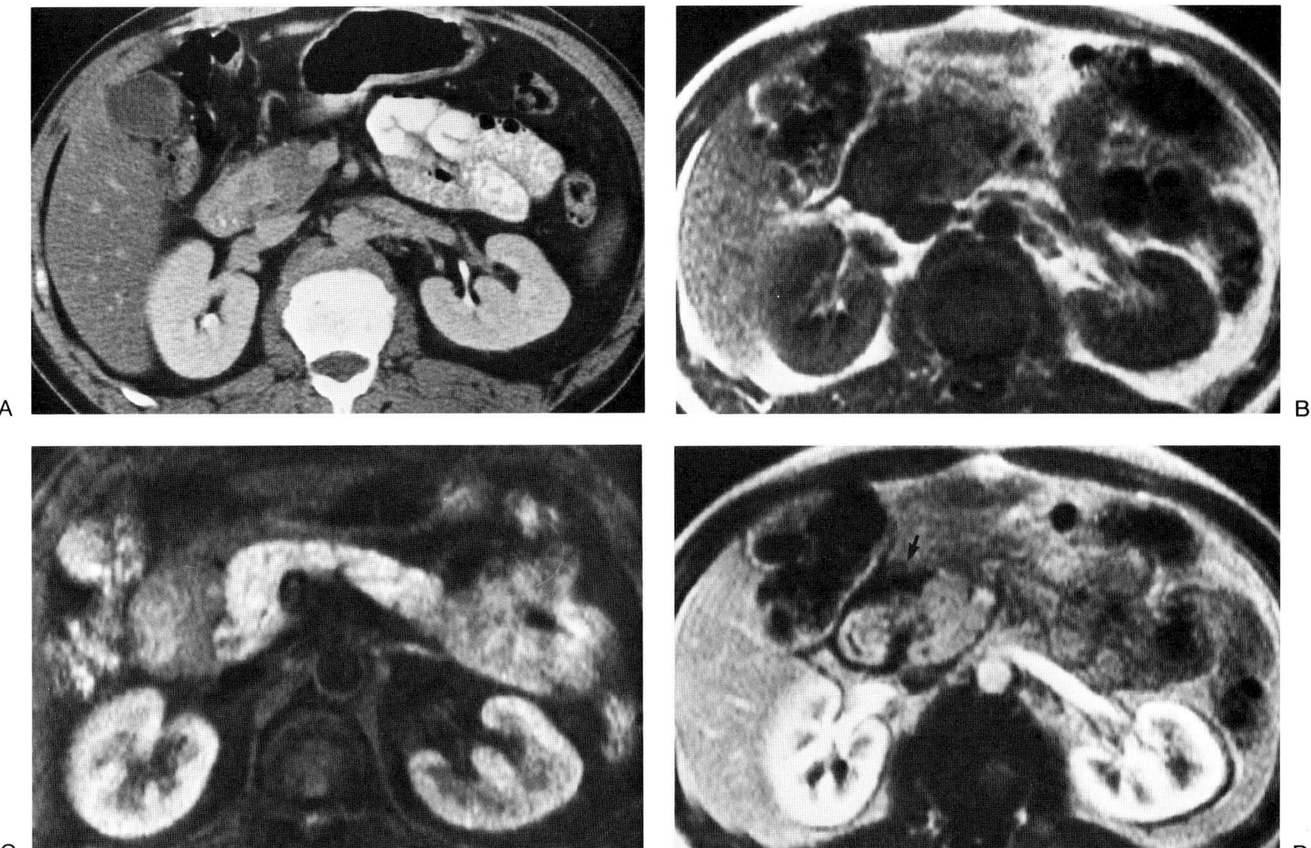

FIG. 18. Acute pancreatitis. Contrast-enhanced CT (**A**), FLASH (**B**), T1FS (**C**), and immediate postcontrast FLASH (**D**) images in a 36-year-old man with acute pancreatitis. The CT image shows diffuse enlargement of the head of the pancreas, compatible with the clinical picture of acute pancreatitis. FLASH demonstrates indistinct low-SI strands surrounding the head of the pancreas in addition to enlargement of the head of the pancreas. The peripancreatic inflammatory changes are better appreciated than on the CT image. The immediate postcontrast FLASH image shows an additional finding of free fluid (*arrow*) around the head of the pancreas and duodenum which was not seen as well on other sequences or on CT. The precontrast fat-suppressed image from a higher level demonstrates normal high SI of the pancreas, suggesting that no fibrosis or devascularization is present. Reprinted with permission from ref. 2.

dynamic contrast-enhanced CT in detecting necrosis because of the higher sensitivity of MRI to Gd-DTPA.

Pseudocyst formation is a common sequela of inflammatory pancreatic disease. Pseudocysts are well shown on MR images after Gd-DTPA enhancement as signal-void oval lesions (Fig. 19).

Complicated Acute Inflammatory Conditions

Hemorrhagic pancreatitis, infected pseudocysts, and pancreatic abscess are acute syndromes related to pancreatic inflammatory disease (42,43). The role of MRI in these conditions is as yet unknown.

Chronic Pancreatitis

Chronic pancreatitis is acquired either as a disease entity distinct from acute pancreatitis or as a complication of repeated attacks of acute pancreatitis. There is a strong association between alcoholism and the development of chronic pancreatitis (32,44). Acute pancreatitis secondary to gallstone disease rarely results in chronic pancreatitis. Chronic pancreatitis is associated with decreased endocrine as well as exocrine function.

An analysis of current generation contrast-enhanced CT images of patients with chronic pancreatitis showed the following features: 66% had dilatation of the main pancreatic duct, 54% had parenchymal atrophy, 50% had pancreatic calcifications, 34% had pseudocysts, 32% had focal pancreatic enlargement, 29% had biliary ductal dilatation, and 16% had densities in peripancreatic fat or fascia. No abnormalities were detected in 7% of patients (45). Focal chronic pancreatitis may be difficult to distinguish from adenocarcinoma in the head of the pancreas, since both entities may cause a focal mass lesion, obstruction of the common bile duct and pancreatic duct,

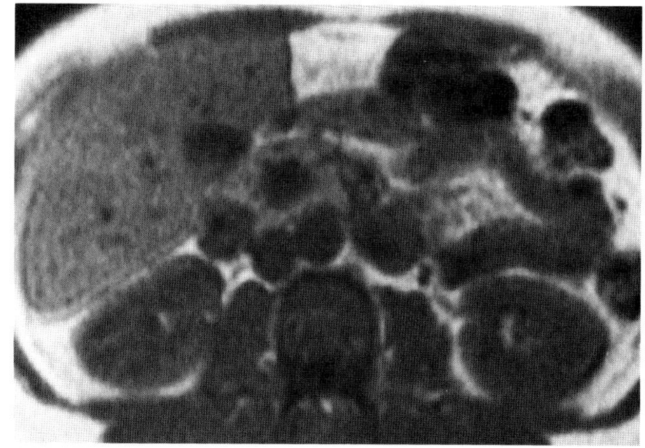
A

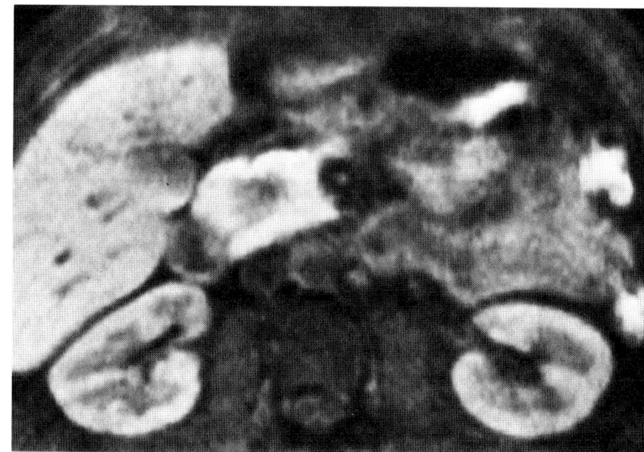
B

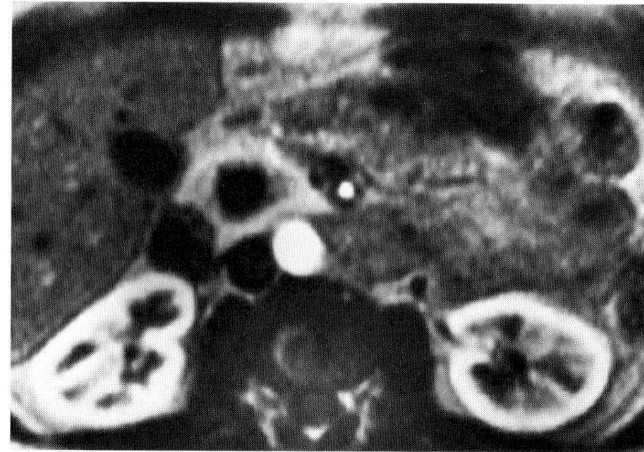
C

FIG. 19. FLASH (**A**), T1FS (**B**), and 1-second postcontrast FLASH (**C**) in a 42-year-old woman with a pseudocyst in the head of the pancreas following acute pancreatitis. The head of the pancreas has a normal SI on T1FS images (B) and enhances in a normal fashion (C). A 2.2-cm low-SI lesion is present in the pancreatic head which is signal void on contrast-enhanced images (C) consistent with a pseudocyst. The findings are compatible with pseudocyst formation following acute pancreatitis.

atrophy of the tail of the pancreas, and obliteration of the fat plane around the superior mesenteric artery (46–48).

MRI may perform better than CT when detecting changes of chronic pancreatitis because MRI detects not only morphological findings but also the presence of fibrosis, which is reflected by a diminished SI on fat-suppressed images (49) (Fig. 20). We performed T1FS and 1-second postcontrast FLASH sequences on a study population of 22 patients, including 13 with chronic calcifying pancreatitis and 9 with presumed acute recurrent pancreatitis. All patients with pancreatic calcifications on CT examination had a pancreas with diminished SI on T1FS and an abnormally low percentage of contrast enhancement on 1-second postcontrast images. Patients with acute recurrent pancreatitis had SI features of the pancreas comparable to findings of normal pancreas. Since fibrosis is a precursor to the development of calcification, MRI may be able to detect chronic pancreatitis at an earlier stage than can CT. Chronic pancreatitis with associated enlargement of the pancreas may be difficult to distinguish from cancer on CT images. MRI can distinguish these entities by demonstrating diffuse low SI on fat-suppressed images and diffuse diminished contrast enhancement on immediate postcontrast images in patients with chronic pancreatitis (Fig. 21). Small pseudocysts are not infrequent and cause focal glandular enlargement, which can be misinterpreted as pancreatic cancer (Fig. 22). Pancreatic pseudocysts occur more frequently in the context of chronic than acute pancreatitis (Fig. 23).

PANCREATIC TRAUMA

CT is the diagnostic tool of choice in evaluating the pancreas after trauma. If MR is used, a breathing-independent sequence such as TurboFLASH may be advisable in an unstable patient.

PANCREAS TRANSPLANTATION

MRI has been advocated in the evaluation of pancreatic transplantation. Dynamic Gd-DTPA enhancement may play a role in determining the presence of rejection (50).

NEW DIRECTIONS

Manganese-DPDP is taken up by the pancreas and results in enhancement of parenchymal tissue (51). The future role of this agent is not known.

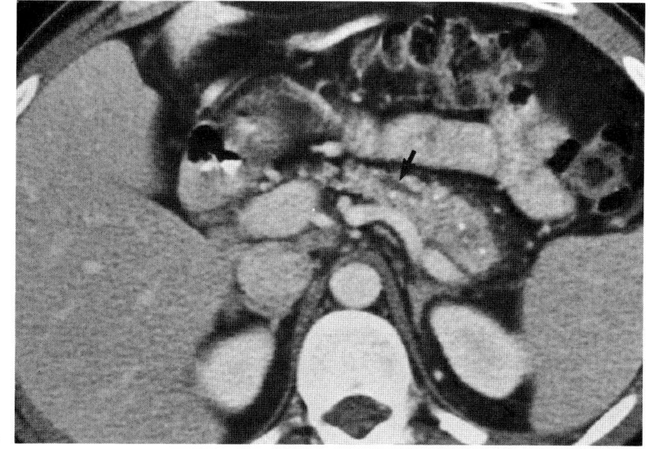

A

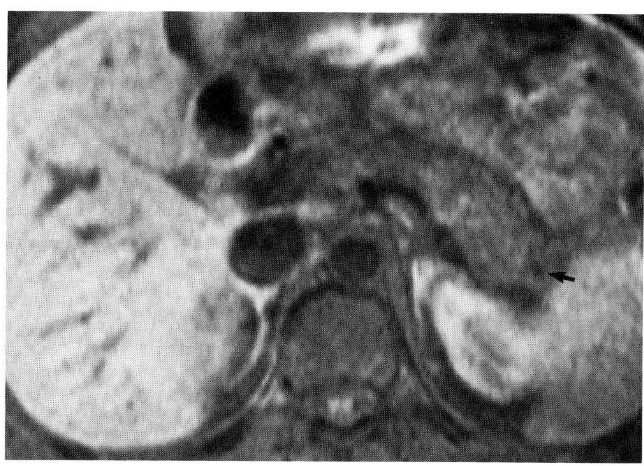

B

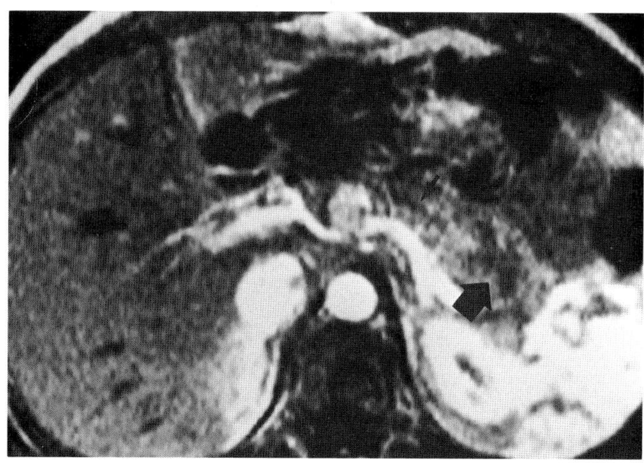

C

FIG. 20. Chronic pancreatitis. Contrast-enhanced 5 mm CT (**A**), T1FS (**B**), and 1-second postcontrast FLASH (**C**) images in a 32-year-old man with chronic pancreatitis. On the CT image calcifications in the pancreas and mild dilatation of the pancreatic duct (*arrow*) are well demonstrated. On the T1FS image the pancreas is of uniform low SI but the signal-void calcifications are difficult to appreciate (*arrow*). On the immediate post-contrast FLASH image, Gd-DTPA enhancement is diminished and the pancreas enhances heterogeneously with a low-SI irregular region consistent with dense fibrosis in the tail (*large arrow*). Mild ductal dilatation can be appreciated (*arrow*). Reprinted with permission from ref. 2.

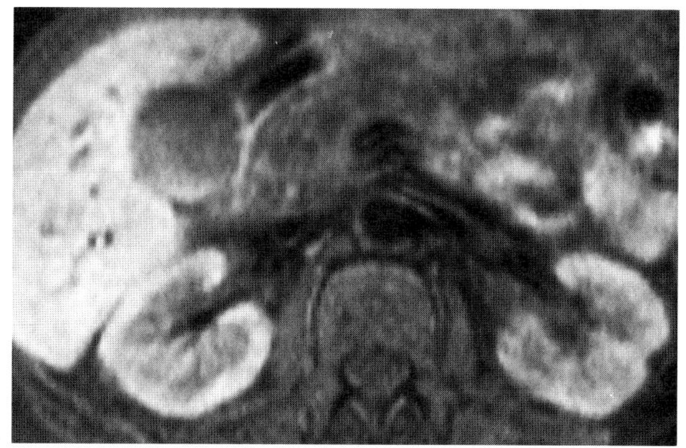

A

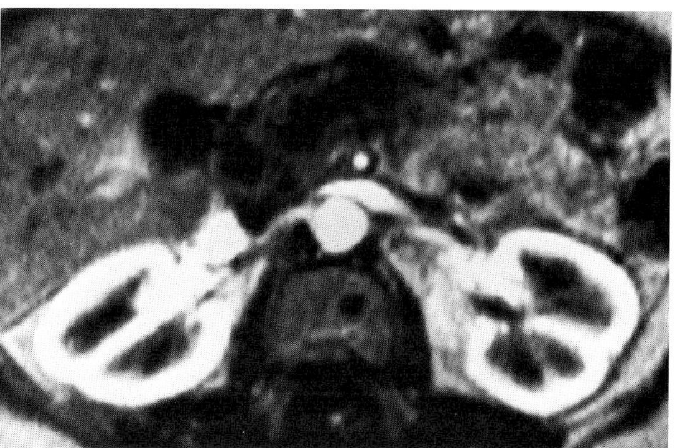

B

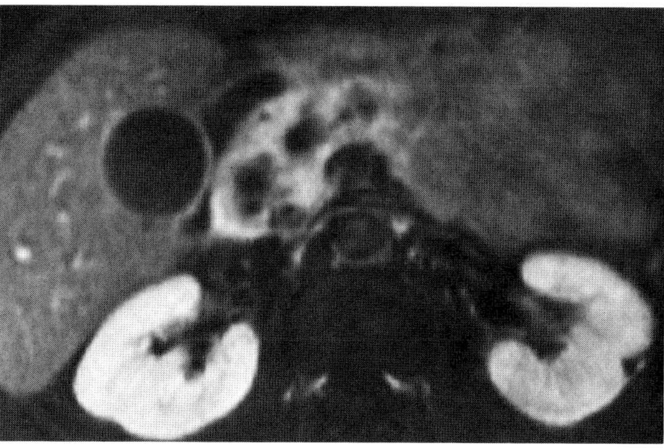

C

FIG. 21. Chronic pancreatitis with focal glandular enlargement. T1FS (**A**), 1-second postcontrast FLASH (**B**), and post-contrast T1FS (**C**) images in a 48-year-old woman with focal enlargement of the head and neck of the pancreas. Low SI of the pancreas on fat-suppressed images (A) and diminished Gd-DTPA enhancement (B) are findings of chronic pancreatitis. Signal-void rounded and tubular structures in the pancreas represent a combination of calcification and common bile and pancreatic ducts (A,B,C).

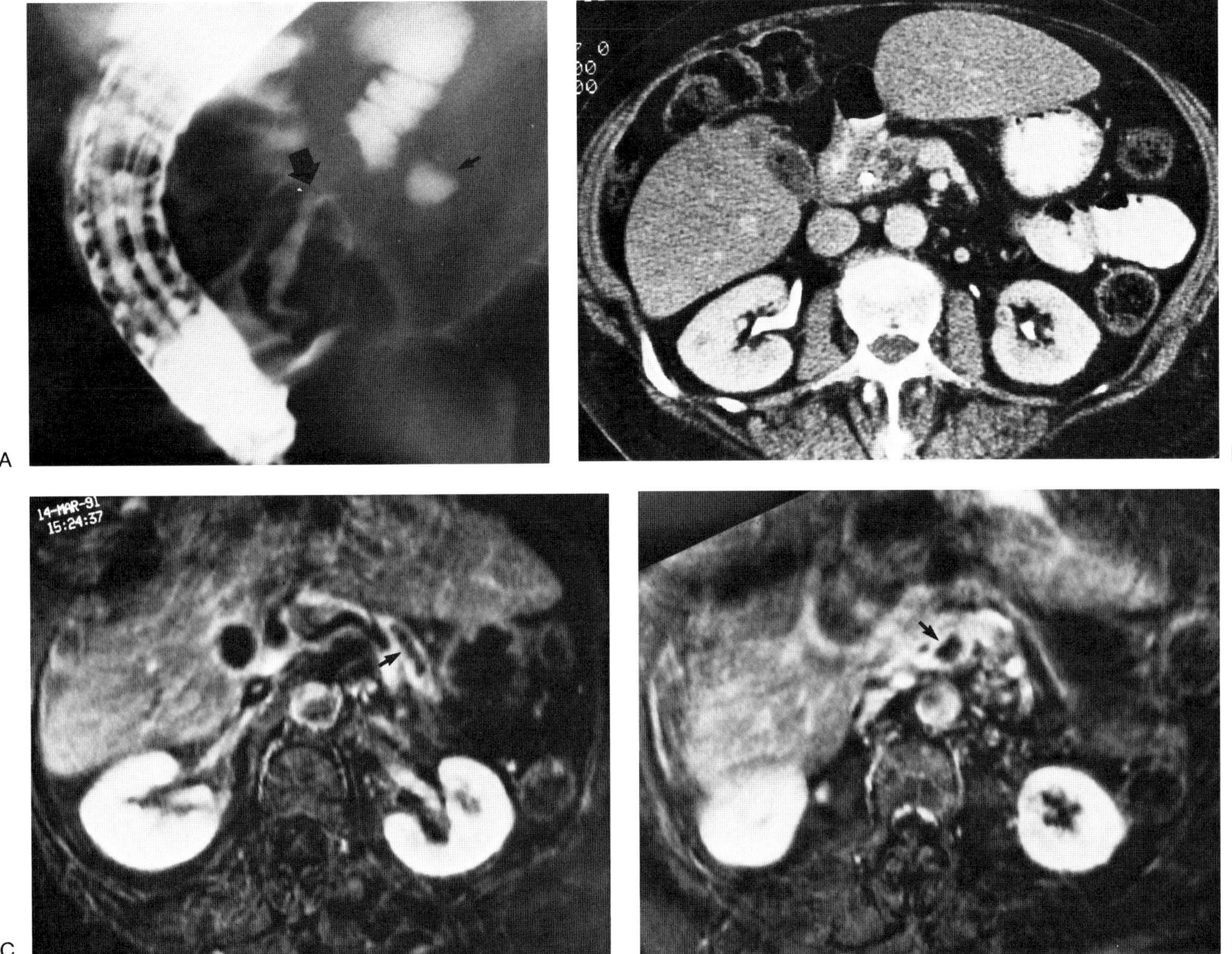

FIG. 22. Chronic pancreatitis with pseudocysts in the head of the pancreas. ERCP (**A**), contrast-enhanced 5-mm CT (**B**), and Gd-DTPA-enhanced T1FS (**C,D**) images. The ERCP study shows irregularity of the common bile duct in the head of the pancreas (*large arrow*) and high-grade obstruction of the pancreatic duct (*arrow*). These findings were interpreted as being secondary to pancreatic cancer. A biliary stent was placed at the time of the ERCP study. On CT images the body and tail of the pancreas were atrophic with dilatation of the pancreatic duct (not shown), and irregular enlargement of the head of the pancreas was interpreted as a finding secondary to pancreatic cancer. On Gd-DTPA-enhanced T1FS, atrophy of the body and tail of the pancreas is apparent with dilatation of the pancreatic duct (*arrow,* C); in the head of the pancreas (D), multiple cysts were identified (*arrow*) with no solid tissue suggestive of cancer. These findings are consistent with chronic pancreatitis with pseudocysts in the pancreatic head. CT-directed biopsy was negative for tumor cells, and the disease did not progress during the 1-year follow-up. Reprinted with permission from ref. 2.

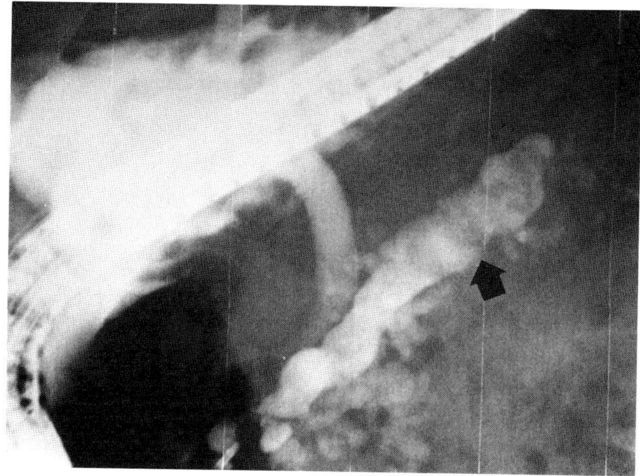
A

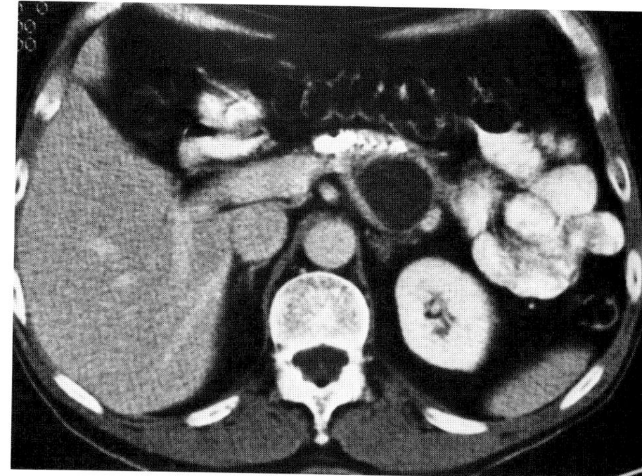
B

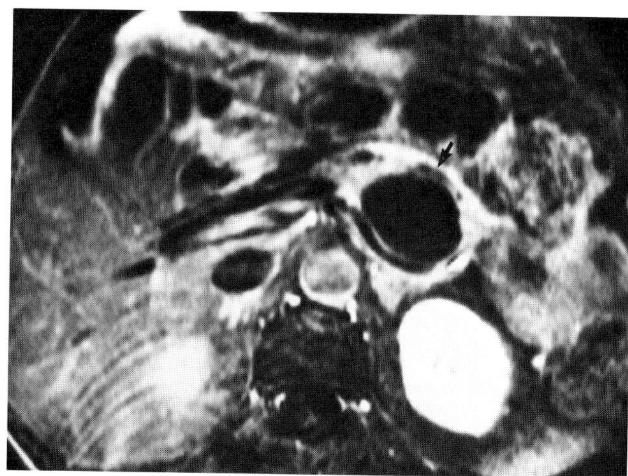
C

FIG. 23. Chronic pancreatitis with pseudocyst. ERCP (**A**), contrast-enhanced 5-mm CT (**B**), and Gd-DTPA-enhanced T1FS (**C**) images. The ERCP study demonstrated dilatation of the pancreatic duct (*arrow,* A) with calcifications throughout the pancreas. No communication between the duct and pseudocyst was shown. The CT image (B) shows extensive calcification along the wall of the pancreatic duct and the pseudocyst arising from the posterior aspect of the body of the pancreas. The MR image demonstrates that the pancreatic duct (*arrow,* C) is anterior in relation to the pseudocyst. Distinction between dilated duct and calcification could not be clearly made. Reprinted with permission from ref. 2.

REFERENCES

1. Mitchell DG, Vinitski S, Saponaro S, Tasciyan T, Burk DL Jr, Rifkin MD. Liver and pancreas: improved spin-echo T1 contrast by shorter echo time and fat suppression at 1.5T. *Radiology* 1991;178:67–71.
2. Semelka RC, Kroeker MA, Shoenut JP, Kroeker R, Yaffe CS, Micflikier AB: Pancreatic disease: prospective comparison of CT, ERCP, and 1.5T MR imaging with dynamic gadolinium enhancement and fat suppression. *Radiology* 1991;181:785–791.
3. Semelka RC, Simm FC, Recht M, Deimling M, Lenz G, Laub GA. MRI of the pancreas at high field strength—a comparison of six sequences. *J Comput Assist Tomogr* 1991;15:966–971.
4. Delhaye M, Engelholm, Cremer M. Pancreas divisum: congenital anatomic variant or anomaly? Contribution of endoscopic retrograde dorsal pancreatography. *Gastroenterology* 1985;89: 951–958.
5. Boring CC, Squires TS, Tong T. Cancer statistics, 1991. *CA Cancer J Clin* 1991;41:19–51.
6. Warshaw AL, Fernández-del Castillo C. Pancreatic carcinoma. *N Engl J Med* 1992;326:455–465.
7. Moossa AR. Pancreatic cancer: approach to diagnosis, selection for surgery and choice of operation. *Cancer* 1982;50:2689–2698.
8. Clark LR, Jaffe MH, Choyke PL, Grant EG, Zeman RK. Pancreatic imaging. *Radiol Clin North Am* 1985;23:489–501.
9. Cubilla AL, Fitzgerald PJ. Cancer of the pancreas (nonendocrine): a suggested morphologic clarification. *Semin Oncol* 1979;6: 285–297.
10. Baron RL, Stanley RJ, Lee JKT, Koehler RE, Levitt RG. Computed tomographic features of biliary obstruction. *AJR Am J Roentgenol* 1983;140:1173–1178.
11. Wittenberg J, Simeone JF, Ferrucci JT Jr, Mueller PR, van Sonnenberg E, Neff CC. Non-focal enlargement in pancreatic carcinoma. *Radiology* 1982;144:131–135.
12. Megibow AJ, Bosniak MA, Ambos MA, Beranbaum ER. Thickening of the celiac axis and/or superior mesenteric artery: a sign of pancreatic carcinoma on computed tomography. *Radiology* 1981;141:449–453.
13. Hosoki T. Dynamic CT of pancreatic tumors. *AJR Am J Roentgenol* 1983;140:959–965.
14. Steiner E, Stark DD, Hahn PF, et al. Imaging of pancreatic neoplasms: comparison of MR and CT. *AJR Am J Roentgenol* 1989;152:487–491.
15. Vellet AD, Romano W, Bach DB, Passi RB, Taves DH, Munk PL. Adenocarcinoma of the pancreatic ducts: comparative evaluation with CT and MR imaging at 1.5T. *Radiology* 1992;183:87–95.
16. Mozell E, Stenzel P, Woltering EA, Rösch J, O'Dorisio TM. Functional endocrine tumors of the pancreas: clinical presentation, diagnosis, and treatment. *Curr Probl Surg* 1990;27:304–385.
17. Thompson NW, Eckhauser FE, Vinik AI, Lloyd RV, Fiddian-Green RD, Strodel WE. Cystic neuroendocrine neoplasms of the pancreas and liver. *Ann Surg* 1984;199:158–164.
18. Tjon A, Tham RTO, Jansen JBMJ, Falke THM, et al. MR, CT, and ultrasound findings of metastatic vipoma in pancreas. *J Comput Assist Tomogr* 1989;13:142–144.
19. Galiber AK, Reading CC, Charboneau JW, et al. Localization of pancreatic insulinoma: comparison of pre- and intraoperative US with CT and angiography. *Radiology* 1988;166:405–408.
20. Semelka RC, Cummings M, Shoenut JP, Yaffe CS, Kroeker MA, Greenberg HM. Islet cell tumors: a comparison of detection by dynamic contrast-enhanced CT and MRI with dynamic gadolinium-enhanced imaging and fat suppression. *Radiology* 1993; 190:799–802.

21. Wank SA, Doppman JL, Miller DL, et al. Prospective study of the ability of computed axial tomography to localize gastrinomas in patients with Zollinger-Ellison syndrome. *Gastroenterology* 1987;92:905–912
22. Frucht H, Doppman JL, Norten JA, et al. Gastrinomas: comparison of MR imaging with CT, angiography, and US. *Radiology* 1989;171:713–717.
23. Compagno J, Oertel JE. Microcystic adenomas of the pancreas (glycogen-rich cystadenomas). *Am J Clin Pathol* 1978;69: 289–298.
24. Zirinsky K, Abiri M, Baer JW. Computed tomographic demonstration of pancreatic microcystic adenoma. *Am J Gastroenterol* 1984;79:139–142.
25. Friedman AC, Lichtenstein JE, Dachman AH. Cystic neoplasms of the pancreas: radiological-pathological correlation. *Radiology* 1983;149:45–50.
26. Minami M, Itai Y, Ohtomo K, Yoshida H, Yoshikawa K, Iio M. Cystic neoplasms of the pancreas: comparison of MR imaging with CT. *Radiology* 1989;171:53–56.
27. Compagno J, Oertel JE. Mucinous cystic neoplasms of the pancreas with overt and latent malignancy (cystadenocarcinoma and cystadenoma): a clinicopathologic study of 41 cases. *Am J Clin Pathol* 1978;69:573–580.
28. Itai Y, Moss AA, Ohtomo K. Computed tomography of cystadenoma and cystadenocarcinoma of the pancreas. *Radiology* 1982;145:419–425.
29. Balthazar EJ, Subramanyam BR, Lefleur RS, Barone CM. Solid and papillary epithelial neoplasm of the pancreas: radiographic, CT, sonographic features. *Radiology* 1984;150:39–40.
30. Wolfman NT, Karstaedt N, Kawamoto EH. Pleomorphic carcinoma of the pancreas: computed-tomographic, sonographic, and pathologic findings. *Radiology* 1985;154:329–332.
31. Zemman RK, Schiebler M, Clark LR, et al. The clinical and imaging spectrum of pancreaticoduodenal lymph node enlargement. *AJR Am J Roentgenol* 1985;144:1223–1227.
32. Durbec JP, Sarles H. Multicenter survey of the etiology of pancreatic diseases: relationship between the relative risk of developing chronic panarthritis and alcohol, protein and lipid consumption. *Digestion* 1978;18:337–445.
33. Kattwinkel J, Lapey A, DiSant'Agnese PA, Edwards WA, Jufty MP. Hereditary pancreatitis: three new kindreds and a critical review of the literature. *Pediatrics* 1973;51:5–69.
34. Lee SP, Nicholls JF, Park HZ. Biliary sludge as a cause of acute pancreatitis. *N Engl J Med* 1992;326:589–593.
35. Donovan J, Sanders RC, Siegelman SS. Collections of fluid after pancreatitis: evaluation by computed tomography and ultrasonography. *Radiol Clin North Am* 1982;20:653–665.
36. Lawson TL. Acute pancreatitis and its complications: computed tomography and sonography. *Radiol Clin North Am* 1983;21: 495–513.
37. Silverstein W, Isikoff MB, Hill MC, Barkin J. Diagnostic imaging of acute pancreatitis: prospective study using CT and sonography. *AJR Am J Roentgenol* 1980;134:497–502.
38. Mendez G, Isikoff MB, Hill MC. CT of acute pancreatitis: interim assessment. *AJR Am J Roentgenol* 1980;135:463–469.
39. Balthazar EJ, Ranson JHC, Naidich DP, Megibow AJ, Caccavale R, Cooper MM. Acute pancreatitis: prognostic value of CT. *Radiology* 1985;156:767–772.
40. Balthazar EJ, Robinson DL, Megibow AJ, Ranson JHC. Acute pancreatitis: value of CT in establishing prognosis. *Radiology* 1990;174:331–336.
41. Johnson CD, Stephens DH, Sarr MG. CT of acute pancreatitis: correlation between lack of contrast enhancement and pancreatic necrosis. *AJR Am J Roentgenol* 1991;156:93–95.
42. Vernacchia FS, Jeffrey RD Jr, Federle MP, et al. Pancreatic abscess: predictive value of early abdominal CT. *Radiology* 1987;162:435–438.
43. Ranson JHC, Balthazar E, Caccavale R, Cooper M. Computed tomography and the prediction of pancreatic abscess in acute pancreatitis. *Ann Surg* 1985;201:656–665.
44. Sarles HG. Chronic calcifying pancreatitis-chronic alcoholic pancreatitis. *Gastroenterology* 1974;66:604–616.
45. Luetmer PH, Stephens DH, Ward EM. Chronic pancreatitis: reassessment with current CT. *Radiology* 1989;171:353–357.
46. Aranha GV, Prinz RA, Freeark RJ, Greenlee HB. The spectrum of biliary tract obstruction from chronic pancreatitis. *Arch Surg* 1984;119:595–600.
47. Lammer J, Herlinger H, Zalaudek G, Hofler H. Pseudotumorous pancreatitis. *Gastrointest Radiol* 1985;10:59–67.
48. Sostre CF, Flournoy JG, Bova JG, Goldstein HM, Schenker S. Pancreatic phlegmon: clinical features and course. *Dig Dis Sci* 1985;30:918–927.
49. Semelka RC, Shoenut JP, Kroeker MA, Micflikier AB. Chronic pancreatitis: MRI features using pre- and postintravenous Gd-DTPA breath hold FLASH and fat suppressed spin echo. *JMRI* 1993;3:79–82.
50. del Pilar Fernandez M, Bernardino ME, Neylan JF, Olson RA. Diagnosis of pancreatic transplant dysfunction: value of gadopentatate dimeglumine-enhanced MR imaging. *AJR Am J Roentgenol* 1991;156:1171–1176.
51. Gehl H-B, Vorwerk D, Klose KC, Günther RW. Pancreatic enhancement after low-dose infusion of Mn-DPDP. *Radiology* 1991;180:337–339.

CHAPTER 7

The Adrenal Glands

Richard C. Semelka and J. Patrick Shoenut

NORMAL ANATOMY

The adrenal glands are paired organs that lie within the perirenal space in close proximity to the anterosuperior aspect of the kidneys. The right adrenal gland is medial to the right lobe of the liver and lateral to the right crus of the diaphragm. The left adrenal gland is seated posterior to the splenic vein and medial to the left crus of the diaphragm.

MR TECHNIQUE

The adrenal glands are well shown on fat-suppressed images with both T1- and T2-weighting. Adrenal glands are relatively high in SI in a background of low-SI (suppressed) fat. Serial dynamic Gd-DTPA-enhanced breath-hold imaging of the adrenals has been advocated as a technique to distinguish benign and malignant adrenal masses. Similarly, T2-weighted images have shown some success in distinguishing benign and malignant adrenal masses. Our preference is to use morphological criteria to distinguish benign and malignant adrenal masses, and the technique most suitable is Gd-DTPA-enhanced fat-suppressed T1-weighted spin echo imaging. We routinely perform immediate postcontrast dynamic breath-hold gradient echo imaging. The appearance of normal adrenal glands using the above-described technique is illustrated in Fig. 1. The demonstration of renal corticomedullary difference on either T1-weighted fat-suppressed spin echo images or immediate postcontrast FLASH images can be helpful to distinguish adrenal from renal tumors (Fig. 2) (1). The multiplanar imaging capability of MRI is also useful to assess large tumors in the region of the upper pole of the kidney to determine intra- or extrarenal origin by imaging in the coronal or sagittal planes (Fig. 3) (2).

MASS LESIONS

Diseases that affect the adrenal glands include benign and malignant tumors and adrenal hyperplasia. Since the adrenal glands perform an endocrine function, adrenal disease can be further categorized as hyperfunctioning or nonhyperfunctioning. Hyperfunctioning disease can result from adrenal hyperplasia or benign or malignant tumors.

Benign Masses

Adrenal Cysts

Adrenal cysts are uncommon. Pseudocysts are the most common clinically detected cysts and usually arise from hemorrhage into a normal adrenal gland (3,4). Endothelial cysts are small lesions and are predominantly lymphogenous in origin. These cysts are asymptomatic and therefore are detected incidentally (3,4). Adrenal cysts are signal void on Gd-DTPA-enhanced MR images (Fig. 4).

Nonhyperfunctioning Adenomas

Adrenal adenomas are the most common adrenal masses and are most frequently nonhyperfunctioning. Incidental adenomas are reported in 2% to 8% of autopsies. Increased incidence has been reported in patients who are elderly, obese, or hypertensive or who have primary malignant neoplasms of bladder, kidney, or endometrium.

R. C. Semelka: Department of Radiology and Magnetic Resonance Services, University of North Carolina at Chapel Hill, Chapel Hill, North Carolina 27599.

J. P. Shoenut: University of Manitoba and Department of Medicine, Saint Boniface General Hospital, Winnipeg, Manitoba R2H 2A6.

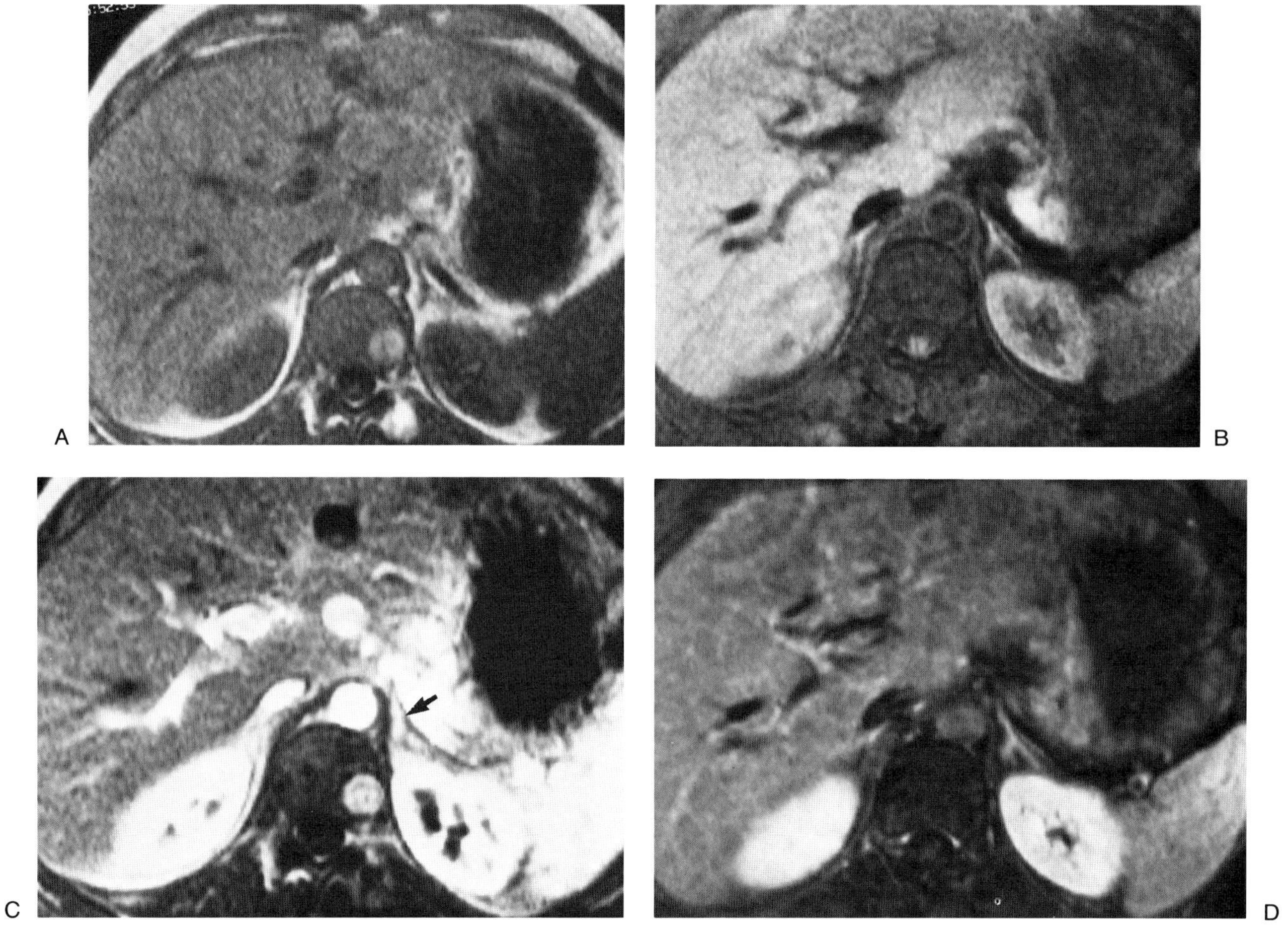

FIG. 1. Normal adrenals. FLASH (130/4.5/80°) (**A**), fat-suppressed spin echo (500/15) (**B**), dynamic Gd-DTPA-enhanced FLASH (130/4.5/80°) (**C**), and Gd-DTPA-enhanced fat-suppressed spin echo (500/15) (**D**) images. Normal adrenals are low in SI on FLASH (A) and relatively high in SI on fat-suppressed spin echo (B). Normal adrenals enhanced substantially in 17% of cases on Gd-DTPA-enhanced FLASH images (*arrow,* C). Uniform signal intensity is present on Gd-DTPA-enhanced fat-suppressed spin echo image (D). Reprinted with permission from ref. 10.

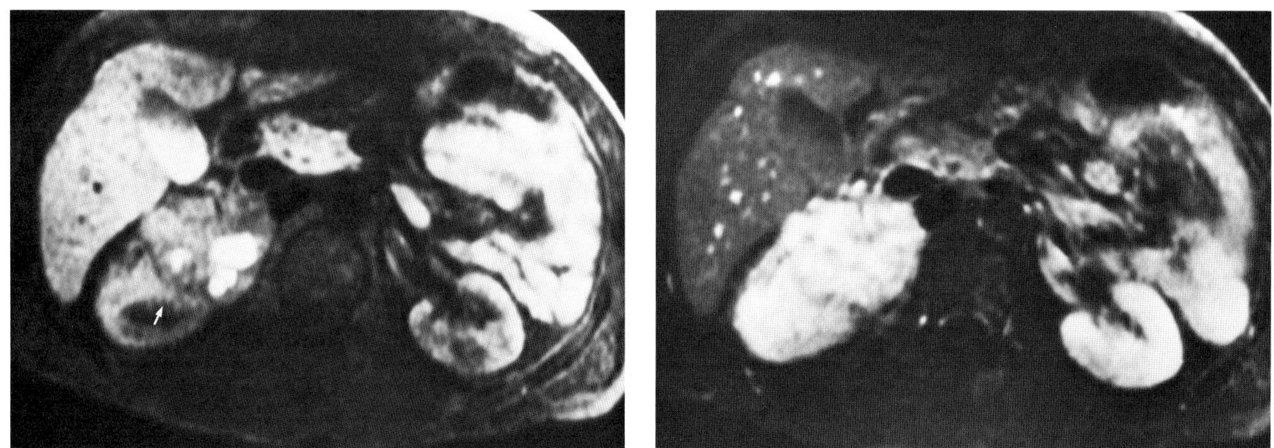

FIG. 2. Pheochromocytoma. T1FS (**A**) and GD-DTPA-enhanced T1FS (**B**) images in a 48-year-old man with a pheochromocytoma. A large tumor mass was identified in the region of the upper pole of the right kidney. Most MR sequences and CT suggested that this lesion was a renal tumor. The T1FS image demonstrates preservation of the ring of renal cortex adjacent to the mass (*arrow*), demonstrating the extrarenal nature of the tumor. A pheochromocytoma with a 7-cm interface with renal cortex was discovered at surgery. The tumor enhanced to a similar extent as renal cortex, resulting in loss of contrast (B).

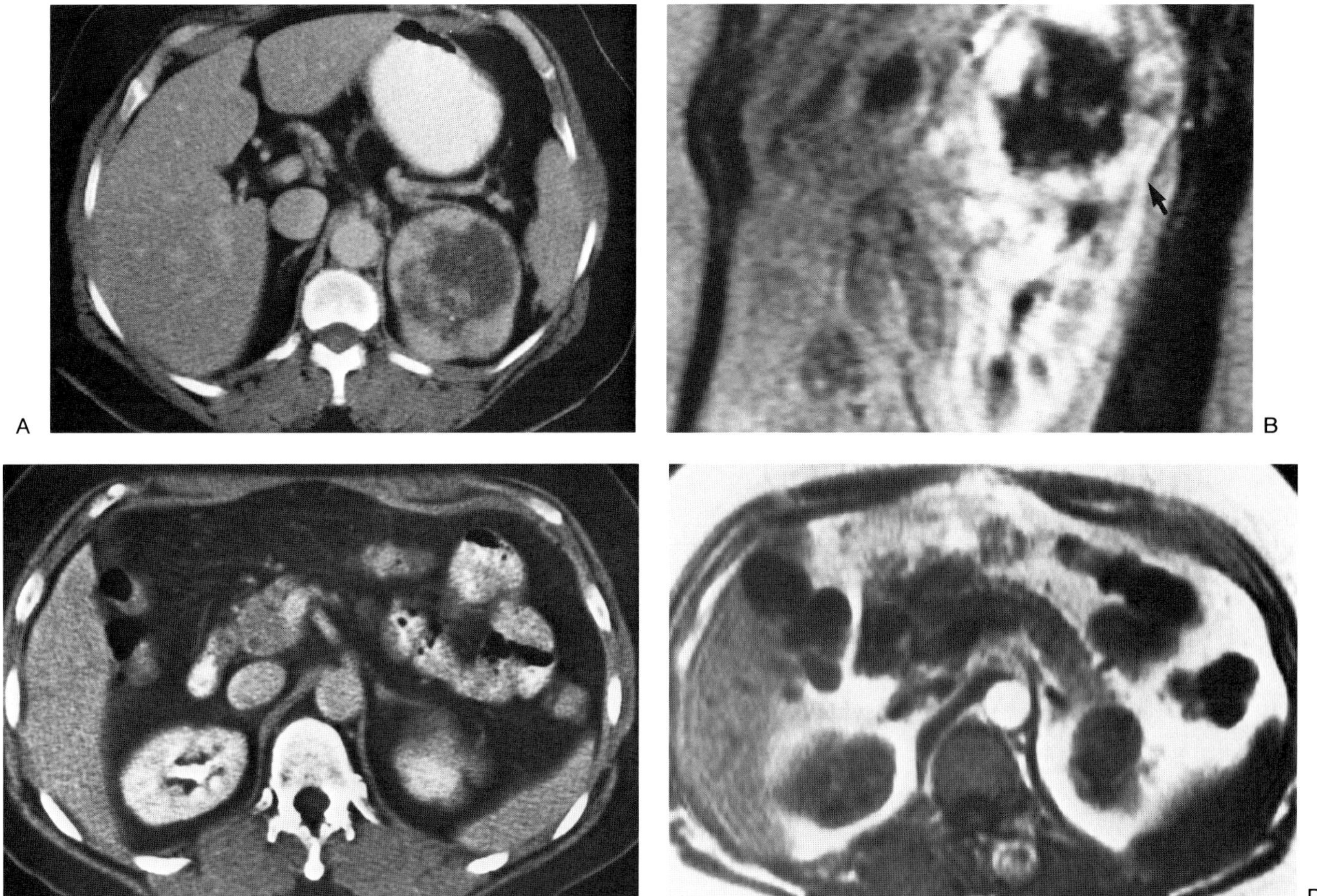

FIG. 3. Renal and adrenal tumors shown on sagittal images. Transverse contrast-enhanced CT (**A**) and sagittal dynamic Gd-DTPA-enhanced FLASH (130/4.5/80°) (**B**) images in a 56-year-old woman with renal cancer. A large mass is identified in the region of the upper pole of the left kidney on CT images (A). Direct sagittal imaging during the capillary phase of enhancement (B) shows that the mass interrupts the ring of renal cortex (*arrow*), with the epicenter of the mass within the expected margin of the upper pole, proving the renal origin of the tumor. In a second patient, a 38-year-old woman with an adrenal tumor, CT (**C**), FLASH (**D**).

Adenomas are oval masses and vary in diameter from 1 to 10 cm, with the majority measuring <4 cm in diameter. The majority of adenomas are low in SI on T2-weighted images (5–9). Contrast enhancement on immediate dynamic images is variable (10). The most reliable features are homogeneity of contrast enhancement and regularity of lesion margins (Fig. 5) (10,11). On serial postcontrast images rapid washout of contrast in adenomas may be a feature differentiating them from malignant adrenal masses (12,13).

Myelolipomas

Myelolipomas are rare benign tumors composed of myeloid, erythroid, and fat elements (14,15). These tumors are usually small and unilateral and typically have a high fat content, which gives them a pathognomonic appearance on CT and MR images (16,17). The amount of fat in these lesions can vary. The diagnosis is virtually certain if the tumor is high in SI on T1-weighted images and suppresses with fat suppression (Fig. 6). On the basis of T1-weighted images alone, the distinction from a hemorrhagic cyst would be difficult.

Aldosteronomas

Aldosteronomas are rare tumors that are responsible for 75% of cases of primary aldosteronism (Conn's syndrome), with adrenal hyperplasia accounting for 25% (18). The clinical presentation includes systemic hypertension with hypokalemia, decreased plasma renin activity, and increased plasma aldosterone. These tumors are typically small, measuring <3 cm in diameter, with tumors smaller than 1 cm common (19,20) (Fig. 7). The

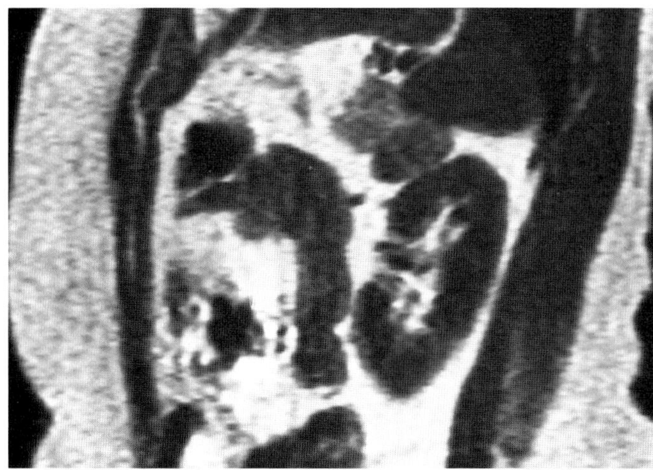
E

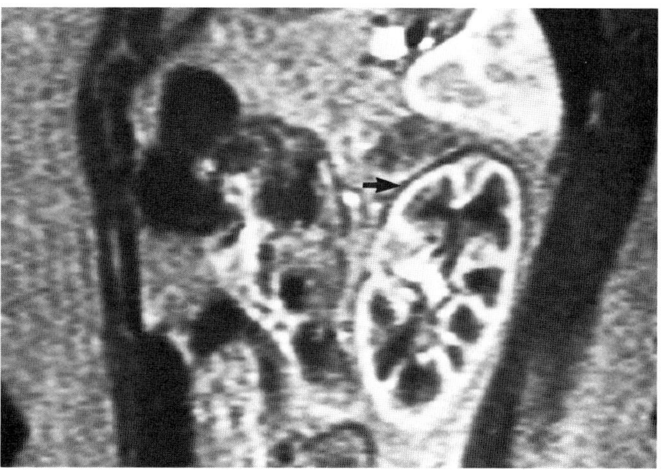
F

G

FIG. 3. (*Continued.*) Sagittal FLASH (**E**), sagittal 1-second postcontrast FLASH (**F**), and GD-DTPA-enhanced T1FS (**G**) images demonstrate a 3-cm mass adjacent to the upper pole of the kidney. Transverse images (C,D,G) suggest that the mass is renal in origin. Sagittal images (E,F) clearly demonstrate the extrarenal origin of the mass. An intact ring of enhancing renal cortex is shown on the 1-second postcontrast image (*arrow,* F).

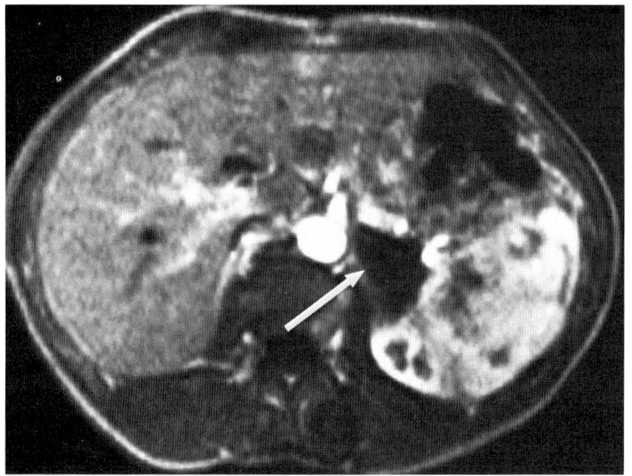

FIG. 4. Adrenal cyst. One-second postcontrast FLASH image in a 42-year-old woman with an adrenal cyst. The cyst arising from the left adrenal is signal void (*white arrow*), and no definable wall is present.

distinction between adenoma and hyperplasia is important, since patients with adenomas will respond to surgical management and patients with hyperplasia are best treated medically (21). Findings on tomographic images may result in diagnostic errors in patients who have a unilateral adenoma but in whom both adrenals have a nodular appearance. Doppman et al. reported on 24 patients with primary aldosteronism in whom CT images suggested the presence of hyperplasia in 6 patients who had a unilateral aldosteronoma (22).

Cortisol-producing Functioning Adenomas

Functioning adrenal adenomas are responsible for approximately 20% of cases of Cushing's syndrome. Most of these adenomas measure >2 cm and are readily detected on CT and MR images (23,24).

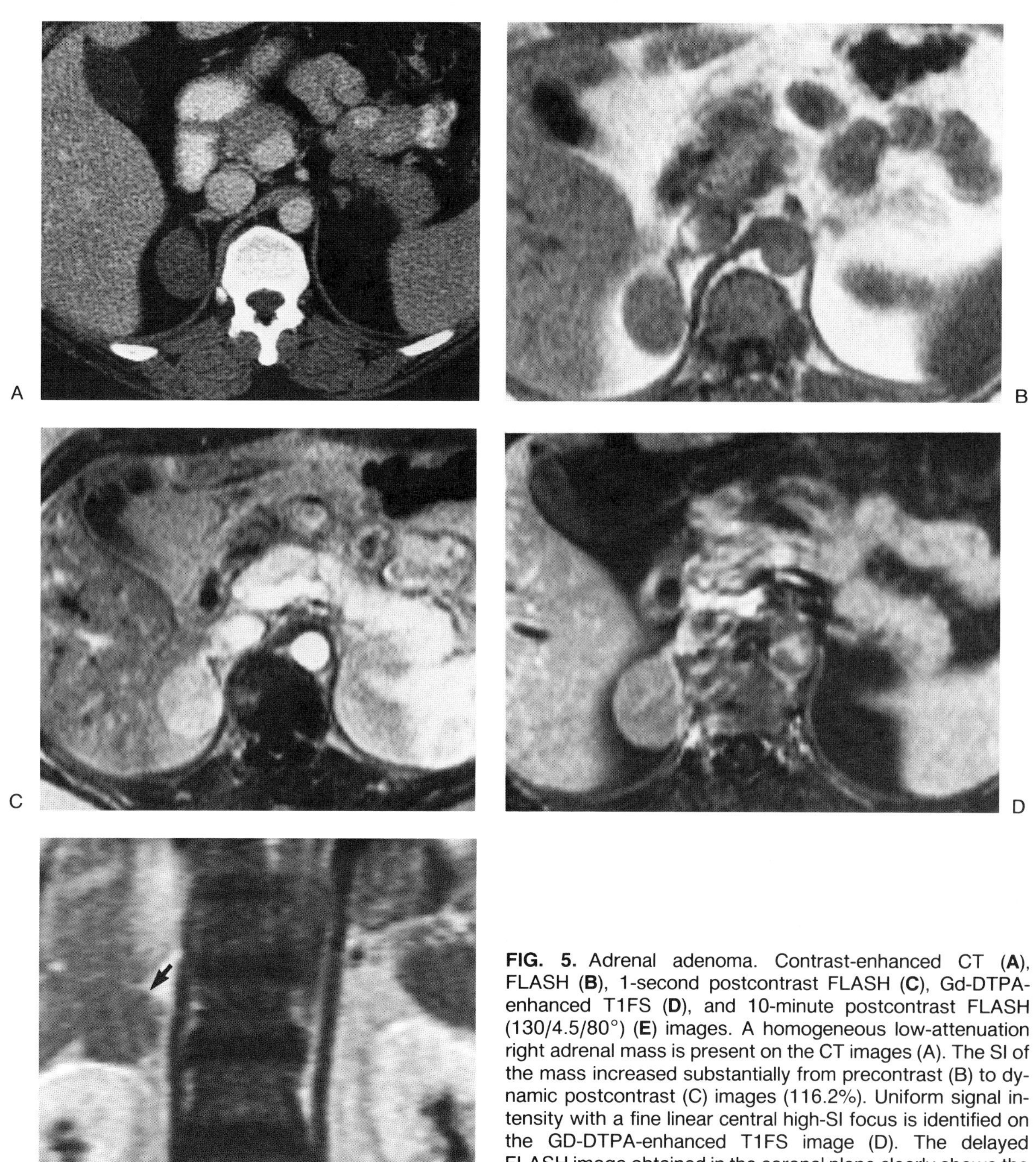

FIG. 5. Adrenal adenoma. Contrast-enhanced CT (**A**), FLASH (**B**), 1-second postcontrast FLASH (**C**), Gd-DTPA-enhanced T1FS (**D**), and 10-minute postcontrast FLASH (130/4.5/80°) (**E**) images. A homogeneous low-attenuation right adrenal mass is present on the CT images (A). The SI of the mass increased substantially from precontrast (B) to dynamic postcontrast (C) images (116.2%). Uniform signal intensity with a fine linear central high-SI focus is identified on the GD-DTPA-enhanced T1FS image (D). The delayed FLASH image obtained in the coronal plane clearly shows the extrarenal location of the mass (*arrow*, E). Reprinted with permission from ref. 10.

Malignant Masses

Metastases

Metastases are the most frequent malignant lesions to involve the adrenal glands. The most common primary tumors are lung, breast, bowel, and pancreas (25–27). Metastatic deposits can vary in size from microscopic involvement to large tumor masses. Metastases are most frequently bilateral, but they may be unilateral. Metastases frequently have irregular margins and enhance in a heterogeneous fashion, although these features are not constant. Direct extension of primary tumors may occasionally be seen. This is most frequently observed in pancreatic or renal cancers. Necrosis is not uncommon in large metastatic deposits (Fig. 8). Hemorrhage is also a

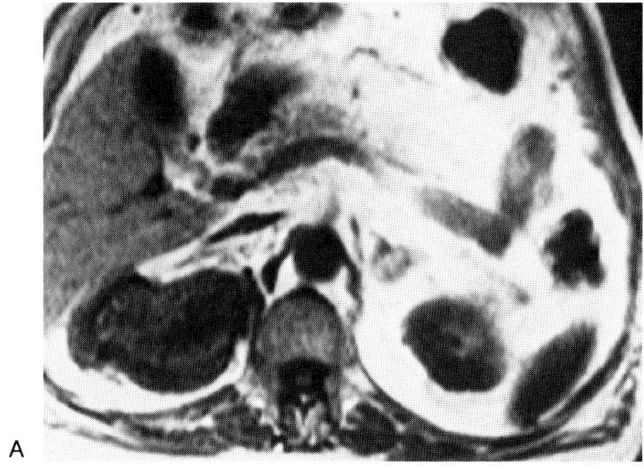
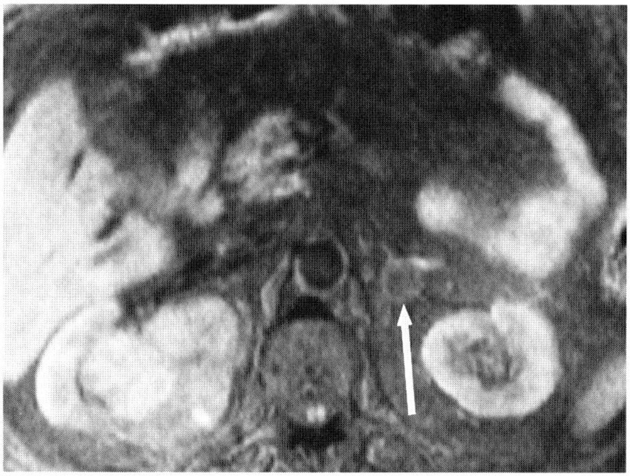

FIG. 6. Myelolipoma. FLASH (130/4.5/80°) (**A**) and T1FS (**B**) images. A high-SI mass in the left adrenal gland on FLASH (A) is attenuated by fat suppression (*white arrow,* B). The CT images (not shown) demonstrated a fat density mass, confirming the diagnosis. A renal cancer of the right kidney is also present.

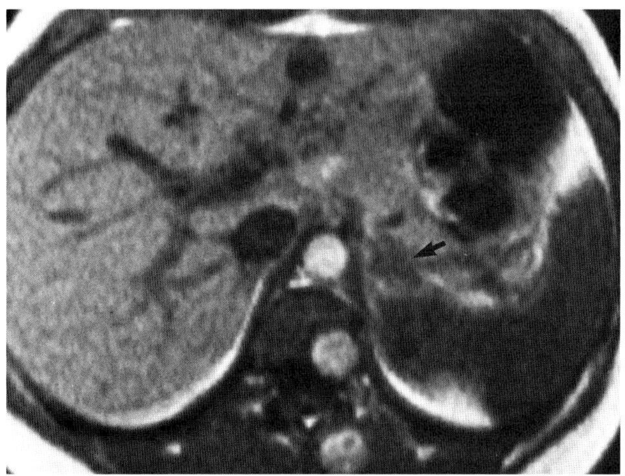
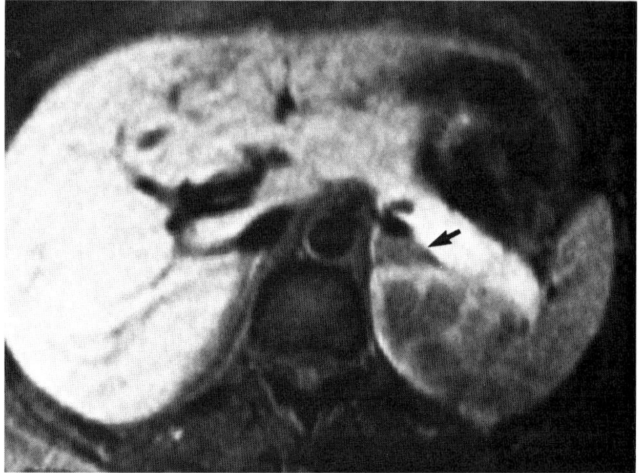

FIG. 7. Aldosteronoma. FLASH (**A**) and T1FS (**B**) images in a 37-year-old woman with an aldosteronoma. A 1-cm mass lesion is present in the left adrenal gland (*arrow,* A). Aldosteronomas are small tumors, usually <3 cm in diameter.

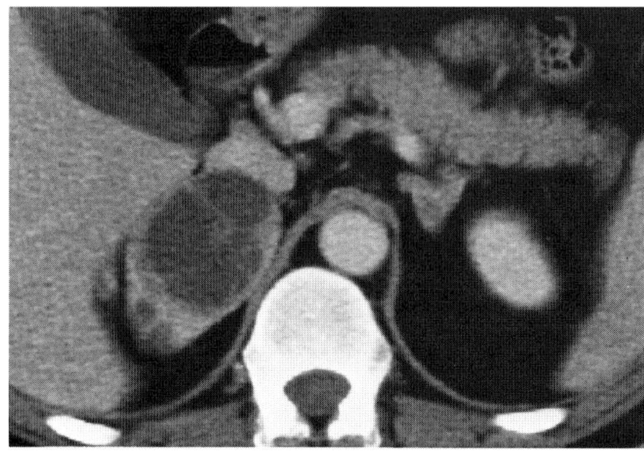
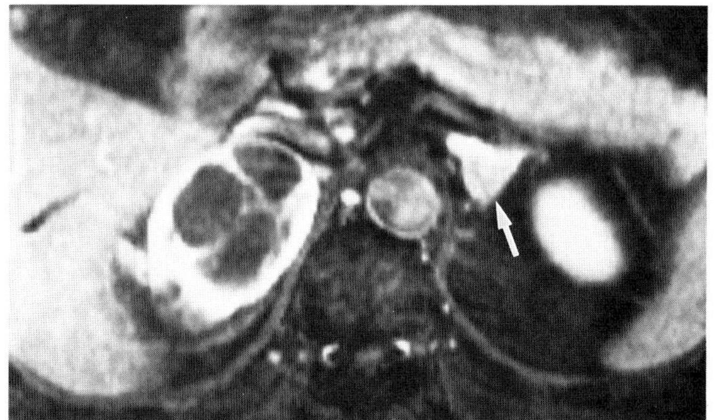

FIG. 8. Adrenal metastases. Contrast-enhanced CT (**A**) and Gd-DTPA-enhanced T1FS (**B**) images in a patient with a renal cell cancer. CT and MR images show a 5-cm right adrenal mass with central necrosis. The left adrenal gland contains a 1.5-cm mass with indeterminate features (*white arrow,* B). A follow-up CT study after 2 months showed enlargement of this mass, confirming the presence of a metastatic deposit. Reprinted with permission from ref. 10.

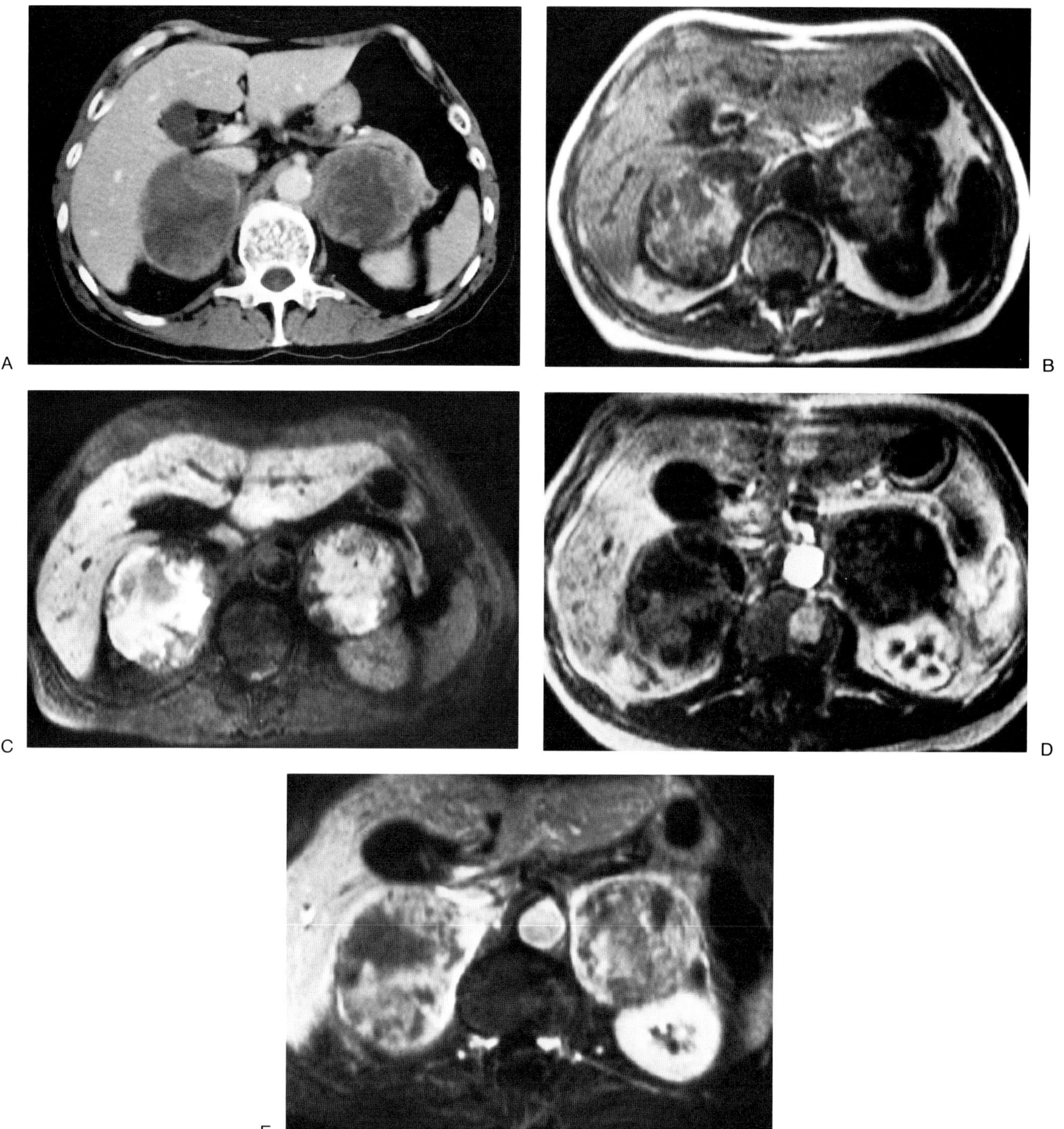

FIG. 9. Hemorrhagic adrenal metastases. Contrast-enhanced CT (**A**), FLASH (**B**), T1FS (**C**), 1-second postcontrast FLASH (**D**), and Gd-DTPA-enhanced T1FS (**E**) images in a patient with colon cancer. The CT image shows bilateral 6-cm adrenal masses with heterogeneous attenuation (A). High-SI tissue apparent on the FLASH images (B) is not attenuated on the fat-suppressed images (C), which is consistent with hemorrhage. The percentage of enhancement of tumor stroma is minimal (13.6% to 25.6%). The Gd-DTPA-enhanced T1FS image shows heterogeneous signal intensity of the masses (E). Reprinted with permission from ref. 10.

feature more typical of malignant than benign masses and is better shown on MR than on CT images (Fig. 9).

The distinction between metastases and adenomas remains problematic for masses measuring <2 cm; therefore, CT-guided biopsies are at present not obviated by MR examination. In patients with no known primary malignant neoplasm, it is considered acceptable management to examine adrenal masses serially to assess change in size. Reassessment at 3 to 6 months and 1 year is performed at many centers (28–30). Herrera et al. have suggested that no change in size in a 3-month interval is sufficient to consider a mass benign (31).

It may be helpful to compare the SI of adrenal masses on T2-weighted images to the SI of either the primary tumor or other metastatic deposits (Fig. 10) to confirm the nature of the adrenal mass (7). T2-weighted images can be a useful adjunct to Gd-DTPA-enhanced breath-hold and fat-suppressed images (8,9). Certain benign lesions do have prolonged T2 values, and therefore T2 information alone is unable to distinguish benign and malignant masses (32).

Pheochromocytomas

Pheochromocytomas are catecholamine-producing tumors that arise from the adrenal medulla in 90% of cases. The remaining 10% occur along the course of sympathetic ganglia, most frequently in a para-aortic or paracaval location, including the organ of Zuckerkandl (located at the aortic bifurcation). Mediastinal and bladder wall tumors account for 2% of pheochromocytomas. Tumors are frequently greater than 3 cm in diameter at presentation (33). Pheochromocytomas are bilateral in 10% of cases and are malignant in about 10% of cases. Extraadrenal tumors are malignant in a greater percentage of cases (40%). Patients present with sustained or paroxysmal hypertension, and nearly all symptomatic patients have elevated urinary catecholamine, vanillylmandelic acid (VMA), and metanephric levels. Patients with multiple endocrine neoplasia Type II, neurofibromatosis, von Hippel-Lindau disease, and multiple cutaneous neuromas have an increased incidence of pheochromocytomas. Seventy-five percent of patients

A

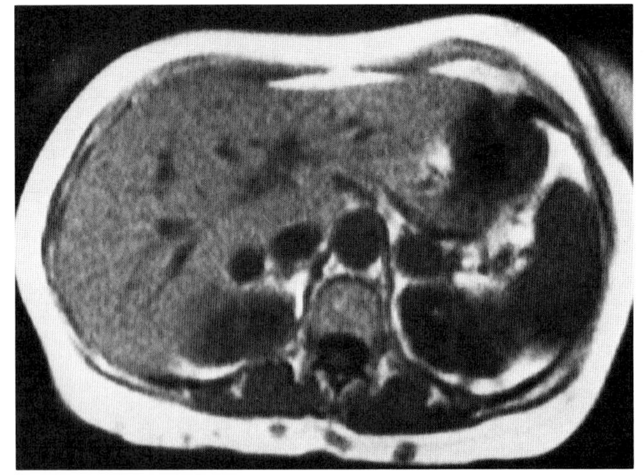

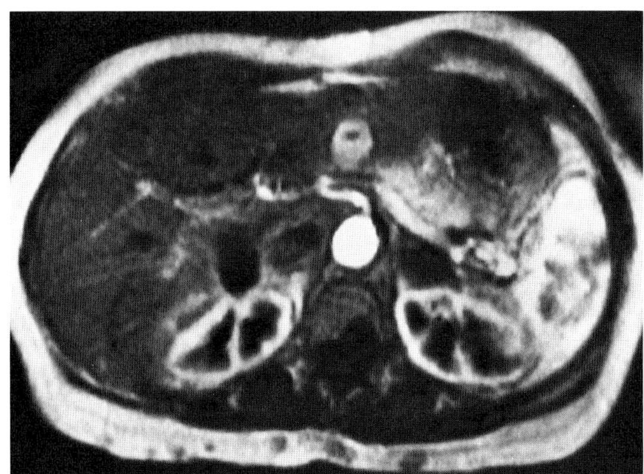

B

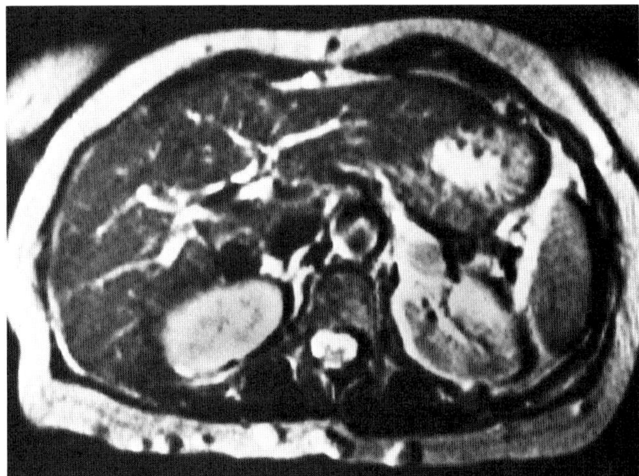

C

FIG. 10. Adrenal metastases. FLASH (**A**), 1-second post-contrast FLASH (**B**), and T2-weighted spin echo (**C**) images in a 56-year-old woman with breast cancer metastases to the adrenal glands and subcutaneous tissue. The adrenal metastases do not enhance substantially with Gd-DTPA on FLASH images and are of low SI on T2-weighted images. These metastatic lesions parallel the SI features of the subcutaneous metastases, which do not enhance substantially with Gd-DTPA and have varying SI on T2-weighted images.

with MEN Type II have bilateral tumors, and tumors are rarely extraadrenal (34). Cystic pheochromocytomas occur, and distinction from cysts may be difficult (35). Pheochromocytomas characteristically have a high SI on T2-weighted images (5) (Fig. 11).

Adrenal Carcinomas

Adrenal cortical carcinoma is a rare aggressive tumor. Tumors usually present when they are large, with over 90% of reported cases exceeding 6 cm in diameter (36,37). Approximately 50% of the tumors are hyperfunctioning, with hypercortisolism and virilization common presentations (38). Metastases are frequently found at presentation, with regional and paraaortic lymph nodes, lungs, and liver common sites. Tumor thrombus into the IVC is common at presentation. Large tumors are frequently necrotic (Fig. 12). Smaller tumors also tend to have greater enhancement of the tumor margin (Fig. 13). Fat-suppressed images help delineate large tumors from adjacent pancreas and kidney. On T2-weighted images tumors have a high SI, which in part reflects the frequent occurrence of central necrosis (2,7,38).

Neuroblastomas

Neuroblastoma is one of the most common solid tumors of children younger than 5 years. Tumors originate from neural crest and sympathetic ganglia. Neuroblastomas most commonly arise from the adrenal medulla. In older patients extraadrenal sites increase in frequency (39). The most common sites of metastatic disease include the skeletal system, lung, liver, and lymph nodes. Extension into the neural canal suggests the diagnosis (Fig. 14).

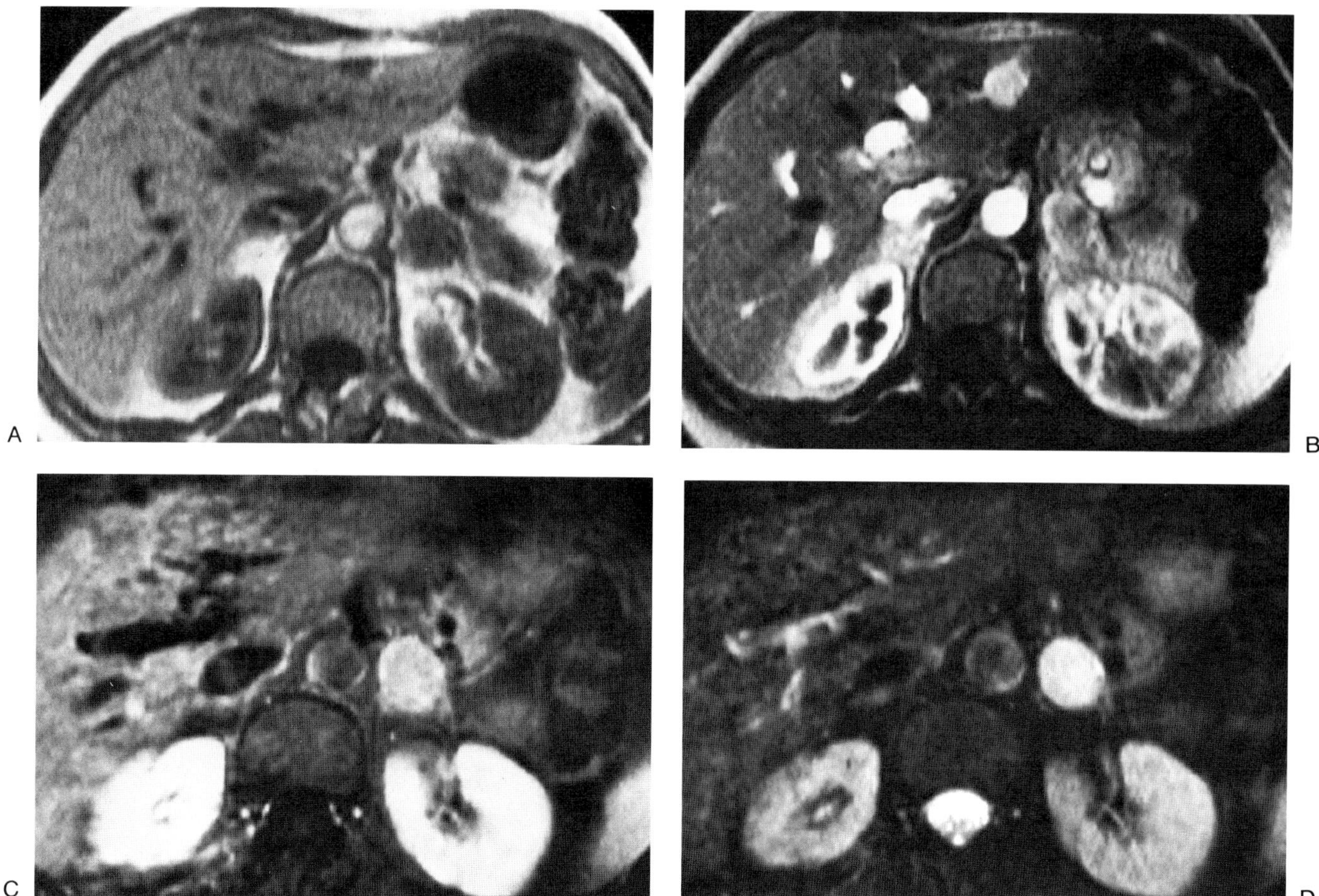

FIG. 11. Pheochromocytoma. FLASH (**A**), 1-second postcontrast FLASH (**B**), Gd-DTPA-enhanced T1FS (**C**), and T2FS (**D**) MR images in a 71-year-old woman with a pheochromocytoma. A well-defined mass in the left adrenal gland shows minimal initial enhancement (B) and relatively homogeneous SI after Gd-DTPA administration (C) and is high in SI on T2-weighted images (D). Pheochromocytomas are characteristically high in SI on T2-weighted images.

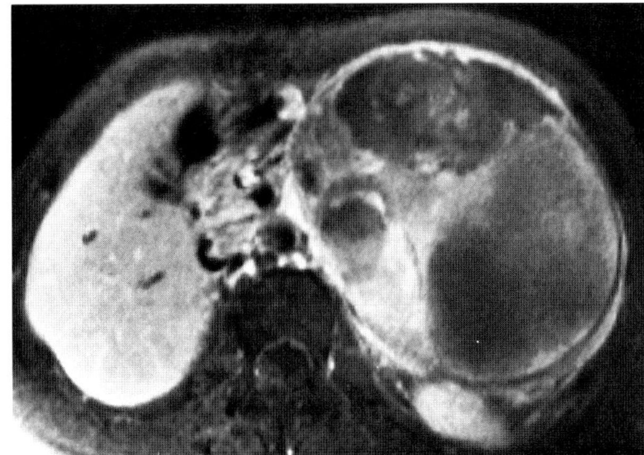

FIG. 12. Adrenal cortical carcinoma. Gd-DTPA-enhanced T1FS image in a 41-year-old woman with adrenal cortical carcinoma demonstrates a 12-cm left adrenal mass, which is largely cystic. Extensive mural nodularity and thick irregular septations are apparent.

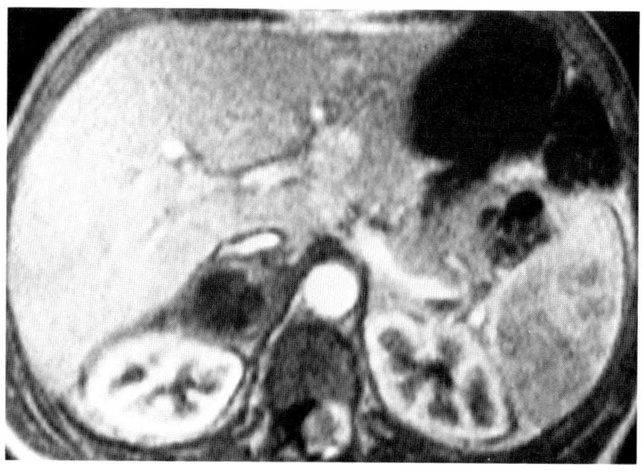

FIG. 13. Adrenal carcinoma. Dynamic Gd-DTPA-enhanced FLASH (130/4.5/80°) image demonstrates a right adrenal mass lesion with moderate peripheral enhancement and central low SI.

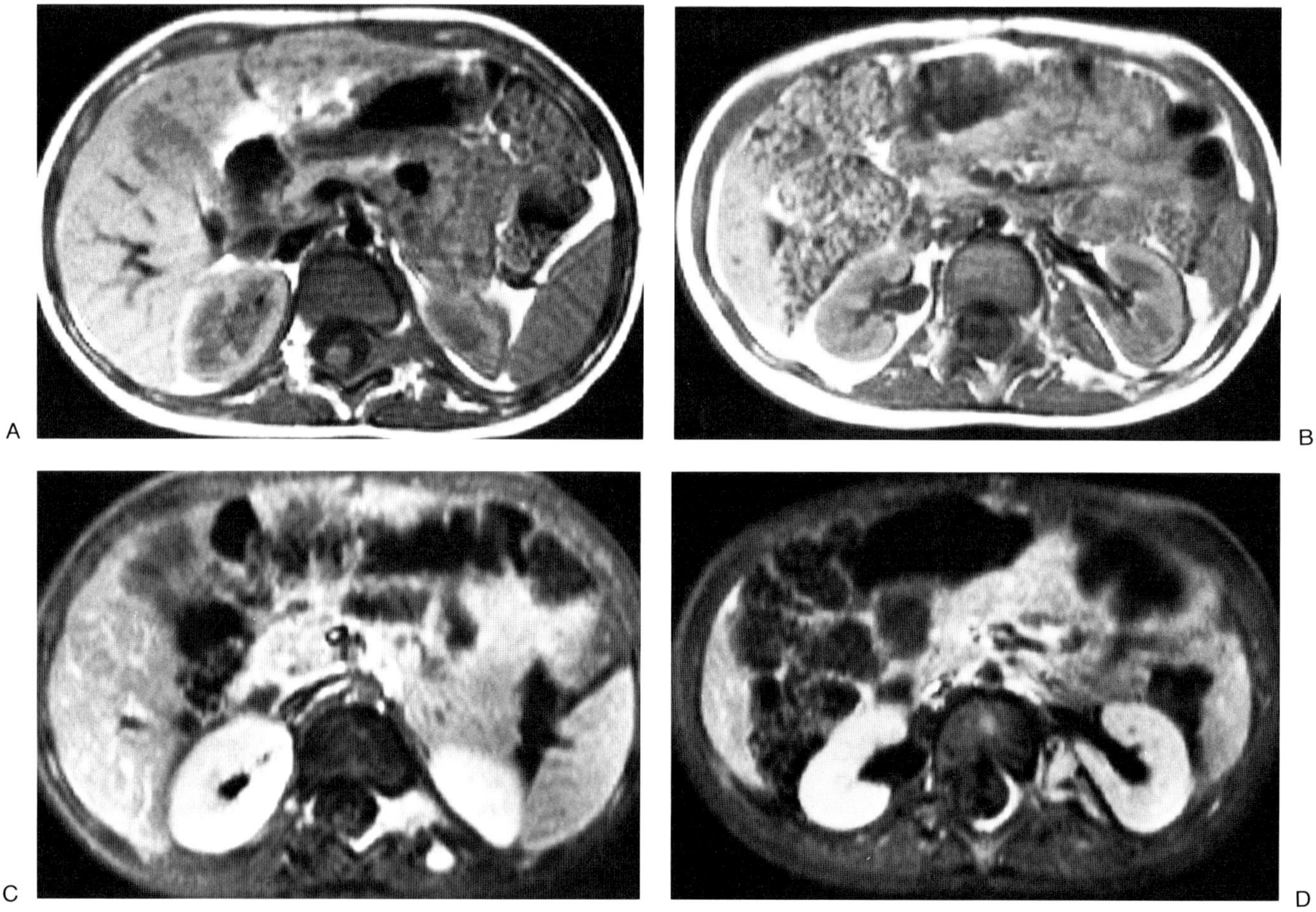

A

B

C

D

FIG. 14. Neuroblastoma. T1-weighted spin echo (**A,B**) and Gd-DTPA-enhanced fat-suppressed spin echo (**C,D**) images in a 3-year-old girl with neuroblastoma. A tumor mass involving the left psoas muscle (B,D) extends into the neural canal, enveloping the dural sac (A,C). The neural origin of the tissue is suggested by the extension into the neural canal. Gd-DTPA-enhanced images (C,D) demonstrate tumor enhancement.

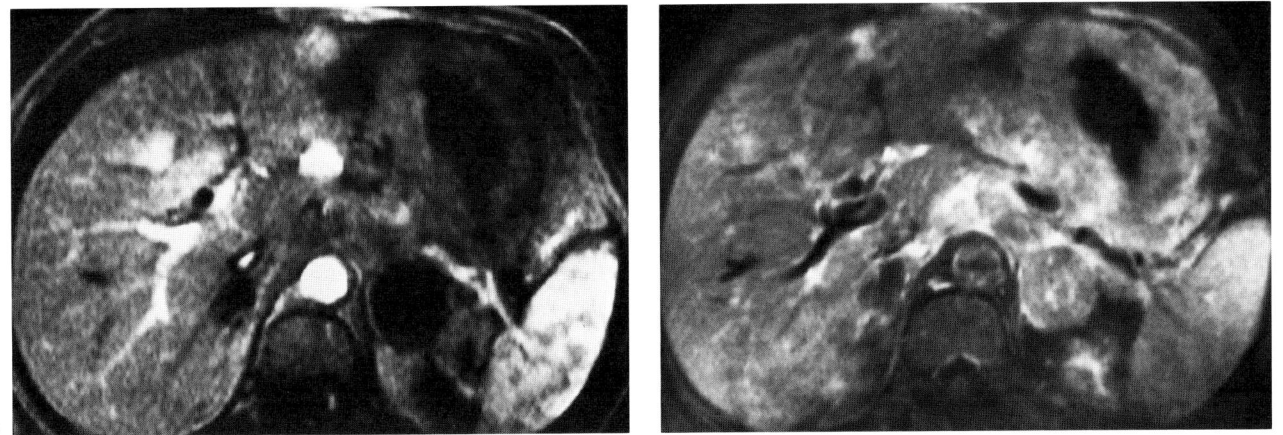

FIG. 15. Lymphoma. One-second postcontrast FLASH (**A**) and Gd-DTPA-enhanced T1FS (**B**) images in a 74-year-old man with non-Hodgkin's lymphoma. A 3-cm mass is present in the left adrenal gland, which shows negligible initial enhancement (A) and central linear high-SI tissue on the later postcontrast image (B). Substantial thickening of the stomach wall is due to associated gastric involvement.

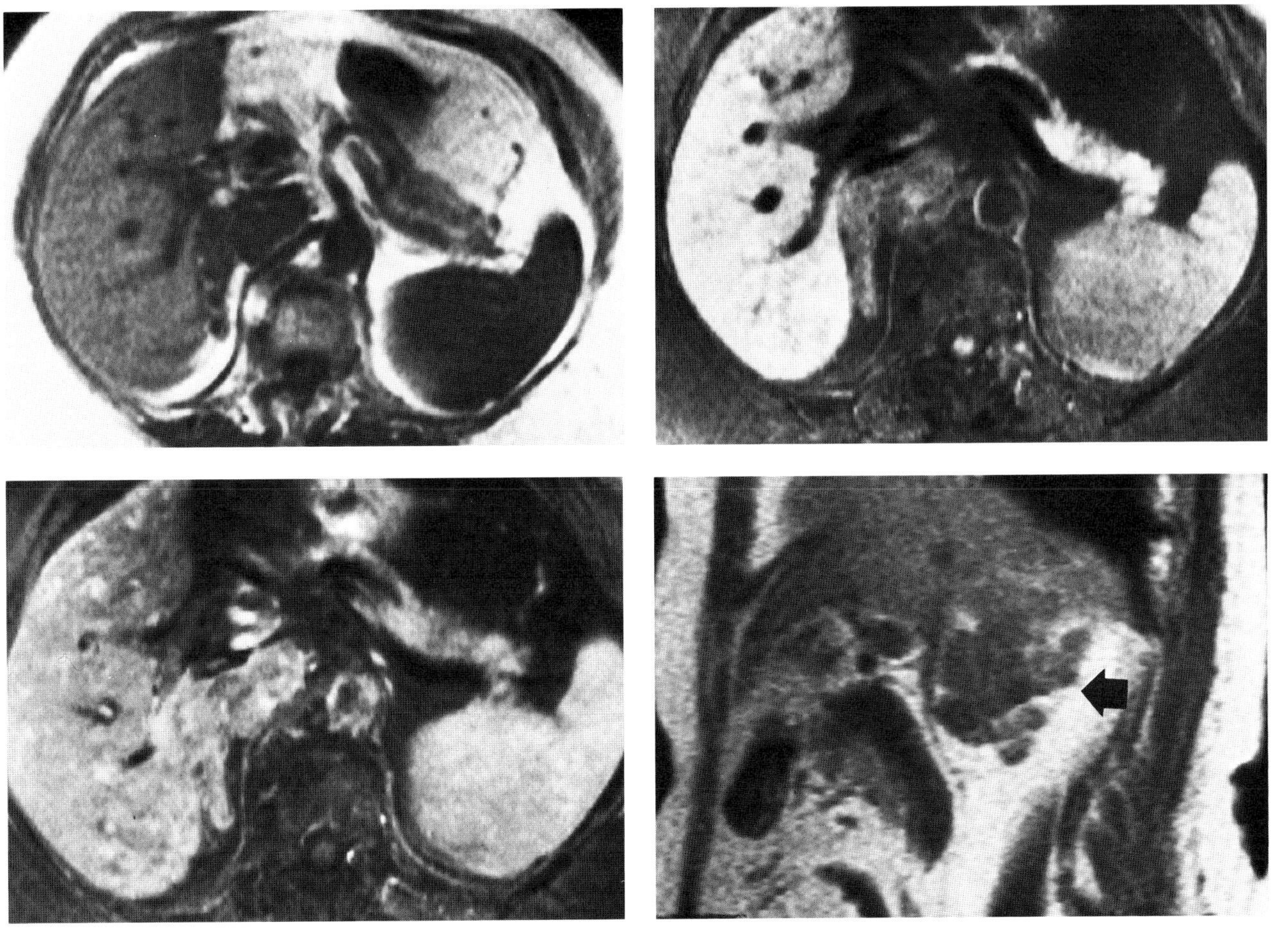

FIG. 16. Macronodular adrenal hyperplasia. FLASH (**A**), T1FS (**B**), Gd-DTPA-enhanced T1FS (**C**), and 10-minute postcontrast sagittal FLASH (**D**) images in a 68-year-old woman with macronodular adrenal hyperplasia. The left adrenal gland had been removed 10 years earlier and had the same histological finding. Multiple 1- to 1.5-cm nodular masses are present within the enlarged adrenal gland. Gd-DTPA enhancement is mildly inhomogeneous (C), and sagittal images demonstrate the "cluster of grapes" appearance (*arrow,* D).

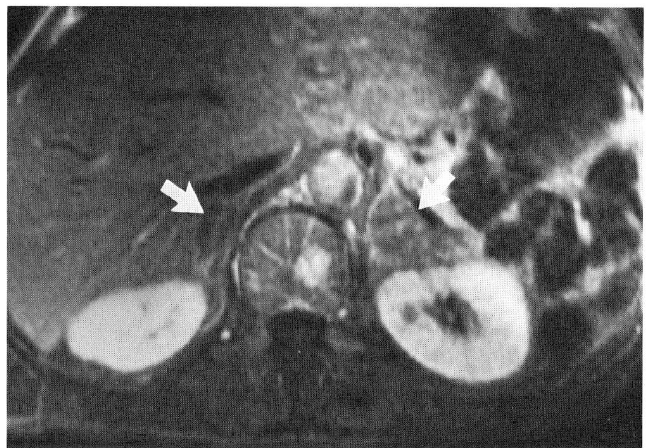

FIG. 17. Tuberculosis. Gd-DTPA-enhanced T1FS image in a 76-year-old man with tuberculous involvement of the adrenal glands. Bilateral enlargement of the adrenal glands is present (*arrows*), with maintenance of adreniform shape.

Lymphoma

Lymphoma occasionally involves the adrenal glands. Non-Hodgkin's lymphoma is the most frequent cell type (40–42). Retroperitoneal lymphadenopathy is frequently an associated finding (41). Contrast enhancement is variable but is usually minimal (Fig. 15).

HYPERPLASIA

Hyperplastic glands usually contain microscopic nodules; however, macroscopic nodules (>2 cm) may be found (Fig. 16) (43). Hyperplasia usually involves both glands, and an adreniform shape is maintained. Unilateral adrenal enlargement may occur. The adrenal glands may also appear normal in size (43).

The majority (70%) of patients with Cushing's syndrome have adrenal cortical hyperplasia secondary to an adrenocorticotropic hormone (ACTH)-producing pituitary microadenoma (Cushing's disease). Adrenal enlargement or hyperplasia is also identified in the context of systematic illness, acromegaly, hyperthyroidism, hypertension, diabetes, and malignant disease.

INFLAMMATORY DISEASES

The adrenal glands may be involved in granulomatous disease, which is most commonly due to tuberculosis, followed by histoplasmosis and rarely blastomycosis (44–47). Diffuse enlargement of both adrenal glands is the most common appearance (Fig. 17). Rarely, massive enlargement may be seen.

ADRENAL HEMORRHAGE

Adrenal hemorrhage occurs secondary to bleeding diathesis, severe stress, blood loss causing hypotension (surgery, childbirth, or sepsis), or trauma (48,49). Acute awareness of adrenal hemorrhage on tomographic images is important in that clinical findings may be nonspecific and fatal, acute adrenal insufficiency may result (50,51). MRI is very sensitive for the detection of adrenal hemorrhage and is superior to CT. Subacute hemorrhage is high in SI on T1-weighted images (52, 53), and the high SI is more conspicuous on fat-suppressed T1-weighted images (Fig. 18).

ADDISON'S DISEASE

Addison's disease results from adrenal insufficiency. The tomographic appearance of the adrenal glands may

A 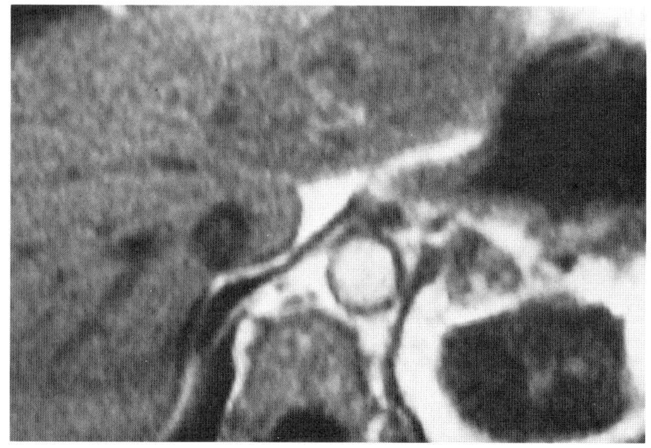

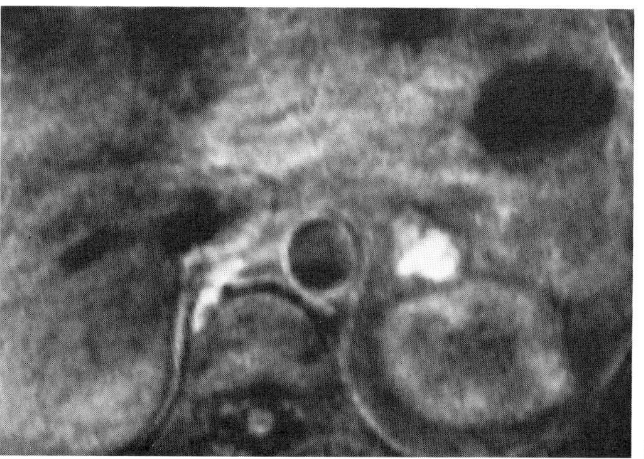 B

FIG. 18. Posttraumatic hemorrhage. FLASH (**A**) and T1FS (**B**) images in a 64-year-old woman who had sustained severe injury of the left upper abdomen in a motor vehicle accident. Enlargement of the left adrenal gland with patchy increased SI is apparent on the FLASH image. On the T1FS image the high SI of blood is more conspicuous.

assist in diagnosing the underlying cause (45,51,54,55). Autoimmune disease or pituitary insufficiency is suggested by the presence of atrophic glands (54,55). Adrenal hemorrhage can be readily detected as high-SI substance in bilaterally enlarged glands (51,52). Enlarged glands without hemorrhage suggest granulomatous disease (45). Metastases rarely cause adrenal insufficiency.

FUTURE DIRECTIONS

Out-of-phase gradient echo images have shown promise as a technique to distinguish benign from malignant adenopathy. Adenomas frequently contain fat and diminish in SI on out-of-phase images, whereas metastases frequently do not contain fat and therefore do not diminish in SI (56). Overlap between benign and malignant masses is still expected (57).

REFERENCES

1. Semelka RC, Hricak H, Stevens S, Finegold R, Tomei E, Carroll P. Combined gadolinium-enhanced and fat-saturation MR imaging of renal masses. *Radiology* 1991;178:803–809.
2. Falke THM, te Strake L, Shaff MI, et al. MR imaging of the adrenals: correlation with computed tomography. *J Comput Assist Tomogr* 1986;10:242–253.
3. Foster DG. Adrenal cysts. *Arch Surg* 1966;92:131–143.
4. Kearny GP, Mahoney EM, Maher E, Harrison JH. Functioning and nonfunctioning cysts of the adrenal cortex and medulla. *Am J Surg* 1977;134:3632–3638.
5. Reining JW, Doppman JL, Dwyer AJ, Johnson AR, Knop RH. Adrenal masses differentiated by MR. *Radiology* 1986;158:81–84.
6. Reinig JW, Doppman JL, Dwyer AJ, Frank J. MRI of indeterminate adrenal masses. *AJR Am J Roentgenol* 1986;147:493–496.
7. Chang A, Glazer HS, Lee JKT, Ling D, Heiken JP. Adrenal gland: MR imaging. *Radiology* 1987;163:123–128.
8. Baker ME, Blinder R, Spritzer C, Leight GS, Herfkens RJ, Dunnick NR. MR evaluation of adrenal masses at 1.5T. *AJR Am J Roentgenol* 1989;153:307–312.
9. Kier R, McCarthy S. MR characterization of adrenal masses: field strength and pulse sequence considerations. *Radiology* 1989;171:671–674.
10. Semelka RC, Shoenut JP, Lawrence PH, Greenberg HM, Maycher B, Madden TP, Kroeker MA: Adrenal masses: evaluation by gadolinium enhancement and fat suppression MRI. *J Magn Reson Imag* (*in press*).
11. Berland LL, Koslin DB, Kenney PJ, Stanley RJ, Lee JY. Differentiation between small benign and malignant adrenal masses with dynamic incremental CT. *AJR Am J Roentgenol* 1988;151: 95–101.
12. Krestin GP, Steinbrich W, Friedmann G. Adrenal masses: evaluation with fast gradient-echo MR imaging Gd-DTPA-enhanced dynamic studies. *Radiology* 1989;171:675–680.
13. Krestin GP, Friedmann G, Fischbach R, Neufang KFR, Allolio B. Evaluation of adrenal masses in oncologic patients: dynamic contrast-enhanced MR vs CT. *J Comput Assist Tomogr* 1991; 15:104–110.
14. Plaut A. Myelolipoma in the adrenal cortex. *Am J Pathol* 1958;34:487–515.
15. Olsson CA, Krane RJ, Klugo RC, Selikowitz SM. Adrenal myelolipoma. *Surgery* 1973;73:665–670.
16. Palmer WE, Gerard-McFarland EL, Chew FS. Adrenal myelolipoma. *AJR Am J Roentgenol* 1991;156:724.
17. Musante F, Derchi LE, Bazzochi M, et al. MR imaging of adrenal myelolipomas. *J Comput Assist Tomogr* 1991;15:111–114.
18. Horton R, Finck E. Diagnosis and localization in primary aldosteronism. *Ann Intern Med* 1972;76:885–890.
19. Geisinger MA, Zelch MG, Bravo EL, Risius BF, O'Donovan PB, Borkowski GP. Primary hyperaldosteronism: comparison of CT, adrenal venography and venous sampling. *AJR Am J Roentgenol* 1983;141:299–302.
20. Ikeda DM, Francis IR, Glazer GM, Amendola MA, Gross MD, Aisen AM. The detection of adrenal tumors and hyperplasia in patients with primary aldosteronism: comparison of scintigraphy, CT, and MR imaging. *AJR Am J Roentgenol* 1989;153:301–306.
21. Grant CS, Carpenter P, Van Heerden JA, Hamberger B. Primary aldosteronism: clinical management. *Arch Surg* 1984;119: 585–590.
22. Doppman JL, Gill JR Jr, Miller DL, et al. Distinction between hyperaldosteronism due to bilateral hyperplasia and unilateral aldosteronoma: reliability of CT. *Radiology* 1992;184:677–682.
23. Dunnick NR, Doppman JL, Gill JR, Strott CA, Keiser HR, Brennan MF. Localization of functional adrenal tumors by computed tomography and venous sampling. *Radiology* 1982;142:429–433.
24. Eghrari M, McLoughlin MJ, Rosen IE, et al. The role of computed tomography in assessment of tumoral pathology of the adrenal glands. *J Comput Assist Tomogr* 1980;4:71–77.
25. Sandler MA, Pearberg JL, Madrazo BL, Gitschlag KF, Gross SC. Computed tomographic evaluation of the adrenal glands in the preoperative assessment of bronchogenic carcinoma. *Radiology* 1982;145:733–736.
26. Vas W, Zylak CJ, Mather D, Figueredo A. The value of abdominal cell carcinoma of the lung. *Radiology* 1981;138:417–418.
27. Nielsen ME Jr, Heaston DK, Dunnick DR, Korobkin M. Preoperative CT evaluation of adrenal glands in non-small-cell bronchogenic carcinoma. *AJR Am J Roentgenol* 1982;139:317–320.
28. Glazer HS, Weyman PJ, Sagel SS, Levitt RG, McClennan BL. Nonfunctioning adrenal masses: incidental discovery on computed tomography. *AJR Am J Roentgenol* 1982;139:81–85.
29. Belldegrun A, Hussain S, Seltzer SE, Loughlin KR, Gittes RF, Richie JP. Incidentally discovered mass of the adrenal gland. *Surg Gynecol Obstet* 1986;163:203–208.
30. Mitnick JS, Bosniak MA, Megibow AJ, Naidich DP. Nonfunctioning adrenal adenomas discovered incidentally on computed tomography. *Radiology* 1983;148:495–499.
31. Herrera MF, Grant CS, van Heerden JA, Sheedy PF, Ilstrung DM. Incidentally discovered adrenal tumors: an institutional perspective. *Surgery* 1991;110:1014–1021.
32. Debatin JF, Spritzer CE, Dunnick NR. Castleman disease of the adrenal gland: MR imaging features. *AJR Am J Roentgenol* 1991;157:781–783.
33. Tisnado J, Amendola MA, Konerding KF, Shirazi KK, Beachley MC. Computed tomography versus angiography in the localization of pheochromocytoma. *J Comput Assist Tomogr* 1980;4:853–859.
34. Thomas JL, Bernardino ME. Pheochromocytoma in multiple endocrine adenomatosis: efficacy of computed tomography. *JAMA* 1981;245:1467–1469.
35. Bush WH, Elder JS, Crane RE, Wales LR. Cystic pheochromocytoma. *Urology* 1985;25:332–334.
36. Dunnick NR, Heaston F, Halvorsen R, Moore AV, Korobkin M. CT appearance of adrenal cortical carcinoma. *J Comput Assist Tomogr* 1982;6:978–982.
37. Henley DJ, Van Heerden JA, Grant CS, Carney JA, Carpenter PC. Adrenal cortical carcinoma—a continuing challenge. *Surgery* 1983;94:926–931.
38. Smith SM, Patel SK, Turner DA, et al. Magnetic resonance imaging of adrenal cortical carcinoma. *Urol Radiol* 1989;11:1–6.
39. Feinstein RS, Gatewood OMB, Fishman EK, Goldman SM, Siegelman SS. Computed tomography of adult neuroblastoma. *J Comput Assist Tomogr* 1984;8:720–726.
40. Paling MR, Williamson BRJ. Adrenal involvement in non-Hodgkin lymphoma. *AJR Am J Roentgenol* 1983;141:303–305.
41. Glazer HS, Lee JKT, Balfe DM, Mauro MS, Griffeth R, Sagel SS. Non-Hodgkin lymphoma: computed tomographic demonstration of unusual extranodal involvement. *Radiology* 1983;149:211–217.
42. Jafri SZ, Francis IR, Glazer GM, Bree RL, Amendola MA. CT

detection of adrenal lymphoma. *J Comput Assist Tomogr* 1983;7:254–256.
43. Korobkin M, White EA, Kressel HY, Moss AA, Montagne JP. Computed tomography in the diagnosis of adrenal disease. *AJR Am J Roentgenol* 1979;132:231–238.
44. Hauser H, Gurret JP. Miliary tuberculosis associated with adrenal enlargement: CT appearance. *J Comput Assist Tomogr* 1986; 10:254–256.
45. Sawczuk IS, Reitelman C, Libby C, Grant D, Vita J, White RD. CT findings in Addison's disease caused by tuberculosis. *Urol Radiol* 1986;8:44–45.
46. Wilson DA, Muchmore HG, Tisdal RG, Fahmy A, Pitha JV. Histoplasmosis of the adrenal glands studied by CT. *Radiology* 1984;150:779–783.
47. Halvorsen RA Jr, Heaston DK, Johnston WW, Ashton PR, Burton GM. Case report: CT guided thin needle aspiration of adrenal blastomycosis. *J Comput Assist Tomogr* 1982;6:389–391.
48. O'Connel TX, Aston SJ. Acute adrenal hemorrhage complicating anticoagulant therapy. *Surg Gynecol Obstet* 1974;139:355–357.
49. Xarli VP, Steele AA, Davis PJ, Buescher ES, Rios CN, Garcia-Bunuel R. Adrenal hemorrhage in the adult. *Medicine* (Baltimore) 1987;57:211–221.
50. Ling D, Korobkin M, Silverman PM, Dunnick NR. CT demonstration of bilateral adrenal hemorrhage. *AJR Am J Roentgenol* 1983;141:307–308.
51. Wolverson MK, Kannegiesser H. CT of bilateral adrenal hemorrhage with acute adrenal insufficiency in the adult. *AJR Am J Roentgenol* 1984;142:311–314.
52. Koch KJ, Cory DA. Simultaneous renal vein thrombosis and bilateral adrenal hemorrhage: MR demonstration. *J Comput Assist Tomogr* 1986;10:681–683.
53. Brill PW, Jagannath A, Winchester P, Markisz JA, Zirinsky K. Adrenal hemorrhage and renal vein thrombosis in the newborn: MR imaging. *Radiology* 1989;170:95–96.
54. Doppman JL, Gill JR Jr, Nienhuis AW, Earll JM, Long JA Jr. CT findings in Addison's disease. *J Comput Assist Tomogr* 1982;6:757–761.
55. McMurry JF Jr, Long D, McClure R, Kotchen TA. Addison's disease with adrenal enlargement on computed tomographic scanning. *Am J Med* 1984;77:365–368.
56. Mitchell DG, Crovello M, Matteucci T, Petersen RO, Miettinen MM. Benign adrenocortical masses: diagnosis with chemical shif MR imaging. *Radiology* 1992;185:345–351.
57. Reinig JW. MR imaging differentiation of adrenal masses: has the time finally come? *Radiology* 1992;185:339–340.

CHAPTER 8

The Kidneys

Richard C. Semelka, J. Patrick Shoenut, and Howard M. Greenberg

NORMAL ANATOMY

The kidneys are paired organs seated in the retroperitoneum in the perinephric space. The renal parenchyma is covered by the renal capsule, which usually is not visible on tomographic images. The perinephric space contains bridging renorenal septae that extend from the kidney to the anterior and posterior (Gerota's) perinephric fascia. The anterior and posterior fascia fuse laterally to form the lateral conal fascia. Superiorly the fascia fuse, while inferiorly they are open, forming a potential communication to the anterior and posterior pararenal spaces. The renal artery, vein, and ureter enter the kidney at the hilum. The kidney is composed of a cortex, medulla, and sinus. The renal sinus contains the renal collecting system, vessels, and fat.

MAGNETIC RESONANCE TECHNIQUE

Gd-DTPA is freely filtered by renal glomeruli and undergoes excretion by the renal tubules with no tubular reabsorption or excretion (1). Gd-DTPA is ideal for studying the kidneys and has an additional property of changing SI based on concentration. When dilute, Gd-DTPA enhances T1 relaxation and renders urine high in SI; when concentrated, Gd-DTPA induces magnetic susceptibility signal loss and causes urine to be low in SI (2–4). The concentrating ability of the kidneys can be evaluated by Gd-DTPA-enhanced MRI, a property that cannot be assessed by dynamic iodine-balanced CT. We routinely use four sequences to examine the kidneys: (a) precontrast T1-weighted breath-hold FLASH, (b) precontrast fat-suppressed T1-weighted spin echo, (c) dynamic capillary phase T1-weighted FLASH, and (d) postcontrast fat-suppressed T1-weighted spin echo (5). Figure 1 illustrates the appearance of normal kidneys with this imaging protocol.

R. C. Semelka: Department of Radiology and Magnetic Resonance Services, University of North Carolina at Chapel Hill, Chapel Hill, North Carolina 27599.

J. P. Shoenut: University of Manitoba and Department of Medicine, Saint Boniface General Hospital, Winnipeg, Manitoba R2H 2A6.

H. M. Greenberg: Department of Radiology, University of Manitoba, Winnipeg, Manitoba R2H 2A6.

NORMAL VARIANTS AND CONGENITAL ANOMALIES

A great variety of anomalies of the kidneys occur. The majority relate to abnormalities of renal position (including renal ascent and rotation), duplication, fusion, and agenesis. Duplication of the collecting system is a relatively common anomaly that can on occasion be difficult to detect on transaxial tomographic images. Pelvic kidney is not uncommon, and the kidney is not infrequently malformed. Intense uptake of Gd-DTPA by renal cortex and the renal corticomedullary organization allows confident diagnosis of this entity (Fig. 2). Horseshoe kidney is the most common fusion abnormality and is readily shown on tomographic images by the fusion of the lower poles of both kidneys across the midline immediately anterior to the vertebral bodies (Fig. 3).

A prominent column of Bertin is frequently observed and can at times pose a difficulty in distinction from a renal mass. On immediate postcontrast images the column enhances to the same extent as renal cortex, and on more delayed images the enhancement of the column remains isointense with cortex, obviating problems with diagnosis.

MASS LESIONS OF THE RENAL PARENCHYMA

Benign Lesions

Cysts

Cysts are the most common renal masses in adults and are usually cortical (6). Cortical cysts are oval, do not

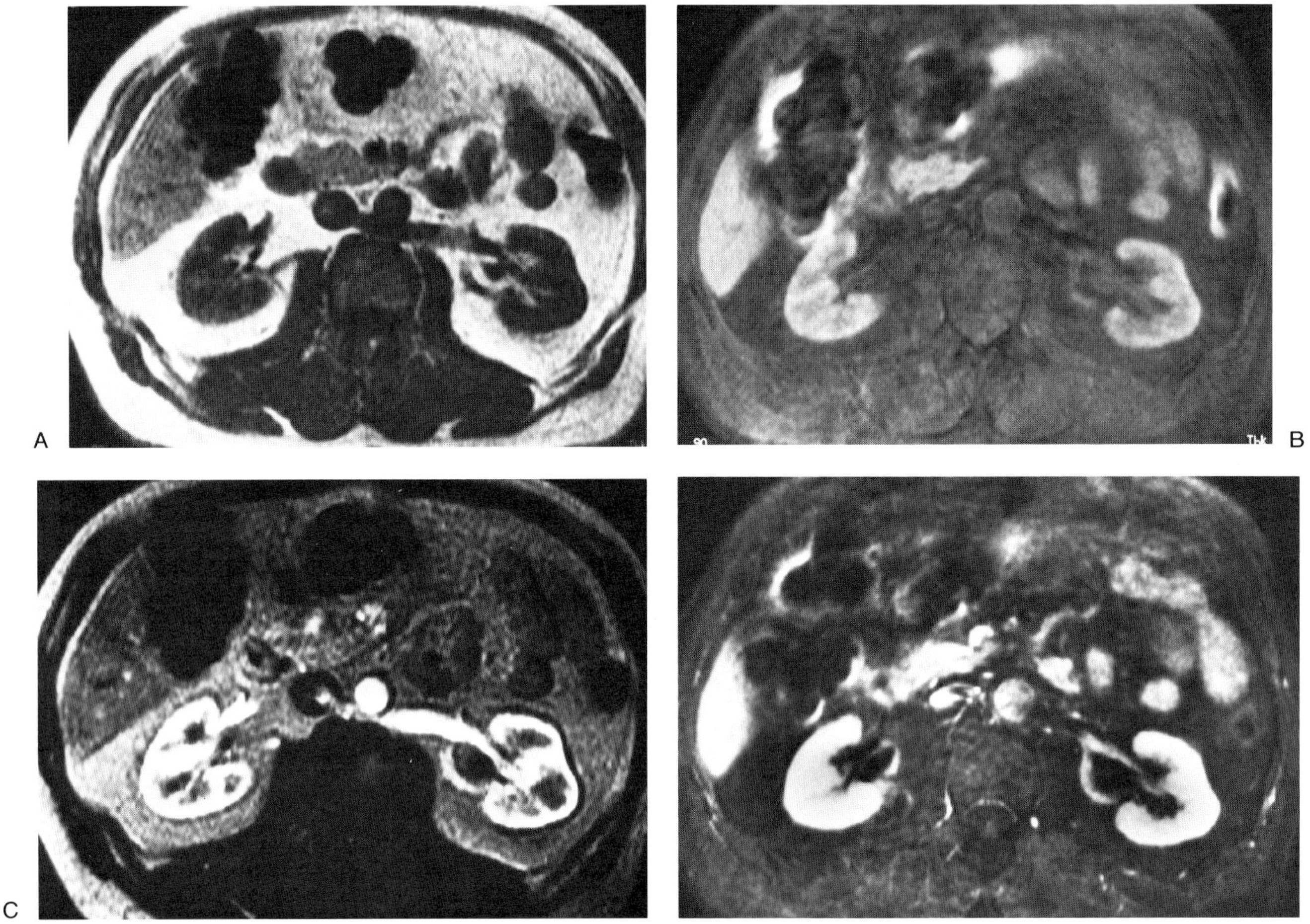

FIG. 1. Normal kidneys. Precontrast FLASH (**A**), precontrast T1FS (**B**), 1-second postcontrast FLASH (**C**), and Gd-DTPA-enhanced T1FS (**D**) images in a 63-year-old man with normal kidneys. Minimal corticomedullary (CM) differentiation is present on precontrast FLASH (A), whereas higher CM differentiation is apparent on precontrast T1FS (B). The highest CM differentiation on the immediate postcontrast FLASH image can be appreciated. Incidental note is made of a retroaortic left renal vein with high Gd-DTPA-enhanced blood draining into the signal-void IVC (*arrow*). High contrast and spatial resolution, very good image quality, and no phase or chemical shift artifact are features of Gd-DTPA-enhanced T1FS (D). Reprinted with permission from ref. 5.

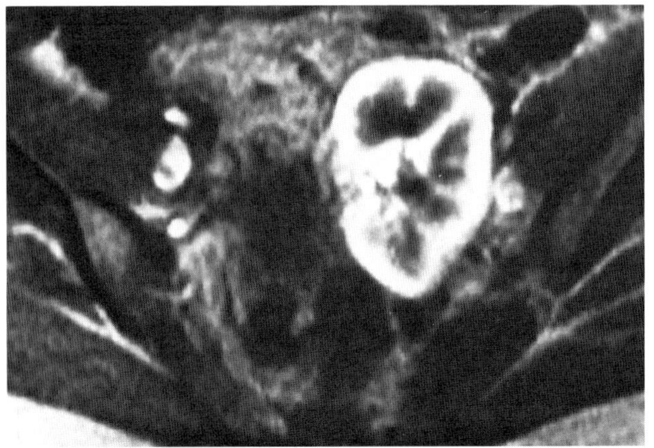

FIG. 2. Pelvic kidney. One-second postcontrast FLASH in a 32-year-old woman with a pelvic kidney. The corticomedullary difference identifies the pelvic mass as a kidney.

enhance with Gd-DTPA, and have a sharp margin with renal parenchyma (5,7). Cysts are considered simple when they contain fluid similar in composition to urine, are signal void on T1-weighted images, and have no definable wall when they extend beyond the renal cortex (Fig. 4). Cysts are considered complicated when they contain blood, septations, or calcifications. Region of interest measurements on pre- and postcontrast T1-weighted images are essential to ensure the lack of contrast enhancement in high-SI cysts. An advantage of MRI over CT in the evaluation of calcified cysts is that calcium is signal void on MRI (7). Densely calcified masses can be evaluated by MRI for tumor enhancement, which is a difficult or impossible determination on CT images.

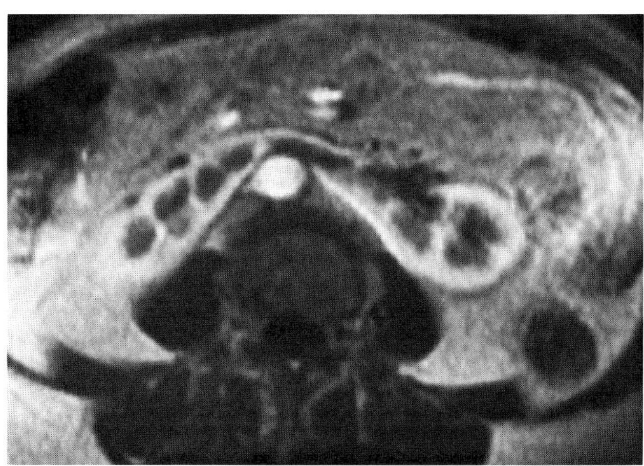
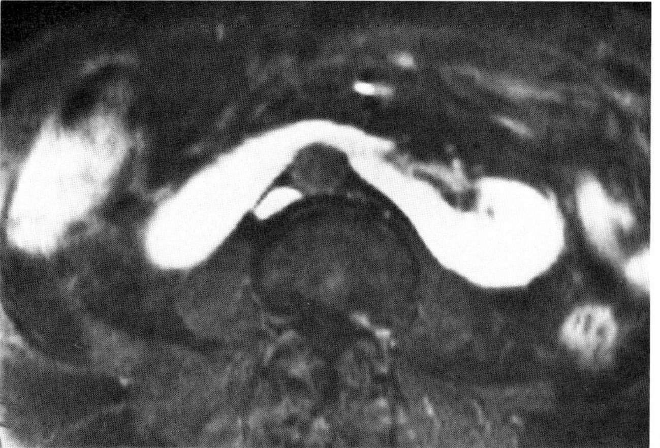

A B

FIG. 3. Horseshoe kidney. One-second postcontrast (**A**) and Gd-DTPA-enhanced T1FS (**B**) MR images in a 54-year-old woman with a horseshoe kidney. The corticomedullary difference on the 1-second postcontrast image and the uniform enhancement on the Gd-DTPA-enhanced T1FS image demonstrate that the isthmus contains functional renal parenchyma.

Parapelvic Cysts

Parapelvic cysts are pseudocysts containing urine-like fluid and may be acquired secondary to prior obstruction and urine leak. At times these lesions may be difficult to distinguish from a dilated renal collecting system. Delayed postcontrast images may be necessary to differentiate high-SI dilute Gd-DTPA urine in the collecting system from low-SI fluid in parapelvic cysts.

Autosomal Dominant Polycystic Kidney Disease

Autosomal dominant polycystic kidney disease is a disease characterized by the progressive development of variously sized renal cysts in both kidneys (8). The disease usually becomes manifest in adult patients, hence the alternate designation of adult polycystic kidney disease. Patients usually present late in the course of the condition with abdominal masses, hypertension, or trauma. Renal failure is a late event. The disease is almost always bilateral, although unilateral disease has been described. There are frequently cysts in other organs, including liver, spleen, and pancreas. Patients are at risk of cerebral hemorrhage from ruptured berry aneurysm.

The typical MR appearance is that of bilaterally enlarged kidneys with multiple renal cysts of varying size distorting the renal architecture. The cysts characteristically have varying SI due to the presence of blood products of varying age (Fig. 5).

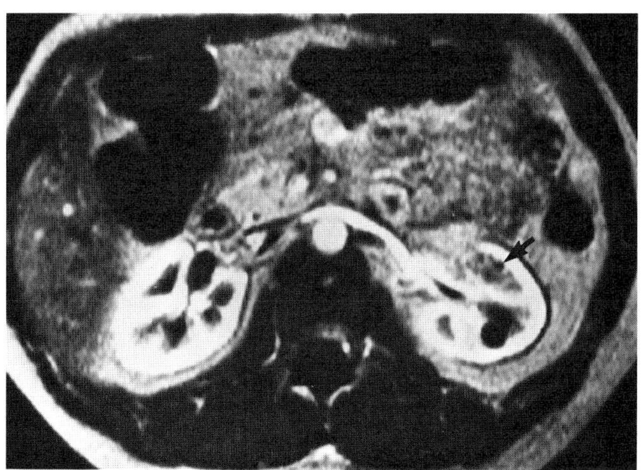
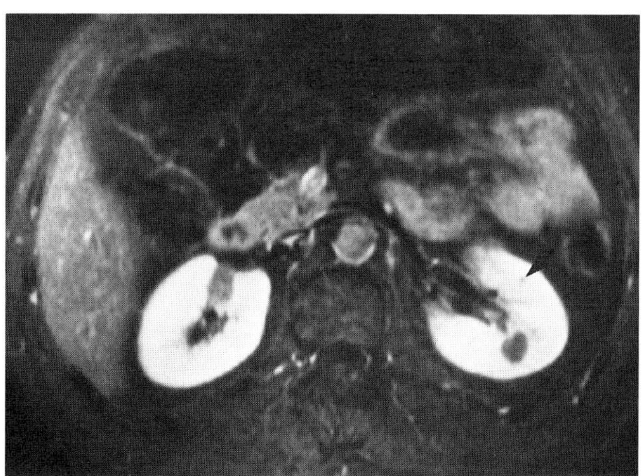

A B

FIG. 4. Renal cysts. Immediate postcontrast FLASH (**A**) and Gd-DTPA-enhanced T1FS (**B**) images in a 47-year-old man with a left renal cancer. Two small, surgically proven cysts are present in the left kidney, the smallest measuring 2 mm (*arrow*), and an 8-mm cyst is present in the right kidney. Cysts are oval, sharply marginated lesions with a signal void on postcontrast FLASH (A) and very low SI on Gd-DTPA-enhanced T1FS (B). Reprinted with permission from ref. 5.

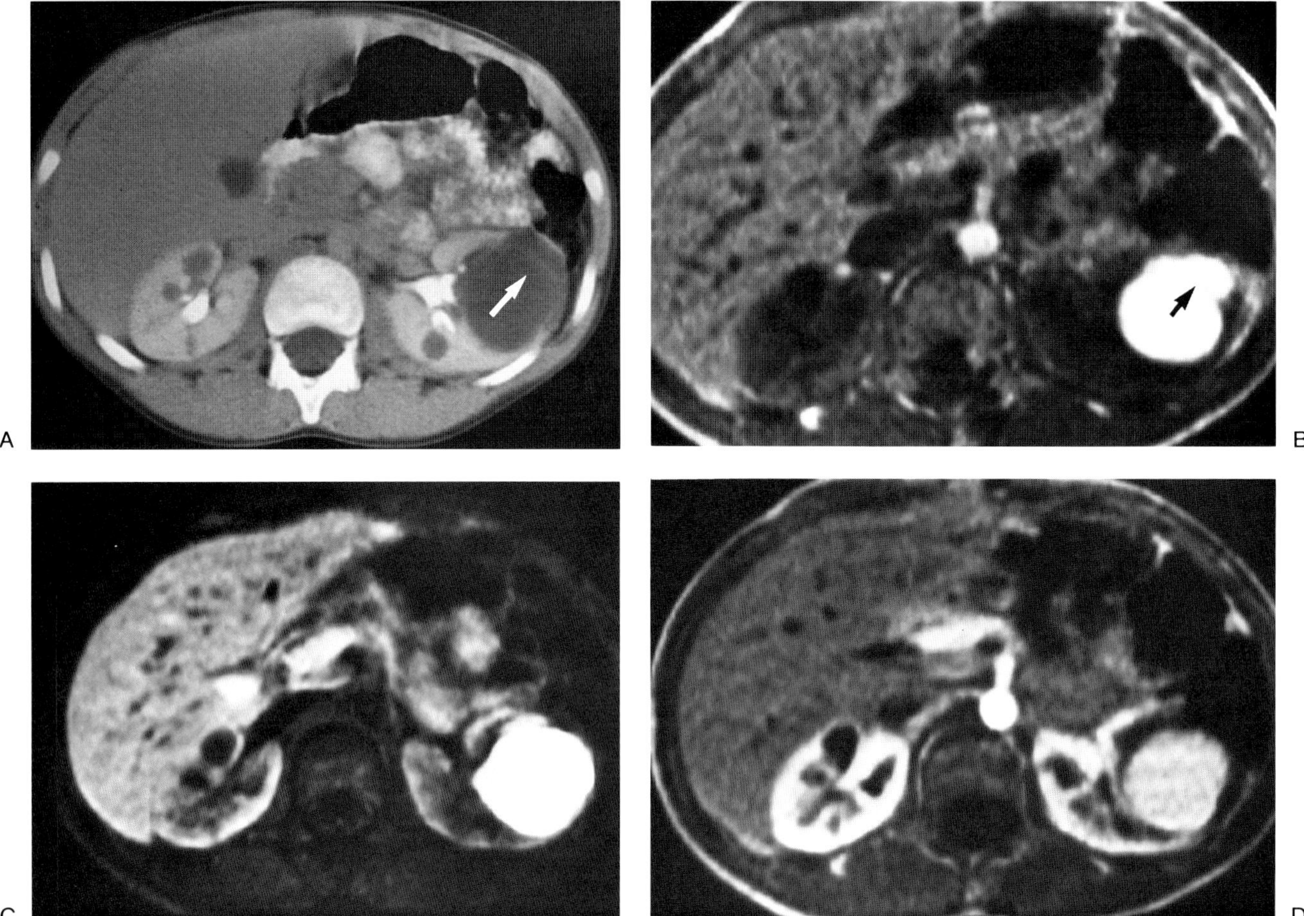

FIG. 5. Autosomal dominant polycystic disease. Contrast-enhanced CT (**A**), precontrast FLASH (**B**), precontrast T1FS (**C**), and 1-second post contrast FLASH (**D**) images in an 8-year-old boy with autosomal dominant polycystic renal disease. A large left renal cyst contains an internal septation on the CT image (*arrow*). Precontrast FLASH (B) shows a high-SI cyst containing a low-SI reticular strand (*arrow*). This cyst does not suppress with fat suppression (C) and does not enhance with Gd-DTPA (D), which is consistent with subacute blood in a hemorrhagic cyst. A signal-void rim is best appreciated on the Gd-DTPA-enhanced FLASH image, which probably represents hemosiderin deposition.

Acquired Cystic Disease of Dialysis

Approximately 50% of patients on long-term hemodialysis develop multiple renal cysts (9–11). The etiology is uncertain but may relate to ischemia or fibrosis. Kidneys are usually atrophic at the time of development of cystic disease. Cysts tend to be located superficially in the renal cortex; in autosomal dominant cystic kidney disease, however, cysts are scattered throughout the parenchyma. Hemorrhage is a frequent complication. The incidence of renal cancer in these patients is high, approximately 7% (11). MRI is well suited for the detection of renal cancer because of good parenchymal enhancement despite diminished renal function (Fig. 6).

Tuberous Sclerosis

Tuberous sclerosis is a neurocutaneous syndrome with autosomal dominant inheritance, although approximately 50% of cases arise from spontaneous mutation. Patients with tuberous sclerosis have an increased incidence of renal cysts and angiomyolipomas (12,13). Angiomyolipomas are frequently multiple and bilateral.

Von Hippel-Lindau Disease

Von Hippel-Lindau disease is a neurocutaneous syndrome with autosomal dominant inheritance. Patients

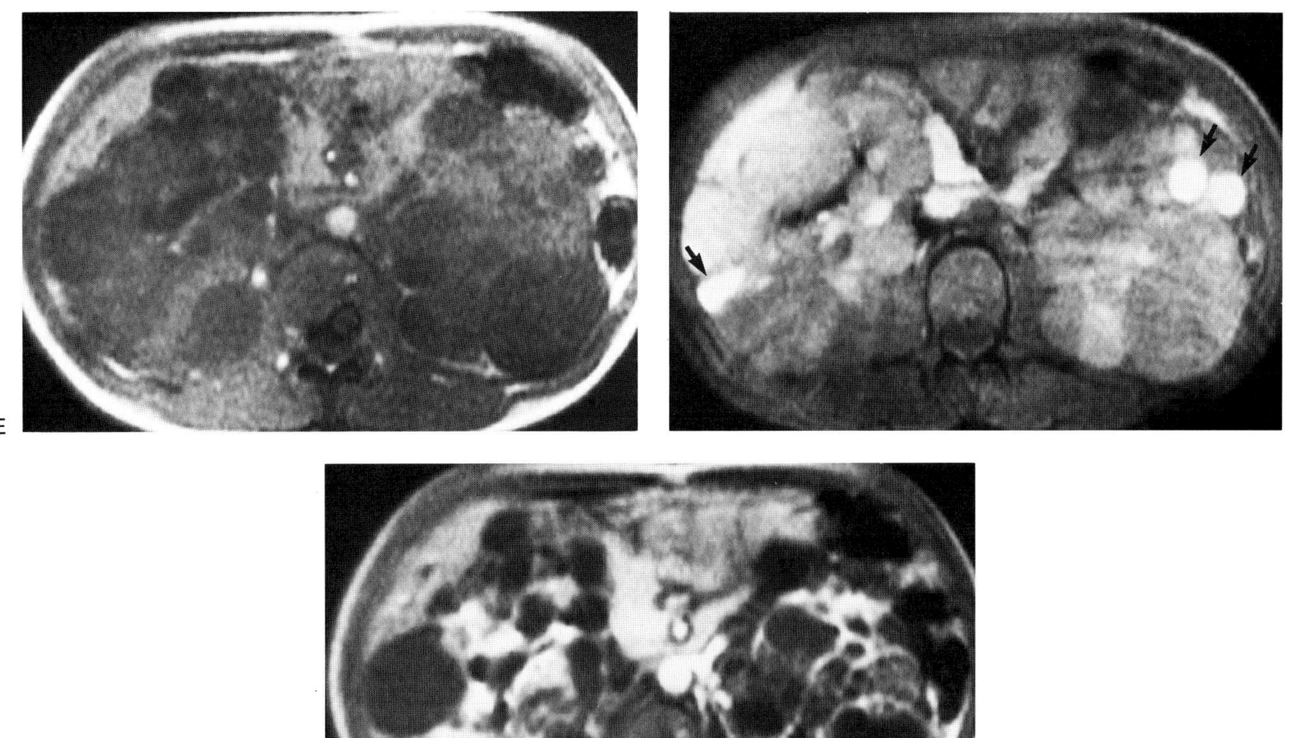

FIG. 5. (*Continued.*) Precontrast FLASH (**E**), T1FS (**F**) and 1-second postcontrast FLASH (**G**) in a 27-year-old woman with advanced changes of autosomal dominant polycystic kidney disease. The kidneys are massively enlarged and contain multiple cysts of varying size scattered throughout the distorted renal parenchyma. Several cysts contain high SI fluid compatible with subacute blood, which are most clearly seen on the T1FS images (*arrows*, F). Parenchymal enhancement is apparent following Gd-DTPA administration compatible with preservation of renal function. Reprinted with permission from ref. 5.

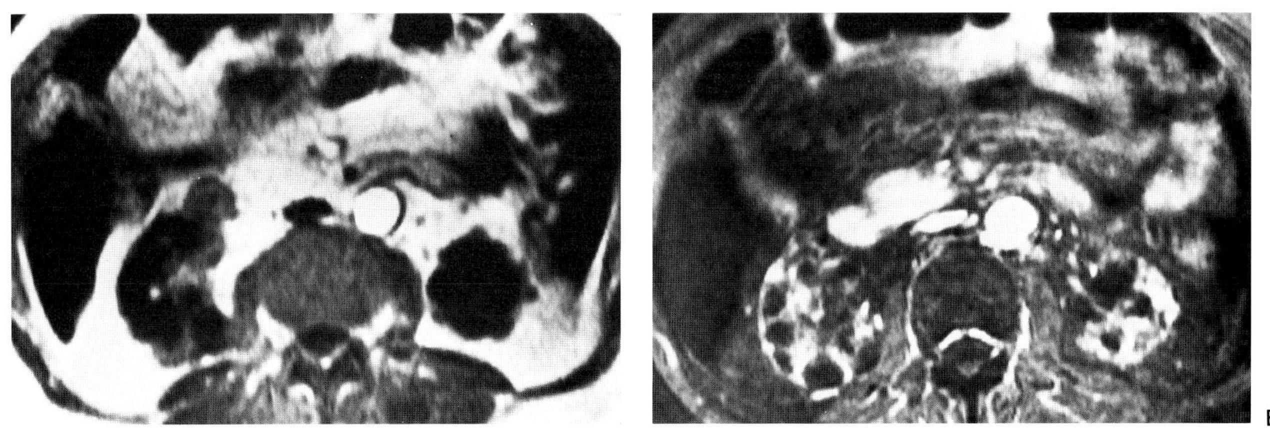

FIG. 6. Acquired cystic disease of dialysis. One-second postcontrast FLASH (**A**) and Gd-DTPA-enhanced T1FS (**B**) images in a 54-year-old man with chronic renal failure on hemodialysis and peritoneal dialysis. The capillary phase of enhancement demonstrates minimal parenchymal enhancement and no corticomedullary differentiation (A). On the Gd-DTPA-enhanced T1FS image, multiple renal cysts are well shown in a background of moderately enhanced atrophic parenchymal tissue (B).

with von Hippel-Lindau disease have an increased incidence of renal cysts, adenomas, and carcinomas (14,15). Carcinomas tend to be multicentric and bilateral.

Multicystic Dysplastic Kidney

Multicystic dysplastic kidney results from a congenital failure of fusion of the metanephrosis and the ureteric bud, resulting in a nonfunctional cystic renal mass. The ureter is typically atretic in this condition.

Autosomal Recessive Cystic Kidney Disease

Autosomal recessive kidney disease presents in infancy or early childhood. The ability of MRI to resolve the 1- to 2-mm cysts found in this condition is not known at present.

Multilocular Cystic Nephroma

Multilocular cystic nephroma is a benign lesion comprising noncommunicating cysts within a fibrous stroma. This lesion is found most frequently in boys 2 months to 4 years old and in adults, predominantly women, older than 40 years. The typical MR appearance is a multicystic renal mass with thick enhancing fibrous septations (Fig. 7).

Medullary Sponge Kidney

Medullary sponge kidney is characterized by multiple cystic cavities in the papillae. Calculi are frequently present in the cystic cavities. The disease is usually bilateral but may be unilateral or segmental. Patients present with calculi, obstruction, infection, or hematuria.

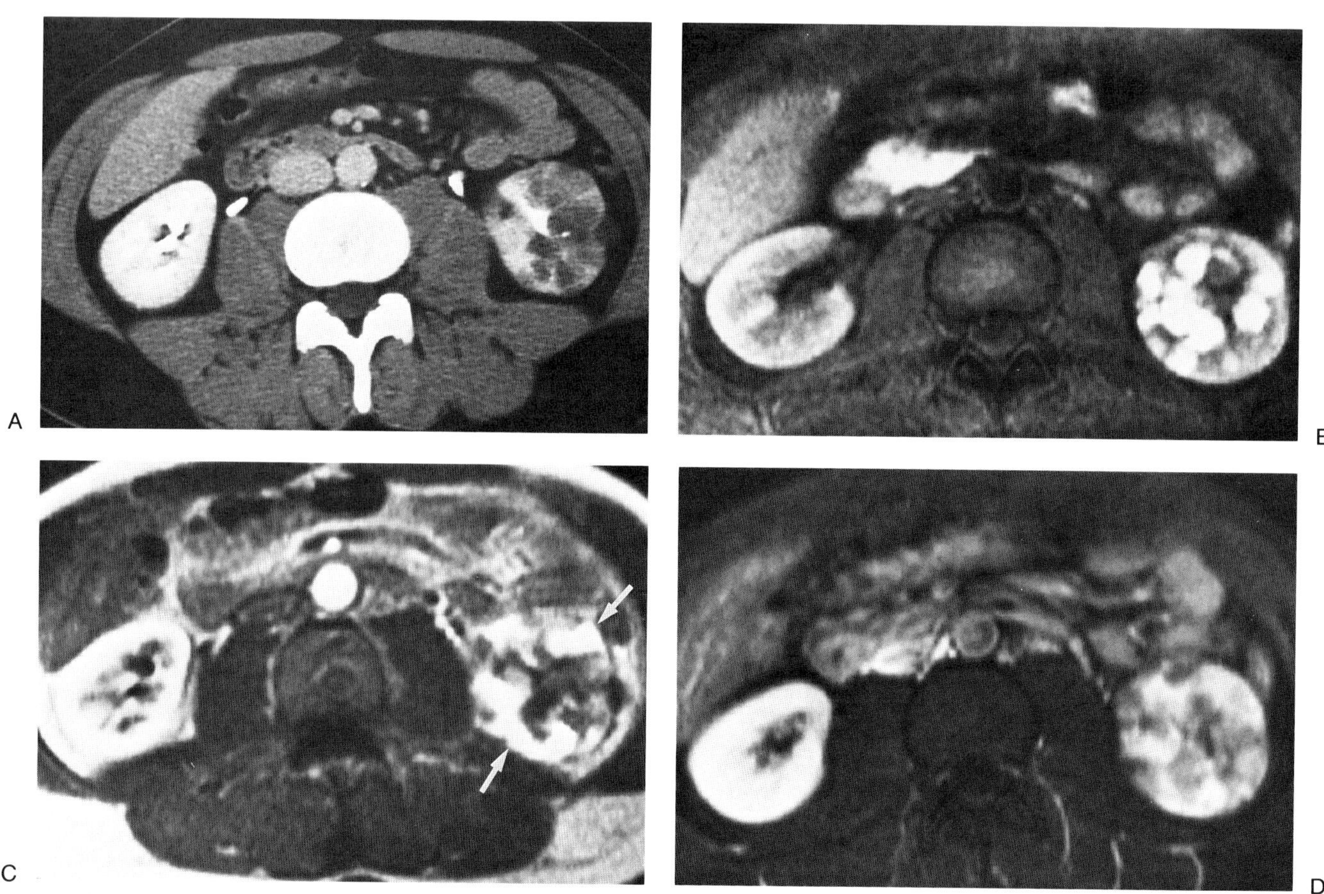

FIG. 7. Multilocular cystic nephroma. Contrast-enhanced CT (**A**), T1FS (**B**), 1-second postcontrast FLASH (**C**), and Gd-DTPA-enhanced T1FS (**D**) images in a 24-year-old man with multilocular cystic nephroma arising from the lower pole of the left kidney. The CT scan demonstrates a multicystic mass arising from the lower pole of the left kidney. The T1FS image demonstrates that many of these cysts are high in SI, which is compatible with either subacute blood or protein. No SI increase of the cysts was identified on the 1-second postcontrast FLASH (C) or the Gd-DTPA-enhanced T1FS (D) images. Fragments of renal cortex enhance in a normal fashion on the 1-second postcontrast image (*arrows,* C).

Medullary Cystic Disease

Medullary cystic disease (nephronopthesis) results in bilateral small kidneys with medullary cysts. Patients present with anemia, azotemia, and salt wasting. Presentation usually occurs between 5 and 20 years of age. The MRI appearance of this condition has not been described.

Arteriovenous Malformations

Arteriovenous malformations (AVMs) are abnormal communications between renal artery and vein which may be congenital or traumatic in origin. These lesions vary in size and may be large. Signal void in AVMs on spin echo images permits ready diagnosis of this entity. Signal from flowing blood can also be high using various refocused MR techniques such as cine MR or using a dynamic Gd-DTPA-enhanced technique.

Angiomyolipomas

Angiomyolipomas are composed of three elements: (a) blood vessels, (b) smooth muscle, and (c) fat. These tumors are virtually always benign. The fat component is usually substantial, permitting characterization on CT images and on combined T1-weighted regular and fat-suppressed images (Fig. 8) (16,17). Lesions as small as 1 cm may be detected and characterized because of the high SI of fat on T1-weighted images which attenuates on fat-suppressed images (Fig. 9). In a small number of cases muscle or vascular components predominate, and distinction from renal cell cancer may be difficult. When the diagnosis, based on imaging findings, is certain and tumors are less than 4 cm in size and asymptomatic, imaging follow-up is adequate management (18).

Adenomas

Renal adenomas are benign tumors of renal cell origin and typically are small, solid neoplasms (19). The rela-

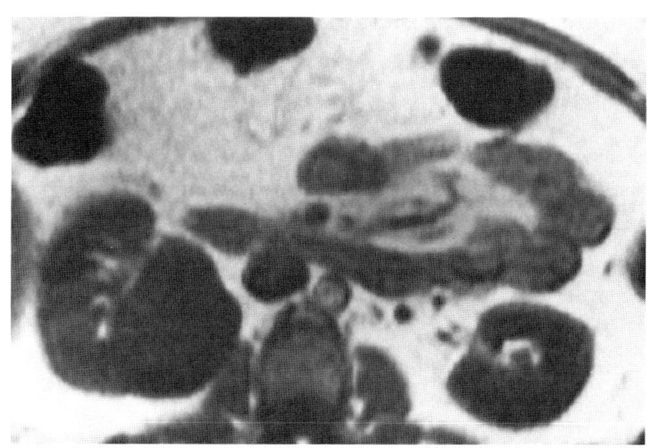

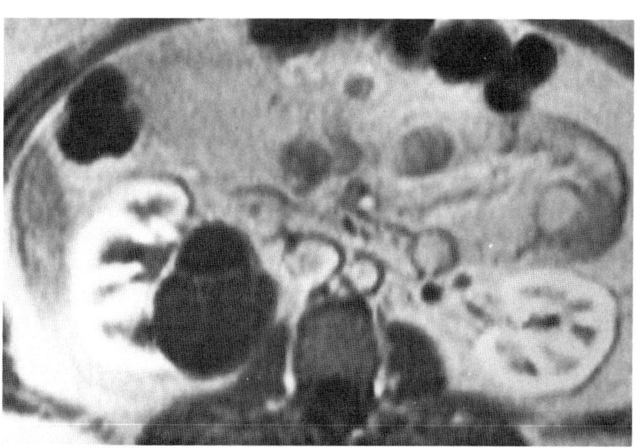

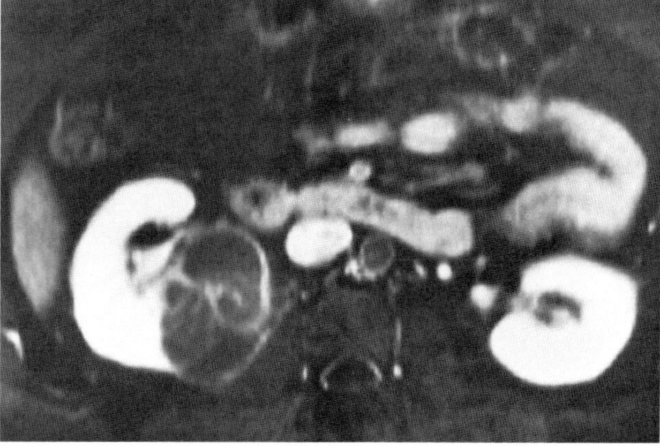

FIG. 7. *(Continued.)* FLASH (**E**), 1-second postcontrast FLASH (**F**), and contrast enhanced T1FS (**G**) MR images in a 46-year-old woman with a multilocular cystic nephroma. A well-defined cystic mass arises from the posterior aspect of the right kidney. Thick, internal septations are present best seen on contrast-enhanced T1FS images. These features are typical for multiocular cystic nephroma.

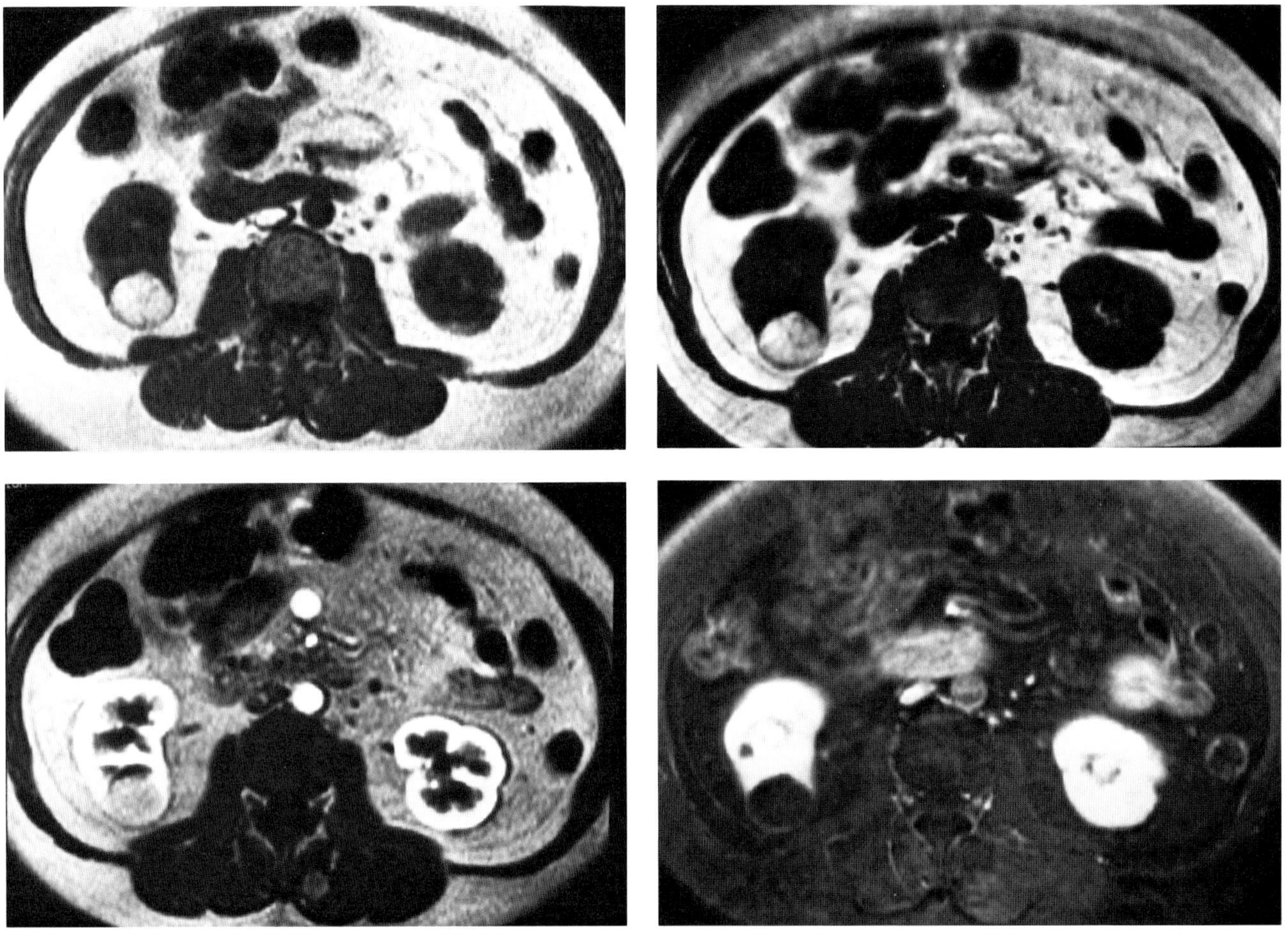

FIG. 8. Angiomyolipoma. Precontrast FLASH (**A**), water-suppressed spin echo (**B**), immediate postcontrast FLASH (**C**), and Gd-DTPA-enhanced T1FS (**D**) images in a 42-year-old woman with a right renal angiomyolipoma. A high-SI lesion on precontrast FLASH (A), which does not suppress with water suppression (B) but does suppress with fat suppression (D), is diagnostic for an angiomyolipoma. The lesion enhances poorly with Gd-DTPA (C) and is a low-SI, sharply marginated lesion on T1FS (D). The appearance of the lesion on T1FS could be mistaken for a renal cyst without information from the precontrast FLASH image. On the Gd-DTPA-enhanced T1FS image, a 4-mm renal cyst is apparent in a lateral location in the right kidney. Reprinted with permission from ref. 5.

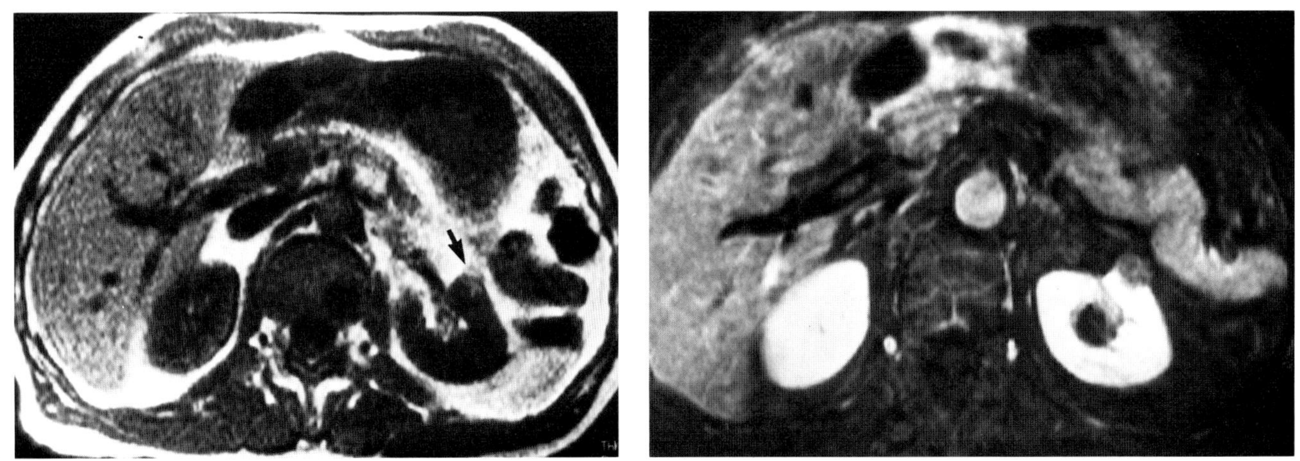

FIG. 9. Small angiomyolipoma. FLASH (**A**) and Gd-DTPA-enhanced T1FS (**B**) MR images in a 64-year-old man with a 1-cm angiomyolipoma. A small, high-SI lesion is apparent arising from the anterior cortex of the left kidney on the FLASH images (*arrow,* A). Fat suppression attenuates the SI of this lesion, and it appears as a well-defined, low-SI lesion on the Gd-DTPA-enhanced T1FS image (B).

TABLE 1. *Renal cancer staging: Robson's classification and TNM*

Robson	Disease extent	TNM
I	Small tumor confined to kidney	T1
II	Large tumor confined to kidney	T2
IIIA	Tumor spread to perinephric fat but within Gerota's fascia	T3a
IIIB	Tumor spread to local lymph nodes	N1–N3
IIIC	Tumor spread to local vessels and lymph nodes	T3b, N1–N3
IVA	Tumor spread to adjacent organs (excluding ipsilateral adrenal)	T4
IVB	Distant metastasis	M1a–d, N4

tionship of adenomas to renal cell carcinomas is unclear. The distinction between adenomas and papillary renal cell cancers is not possible on tomographic techniques (20). The role of imaging in patients with small solid tumors is to reassess these lesions serially to detect tumor growth that would suggest malignancy (21–24). A recommended interval between serial scans is not presently established, but it may be reasonable to follow a mass at 3 months, 6 months, 1 year, and yearly thereafter.

Oncocytomas are an uncommon type of renal adenoma. Their pathognomonic diagnostic feature is a spoke-wheel arterial vasculature on angiographic studies. These lesions frequently possess a central scar (25).

Malignant Masses

Renal Cell Carcinomas

Renal cell carcinoma is the most common renal neoplasm. The incidence is over 25,000 with a mortality over 10,000 annually in the United States (26). The peak age of incidence is 50 to 60 years, with a male to female ratio of 2:1 (26). Tumors are usually solitary. In approximately 5% of patients, tumors are multiple. Tumors tend to become symptomatic when they are large and in an advanced stage. Renal cell cancer is associated with a myriad of presenting features, including paraneoplastic phenomena.

Staging of renal cell cancer can be performed by either Robson's or the tumor, node, metastasis (TNM) classification (Table 1). Both MRI and current generation CT scanners are able to detect renal cancers that measure 1 cm in diameter (Fig. 10).

Conventional MR sequences have been useful in the evaluation of renal tumors to assess the presence of tumor thrombus or the extension of tumor to adjacent organs (27). Thrombus is well shown on spin echo images because of high contrast between tumor thrombus and signal-void blood on spin echo sequences (27–32). MRI using gadolinium enhancement breath-hold techniques and fat suppression is superior to CT in differentiating cysts from solid tumors because of the increased sensitivity of MRI for Gd-DTPA (5,7,33) (Fig. 11). Indeterminate renal lesions should be evaluated by MRI.

The typical appearance of renal cell cancer is an irregular mass with ill-defined margins with the renal paren-

A 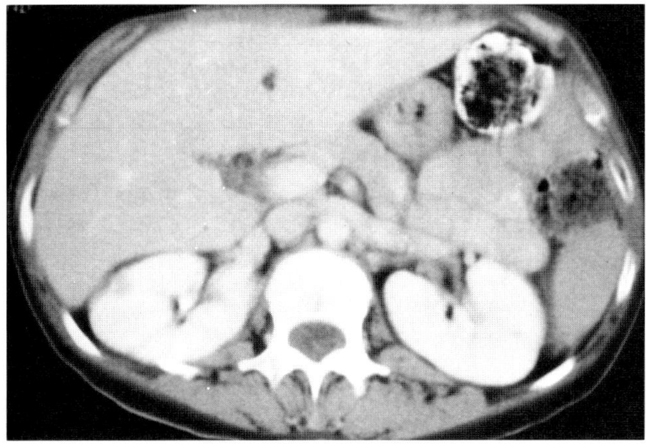

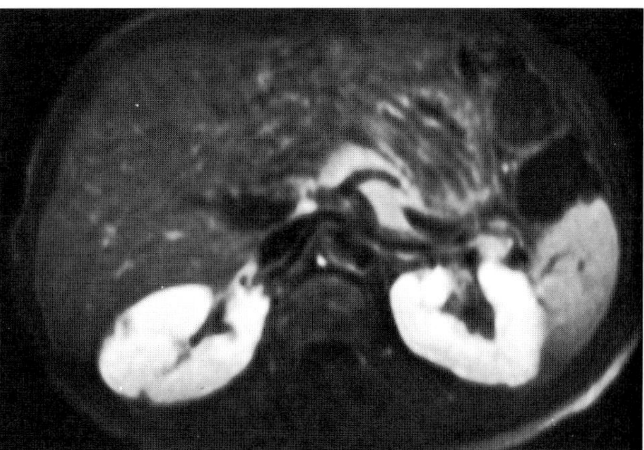 B

FIG. 10. Small renal cell cancer. Contrast-enhanced CT (**A**) and T1FS (**B**) images in a 56-year-old man demonstrate a 1-cm renal cancer arising from the lateral aspect of the right kidney. A small focus of enhancing tissue is noted in the center of the tumor, which confirms that the lesion is not a cyst.

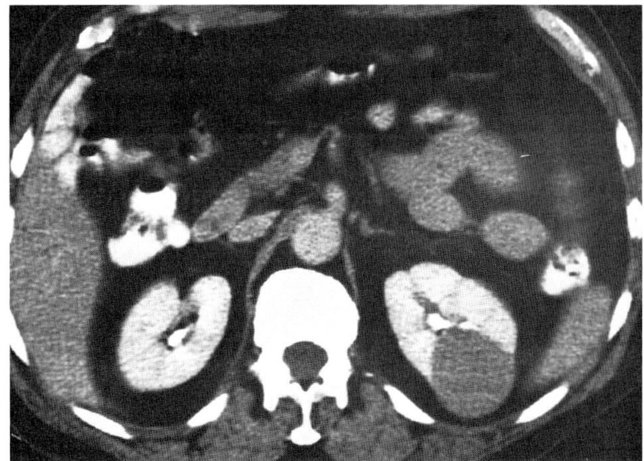

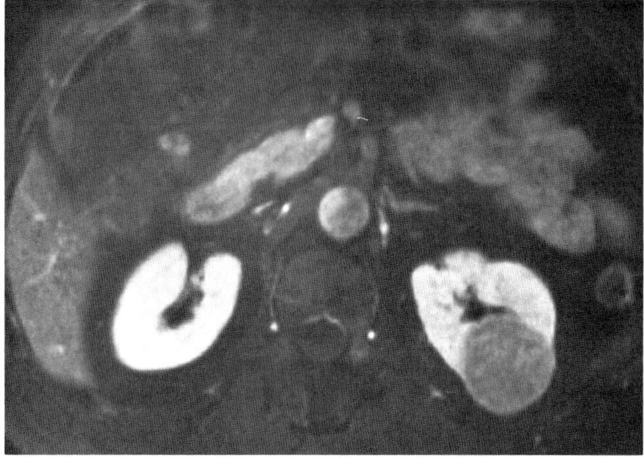

A B

FIG. 11. Hypovascular renal cell cancer. Contrast-enhanced CT (**A**) and Gd-DTPA-enhanced, fat-suppressed MR (**B**) images in a 56-year-old man with a hypovascular renal cell cancer. No enhancement and no internal architecture is identified in the sharply marginated left renal mass on the CT image. MR images demonstrate internal enhancement consistent with a tumor. Reprinted with permission from ref. 37.

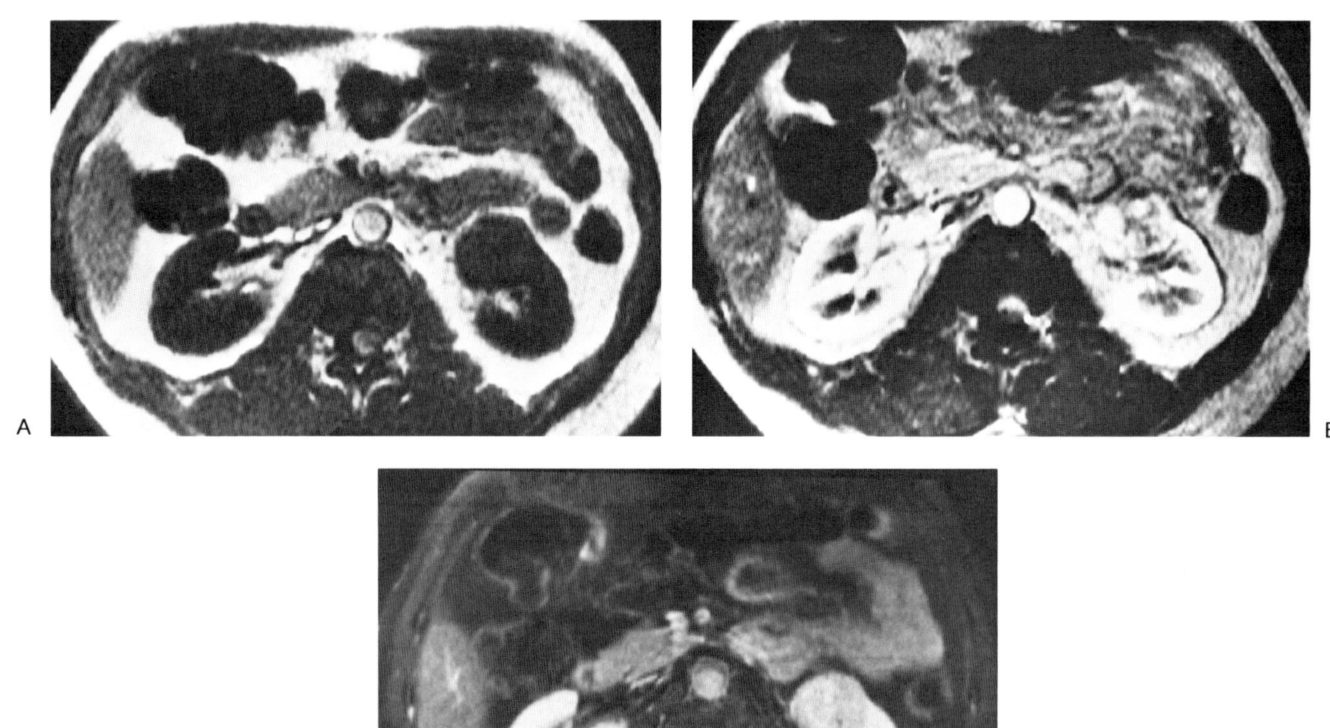

A B C

FIG. 12. Stage I renal cell cancer. Precontrast FLASH (**A**), immediate postcontrast FLASH (**B**), and Gd-DTPA-enhanced T1FS (**C**) images in a 47-year-old man with a Stage I renal cell cancer reveal a 3.5-cm tumor in the left kidney. The homogeneous, slightly hypointense mass on the precontrast image (A) enhances in a heterogeneous fashion after contrast enhancement (B) and is hypointense relative to renal cortex on Gd-DTPA-enhanced T1FS (C). Although the tumor is well demonstrated on the postcontrast FLASH image, the tumor margins are not as well defined as on postcontrast T1FS. Reprinted with permission from ref. 5.

chyma, heterogeneous enhancement on immediate postcontrast images, and diminished enhancement on more delayed postcontrast images (Fig. 12). Tumors are frequently hypervascular and demonstrate increased SI on immediate postcontrast images, usually in a heterogeneous fashion, although homogeneous enhancement does occur. Homogeneously enhancing small tumors may be difficult to distinguish from renal cortex on immediate postcontrast images (Fig. 13).

Tumor size is not a reliable criterion for the diagnosis of renal cancer or for distinguishing cancer from adenoma (20–24). Renal cell cancers occasionally show no change in size over intervals of more than 1 year (22). Any solid renal tumor that is nonfatty should be considered a possible renal cell cancer and should at a minimum be followed by serial imaging.

Cancers that are completely intraparenchymal are Stage I cancers. Based on imaging features the distinction between Stage I and Stage II cancers cannot be reliably made on tumors that extend beyond the cortical margins. Large exophytic tumors can be Stage I, and tumors with a small extrarenal component can be Stage II. Surgical management is identical for Stage I and II disease, so differentiation by imaging is not essential. Stage I and II renal cell cancers are associated with a high survival rate, since the tumor is amenable to complete resection.

Stage IIIa renal cancer is defined by tumor extension into the renal vein, which frequently extends into the IVC (Fig. 14). MRI has been recognized as superior to CT in determining the presence of thrombus before the use of intravenous Gd-DTPA. In our experience, modern generation CT is not substantially inferior to MRI in detecting the presence of thrombus. The superiority of MRI lies in detecting the superior extent of thrombus and in determining whether thrombus enhances to distinguish tumor from blood thrombus (Fig. 15). Zeman et al. reported that, on thin-section CT images, tumor thrombus was correctly detected in 18 of 19 patients, but only three of these thrombi demonstrated appreciable enhancement (34). A gradient echo technique that refocuses the signal of flowing blood (e.g., GRASS) has been

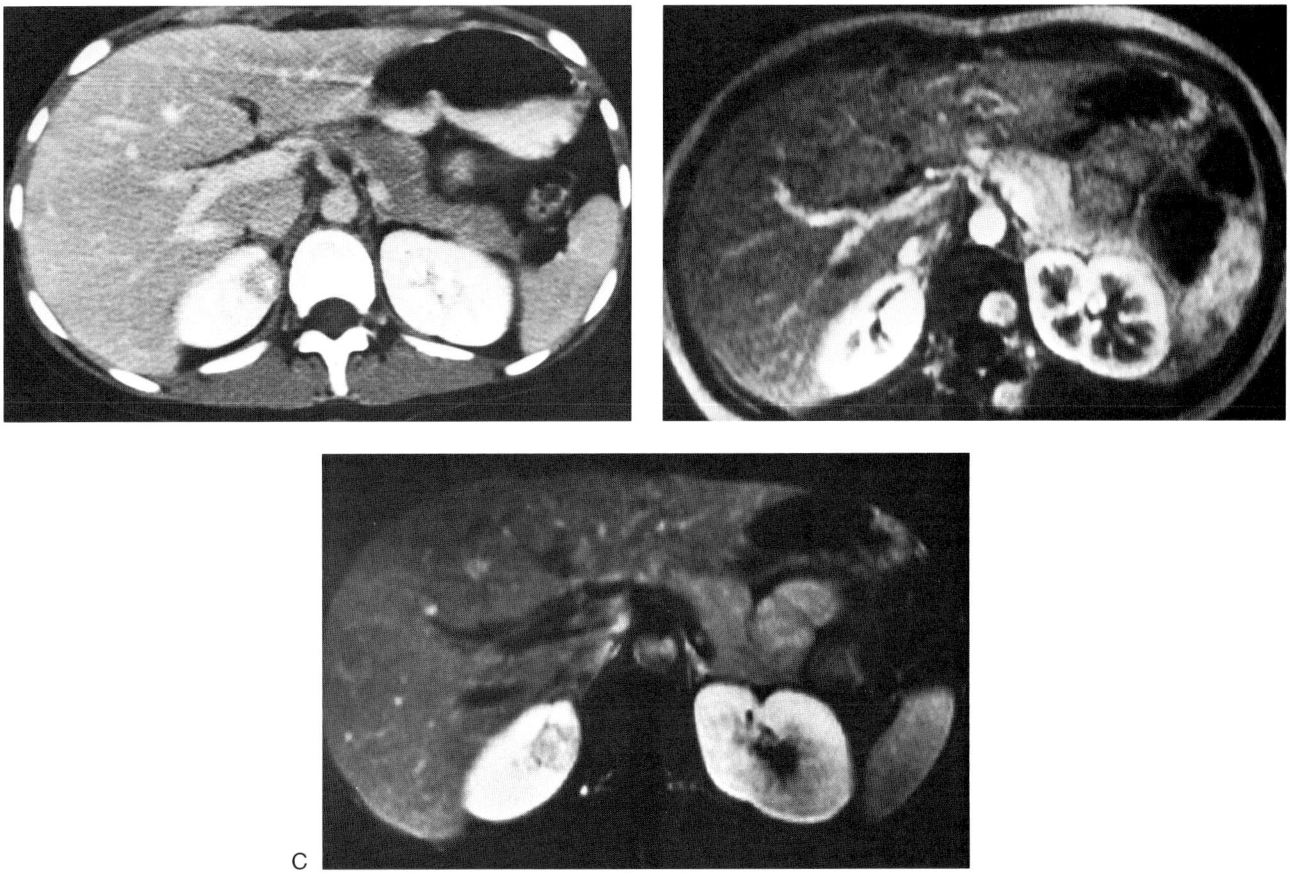

A

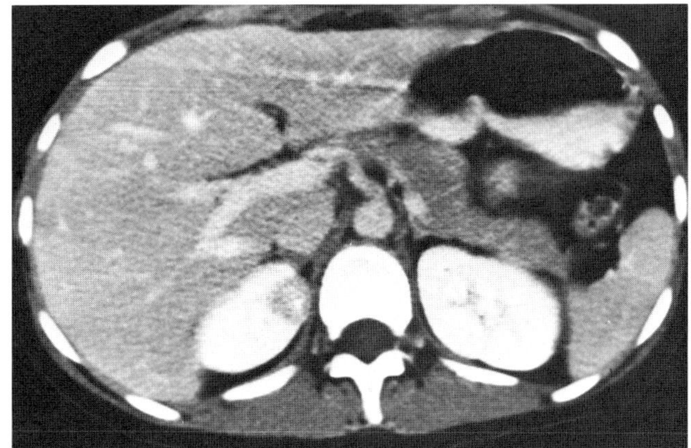

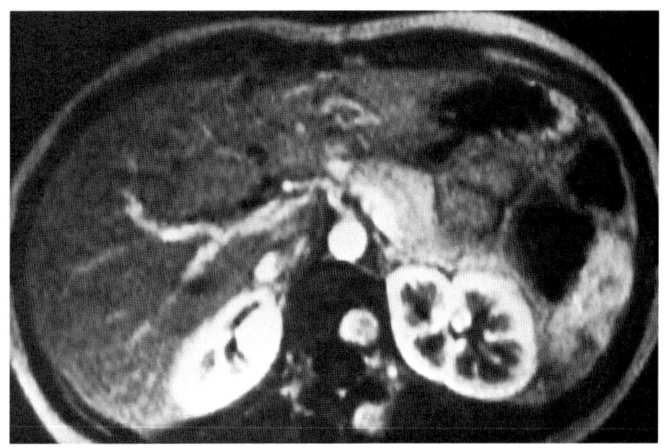

B

C

FIG. 13. Renal cell cancer. Contrast-enhanced CT (**A**), dynamic Gd-DTPA-enhanced FLASH (**B**), and Gd-DTPA-enhanced, fat-suppressed spin echo (**C**) images in a 21-year-old woman with renal cancer. Contrast-enhanced CT and fat-suppressed spin echo images demonstrate a 2-cm, low-attenuation/SI mass arising from the upper pole of the right kidney. A uniform tumor blush with SI comparable to that of renal cortex was present on the dynamic FLASH images. Reprinted with permission from ref. 37.

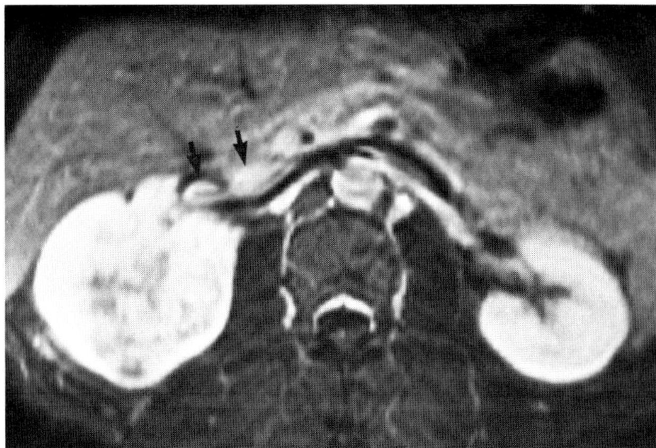

FIG. 14. Stage IIIa renal cancer. Gd-DTPA-enhanced T1FS image in a 65-year-old man with a Stage IIIa renal cell cancer of the right kidney. Enhancing tumor thrombus can be appreciated extending along the right renal vein into the IVC (*arrows*). Reprinted with permission from ref. 5.

proposed as another method to evaluate tumor thrombus (35).

Stage IIIb renal cancer is defined by the presence of malignant nodes. MRI is occasionally able to detect necrosis in lymph nodes, shown by irregular low-SI centers, which may not be identified on CT images (Fig. 16). In the presence of a necrotic primary tumor, necrosis of lymph nodes may be specific for nodal involvement. The presence of enlarged lymph nodes does not necessarily indicate Stage IIIb or IIIc disease, as adenopathy may also be benign. Studer et al. reported that 58% of 163 patients with renal cell cancer had enlarged hyperplastic lymph nodes (36). Stage IIIc indicates tumor extension into the renal vein and nodal involvement.

Stage IV disease extends to local or distant sites. Renal cancer metastasizes to lung, adrenal glands, mediastinum, axial skeleton, and liver. Lung metastases are the most common.

Multiple bilateral renal tumors occur in <5% of patients with renal cancer. In these patients tumor seeding of cysts may result in cystic renal cell cancer (Fig. 17). Cysts in patients with multiple bilateral renal cancers should be viewed with suspicion.

Recent reports have shown that MRI is slightly superior to CT in the detection, characterization, and staging of renal cancer (5,7). Whether this justifies the routine use of MRI in the investigation of renal masses is unclear. There are, however, definite indications for the use of MR, which include (a) allergy to iodine contrast, (b) indeterminate or calcified renal masses, and (c) renal failure (37–40). The greater enhancement of renal parenchyma in patients with renal failure, the smaller volume of contrast, and the lesser renal toxicity justify the routine performance of Gd-DTPA-enhanced MRI in these patients (Fig. 18) (39). There may be no indication to perform noncontrast CT alone in the investigation of renal masses.

Early detection of renal cancer is critical to improve the patient's survival (21,41,42). Because of the ability of MRI to detect renal tumors as small as 1 cm in diameter, the role of MRI in detecting and characterizing renal masses seems important. This is particularly true as kidney-sparing surgery is becoming a more prevalent practice (43–46).

Wilms' Tumor

Wilms' tumor is a rare solid tumor of the kidney found in children; the peak age of occurrence is 2 years,

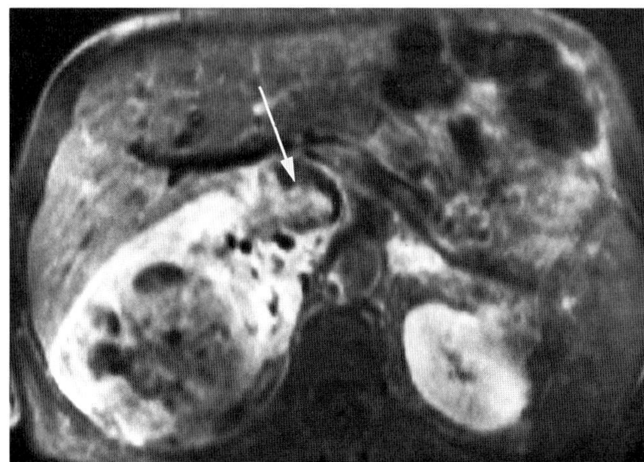

A

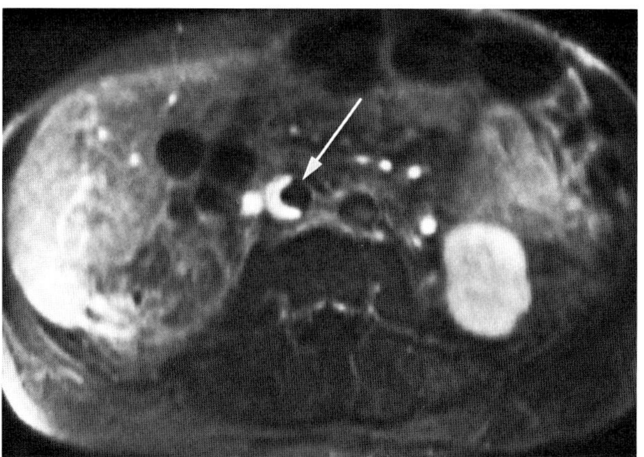

B

FIG. 15. Tumor and blood thrombus. Gd-DTPA-enhanced T1FS images of the IVC at the level of the entry of the right renal vein (**A**) and below the renal vessels (**B**). Enhancing tumor thrombus is appreciated extending from the right renal vein into the IVC (*arrow,* A). Thrombus in the IVC below the renal vessels does not enhance and is signal void, consistent with blood thrombus (*arrow,* B). Reprinted with permission from ref. 37.

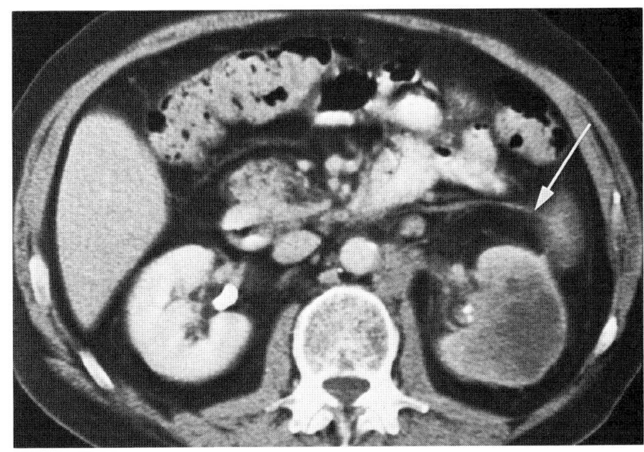

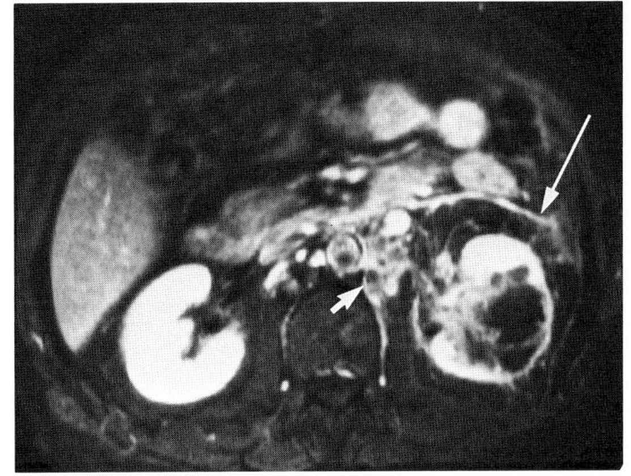

A B

FIG. 16. Stage IIIb renal cancer. Contrast-enhanced CT (**A**) and Gd-DTPA-enhanced T1FS (**B**) images in a 63-year-old man with Stage IIIb renal cell cancer. Enlarged nodes are apparent in a paraaortic location on the CT scan. On the postcontrast T1FS image, the nodes enhance in a heterogeneous fashion with central low SI (*short arrow,* B), similar in appearance to the primary tumor. Note the thickening of Gerota's fascia (*long arrows,* A, B), which is shown on both the CT and the MR images. Reprinted with permission from ref. 5.

and 75% of Wilms' tumors occur before age 5 (47). Wilms' tumor has a triphasic histology composed of blastemal, epithelial, and stromal elements. Focal hemorrhage and necrosis are common. The lesions are usually solitary but may be multiple in 5% to 10% of cases. Tumors present as large masses; in contrast to neuroblastomas, which calcify in 50% of cases, Wilms' tumors calcify in only 5% of cases. Unilateral Wilms' tumor is associated with a 40% incidence of nodular blastema, whereas multifocal Wilms' tumor has a 100% incidence of nodular blastema. Associated congenital abnormalities include aniridia, hemihypertrophy, and Beckwith-Wiedemann and Drash syndromes. Metastases to the lungs, liver, and lymph nodes occur. Wilms' tumor rarely may be highly cystic. Wilms' tumor appears as a tumor mass arising from the kidney, with an appearance indistinguishable from renal cell cancer (Fig. 19). Age constitutes a criterion for suggesting the diagnosis. The most common renal malignant neoplasm in the pediatric patient is Wilms' tumor. A transition occurs in the midteens, after which renal cell cancer is the most common renal tumor.

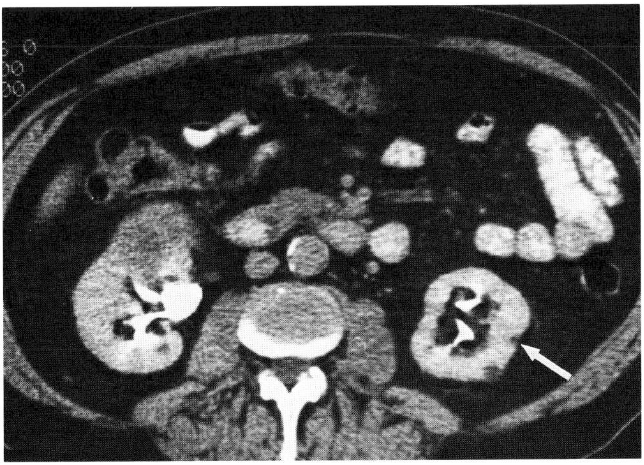

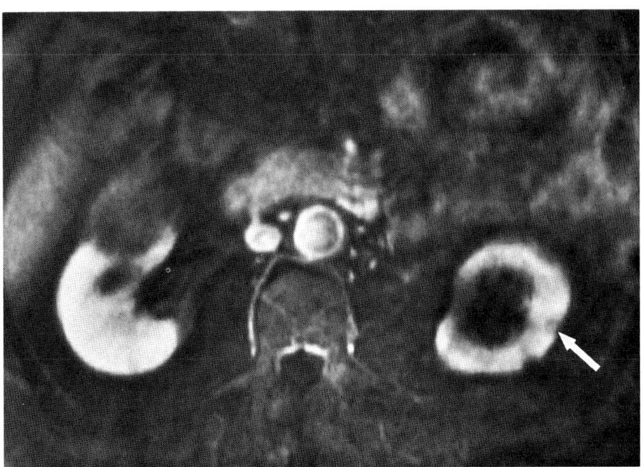

A B

FIG. 17. Purely cystic renal cell cancer. Contrast-enhanced CT (**A**) and Gd-DTPA-enhanced T1FS MR (**B**) images demonstrate two 5-mm subcapsular lesions in the lower pole of the left kidney in a patient with multiple bilateral renal cell cancers. These lesions were interpreted as cysts on both CT and MR images; however, at histopathological examination a thin lining of tumor cells was found in part of the cyst walls. In retrospect, the SI of one of the cysts was slightly higher than that of a usual simple cyst on the MR image (*white arrow,* A, B). Also apparent on this image is a renal cell cancer arising from the right kidney.

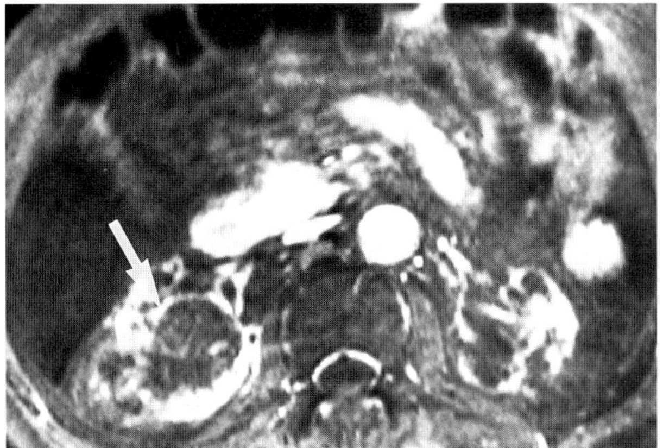

FIG. 18. Renal cell cancer superimposed on chronic renal failure. Gd-DTPA-enhanced T1FS image in a 64-year-old man with chronic renal failure and a 4-cm hypovascular renal cancer (*arrow*) arising from the right kidney.

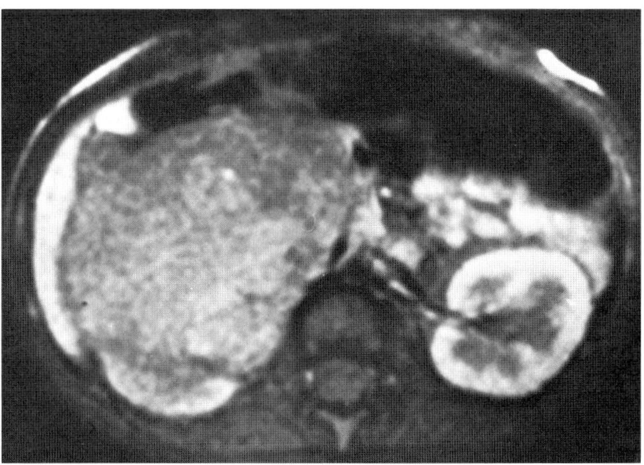

FIG. 19. Wilms' tumor. T1FS image in a 4-year-old boy with a large Wilms' tumor arising from the right kidney.

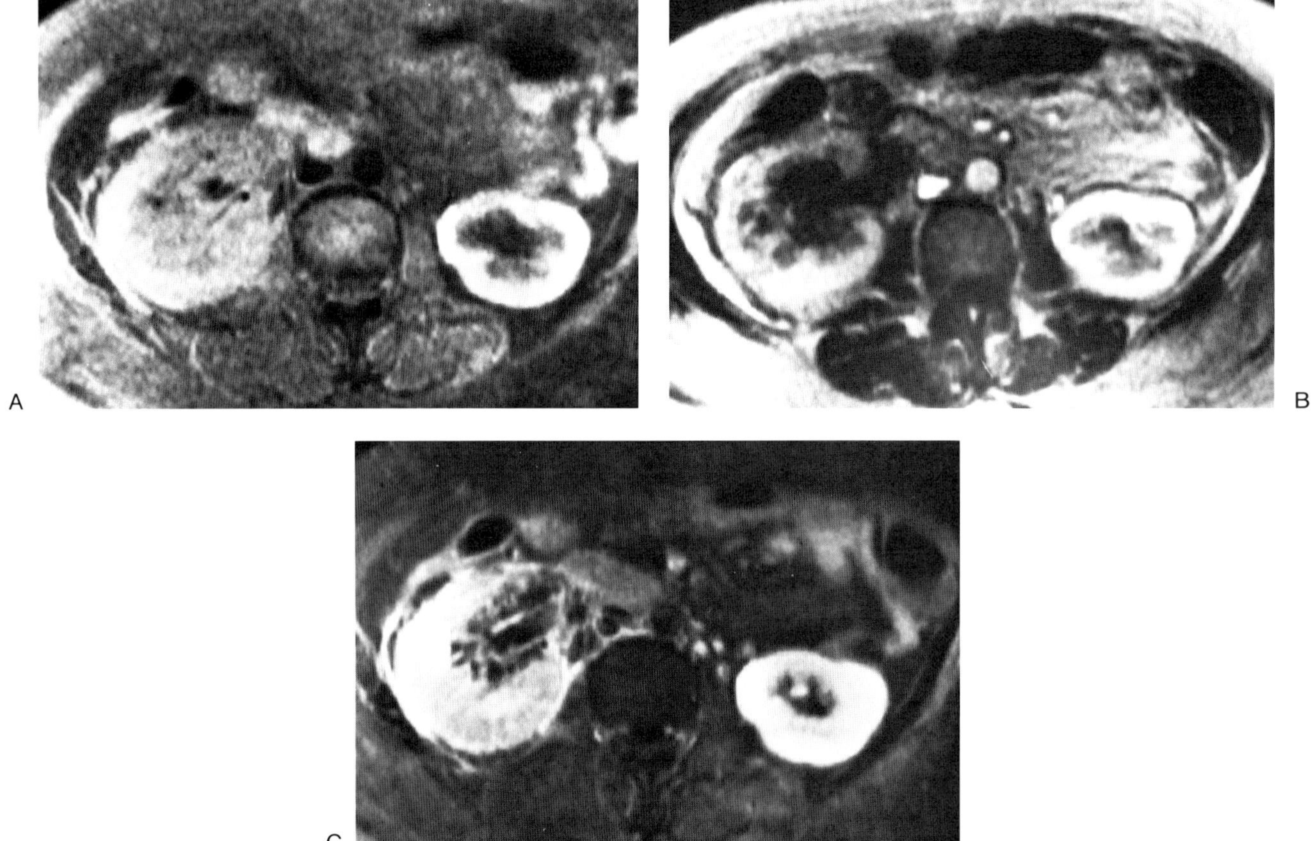

FIG. 20. Lymphoma. T1FS (**A**), 1-second postcontrast FLASH (**B**), and Gd-DTPA-enhanced T1FS (**C**) images in a 65-year-old woman with diffuse lymphomatous involvement of the right kidney. Generalized renal enlargement with loss of corticomedullary differentiation on T1FS (A) and dynamic Gd-DTPA-enhanced (B) images is present. Multiple low-SI lesions are noted in the renal medulla on postcontrast images (B,C) which probably represent lymphomatous deposits.

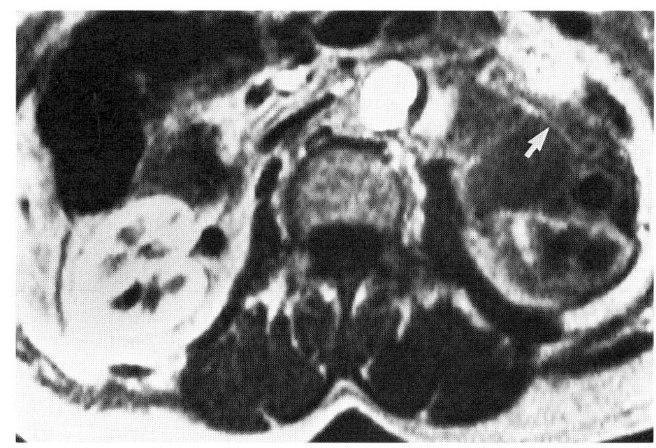

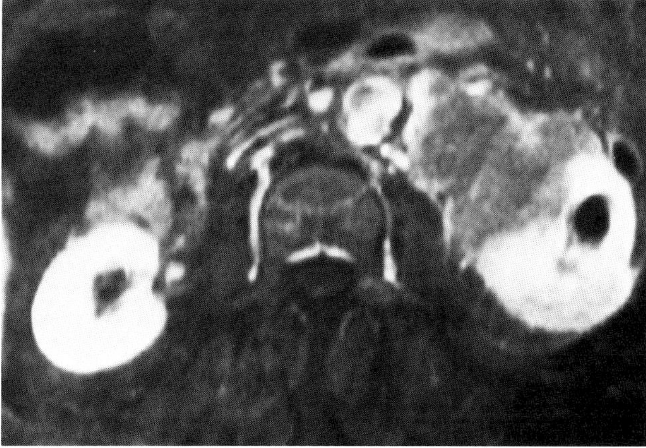

FIG. 21. Lymphoma. One-second postcontrast FLASH (**A**) and Gd-DTPA-enhanced T1FS (**B**) images in a 54-year-old man with a solitary mass of lymphoma arising from the left kidney. A large tumor mass extends from the renal sinus to the left periaortic space. Diminished contrast enhancement of the renal cortex of the involved kidney on the 1-second postcontrast image reflects compromised renal arterial flow. An attenuated left renal artery is identified (*arrow,* A). The tumor is relatively homogeneous and low in SI on the Gd-DTPA-enhanced T1FS image. The combination of vascular compromise and a homogeneous, poorly enhancing tumor is characteristic of lymphoma and uncommon for a renal cell cancer.

Lymphoma

Lymphomatous involvement of the kidneys is generally multifocal and part of widespread disease; however, isolated focal involvement of the kidney does occur (48,49). Non-Hodgkin's lymphoma more commonly involves the kidneys than does Hodgkin's disease. A variety of patterns of involvement occur. In descending order of frequency, they are (a) enlargement with maintenance of reniform shape, (b) multiple bilateral nodules, (c) direct invasion from adjacent disease, (d) solitary renal mass, and (e) perinephric involvement (48,49).

Renal parenchyma lacks lymphoid tissue so primary renal lymphoma usually occurs secondary to occult disease or arises from the retroperitoneum adjacent to the renal sinus. Lymphomatous masses tend to enhance in a diminished fashion after dynamic administration of Gd-DTPA. This differentiates lymphoma from renal cell cancer, which usually has regions of increased enhancement. Diffuse renal involvement with lymphoma results in generalized increase in renal size with loss of corticomedullary differentiation on both precontrast and dynamic postcontrast images (Fig. 20). A large tumor mass of lymphoma has a different appearance than renal cell cancer as there is a greater tendency toward tumor encasement of the renal artery, resulting in compromised renal blood flow and generally diminished enhancement (Fig. 21).

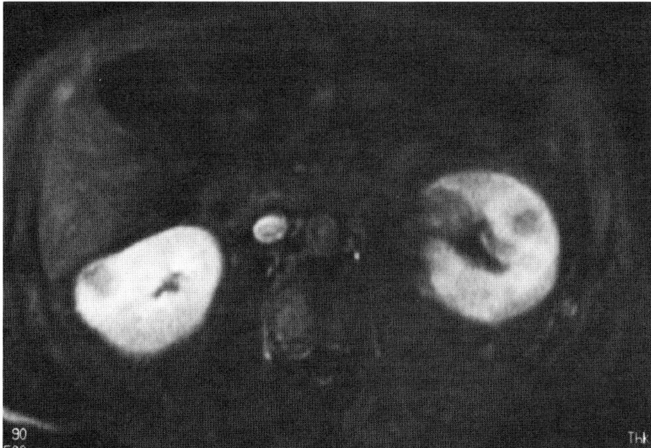

FIG. 22. Renal metastases. GA-DTPA enhanced T1FS image from a 72-year-old man with adenocarcinoma of the lung with extensive metastatic disease. Renal metastases are shown as multiple bilateral poorly enhancing renal masses.

Metastases

Metastases to the kidney are a late manifestation of advanced disease. Lung and breast cancer are the two most common primary tumors. Metastases usually appear as multiple bilateral renal masses (Fig. 22). Tumor masses (chloromas) from leukemic involvement can occur and are more common in children.

DISEASES OF THE RENAL COLLECTING SYSTEM

Mass Lesions

Benign Lesions

A variety of benign lesions affect the urothelium, including fibroepithelial polyp, pyelitis cystica, cholestea-

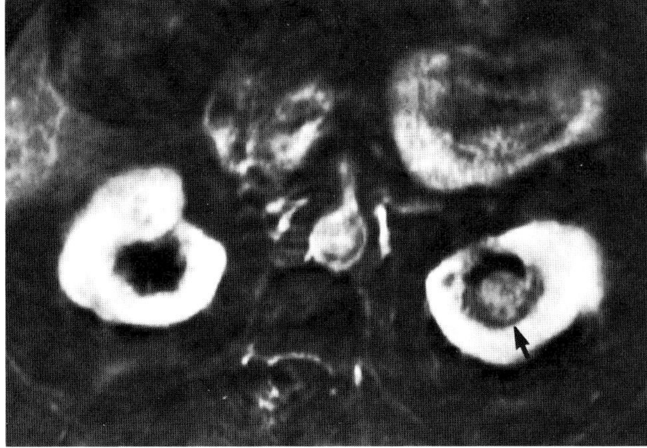

FIG. 23. Transitional cell cancer. Gd-DTPA-enhanced T1FS images in 51-year-old man with a transitional cell cancer arising from a superior pole calyx in the left kidney. A rounded, 2-cm tumor is identified (*arrow*) and has diminished contrast enhancement.

toma, leukoplakia, and malakoplakia. The MR appearances of these lesions have not been defined.

Transitional Cell Cancer

Transitional cell cancer (TCC) is the most common malignant neoplasm of the urothelium, accounting for >90% of tumors. Squamous cell cancer accounts for 8%, and adenocarcinoma <1%. TCC represents 8% of all renal tumors. TCC rarely occurs in patients younger than 30 years and affects male patients more than female patients at a ratio of 3:1. Risk factors include the use of analgesics, tobacco, or caffeine; chronic infection; and urolithiasis.

Tumors tend to appear as eccentric filling defects in the renal pelvis (Fig. 23) (50,51). On occasion they may cause concentric wall thickening (Fig. 24) (50,51). Tumors usually spread superficially but rarely may be large

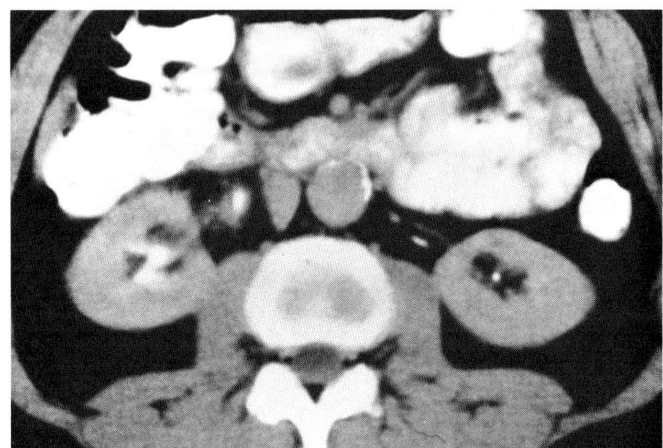

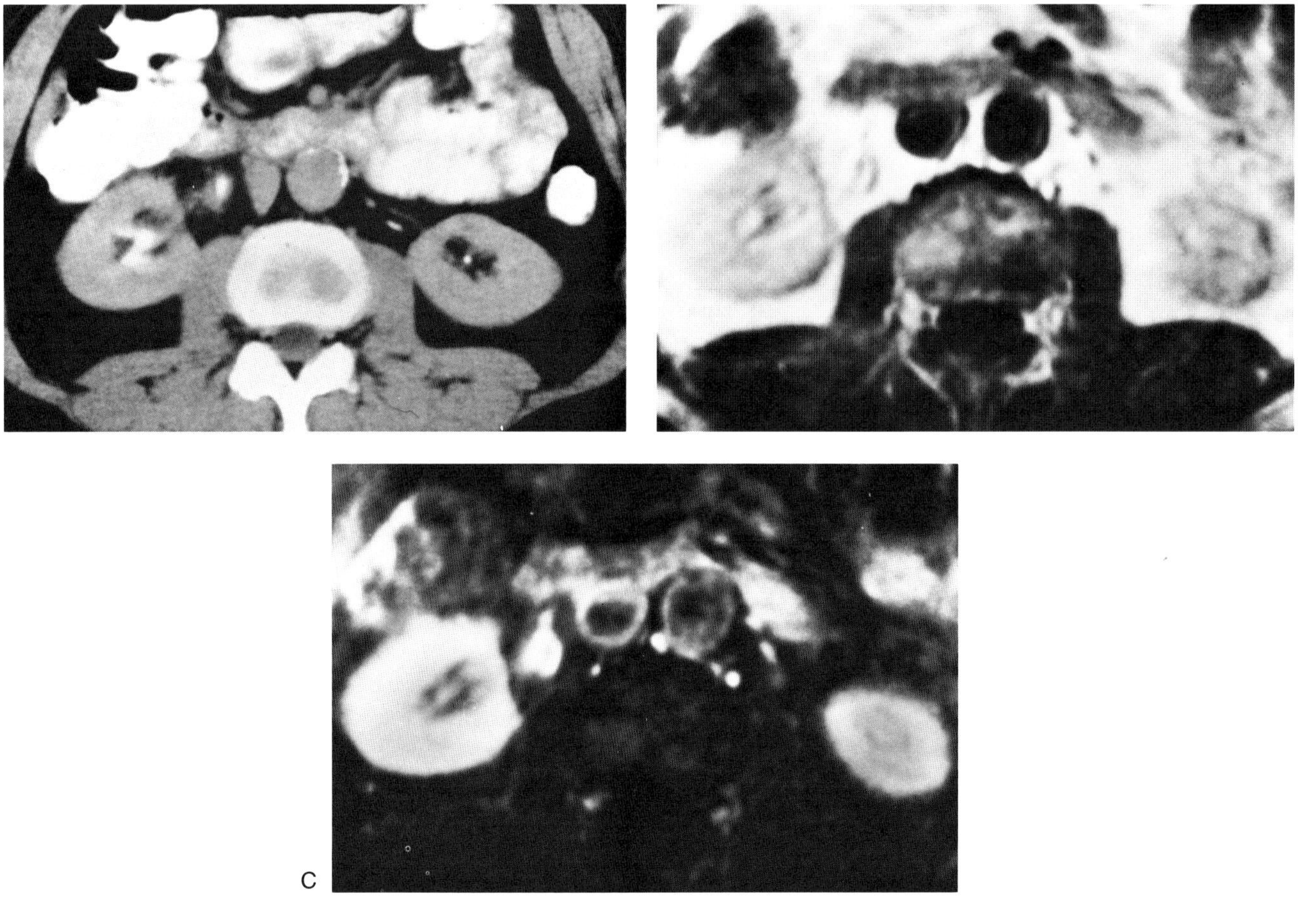

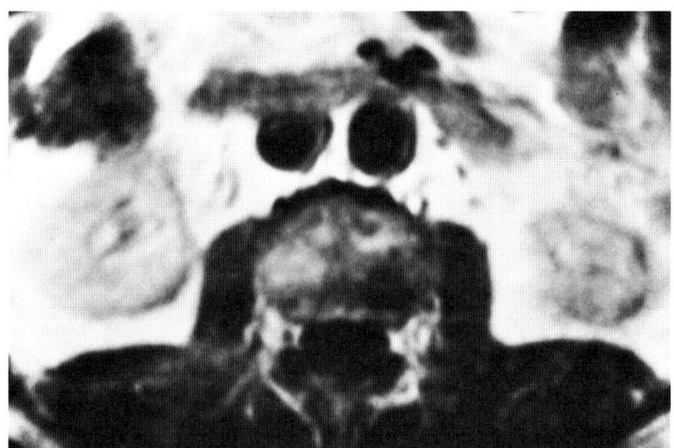

FIG. 24. Transitional cell cancer. Contrast-enhanced CT (**A**), contrast-enhanced T1-weighted spin echo (**B**), and Gd-DTPA-enhanced T1FS (**C**) images in a 52-year-old woman with transitional cell cancer of the proximal right ureter. The CT study demonstrates irregular circumferential thickening of the proximal ureter. Gd-DTPA-enhanced spin echo demonstrates thickening and enhancement of the ureter. Increased wall thickness and enhancement of the proximal ureter are more conspicuous with the removal of the competing high SI of fat (C).

focal masses. TCC has a propensity to invade renal parenchyma, but invasion may be difficult to detect. Although these tumors are hypovascular, they may be high in SI on Gd-DTPA-enhanced T1FS MR images, presumably because of abnormal clearance of contrast from the extracellular space. Tumors tend to invade locally with spread to adjacent lymph nodes. There is a great propensity for the tumor to be multifocal (30% to 50% of cases) and bilateral (15% to 25%); thus, evaluation of the entire urothelium with retrograde pyelography is essential.

Metastases

Metastases to the urothelium can resemble primary tumors in appearance. The most common metastatic tumors are melanoma, breast cancer, and ovarian cancer.

Filling Defects in the Collecting System

Calculi are the most common filling defects in the renal collecting system. Calcium oxalate stones are the most common form of renal calculi in North America, accounting for approximately 65% of cases (52). Regardless of calcium composition all renal calculi are signal void on MR images. MRI has not been used to detect renal calculi because T1-weighted sequences, which have the clearest anatomical display, have signal-void urine, which makes the detection of signal-void calculi difficult. MRI can be sensitive to the detection of calculi if the examination is tailored accordingly. In well-hydrated patients the signal intensity of Gd-DTPA-containing urine will be high in the renal pelvis 2 to 30 minutes after contrast administration. Signal-void calculi 1 to 2 mm in diameter can be detected in a background of high-SI urine (Fig. 25). Obstruction by calculi causes alteration in renal parenchymal enhancement and in the transit of contrast material within the kidney, which is well shown on MR images (see under "Renal Function," below).

Other filling defects, such as blood clots or fungus balls, are also well depicted on MR images. They are shown as nonenhancing mass lesions seated in the contrast-filled collecting system (Fig. 26).

Obstruction

Changes of acute and chronic obstruction are demonstrated on MR images. In acute obstruction, kidney size is enlarged and contrast persists in the renal parenchyma for a prolonged period, resulting in a prolonged nephrogram phase. Corticomedullary differentiation is diminished (2). In chronic obstruction the kidney decreases in size and renal perfusion diminishes (2). As in chronic ischemia the kidney is small, has a smooth contour, and has decreased contrast enhancement. The collecting system generally remains dilated, which permits distinction from chronic ischemia (Fig. 27).

Ischemia

Vascular diseases of the kidney most commonly are thromboembolic in origin because of underlying atherosclerotic disease; however, vasculitis may have an underlying immunologic cause. Acute and chronic renal ischemia is well shown on MR images. Relative renal blood flow between the kidneys can be readily appreciated on immediate post-Gd-DTPA-enhanced dynamic MR images. Relative quantification of renal blood flow can

A 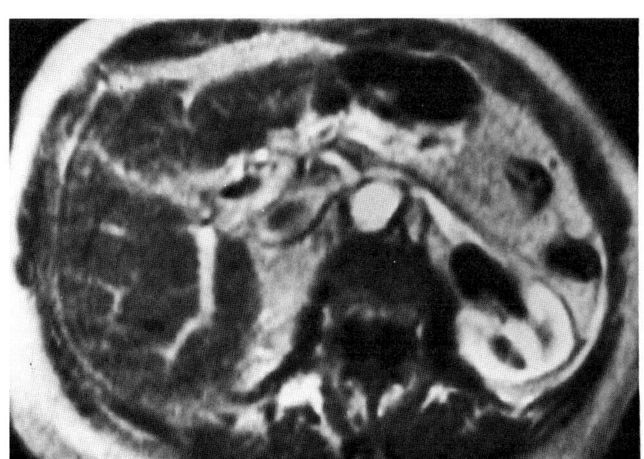

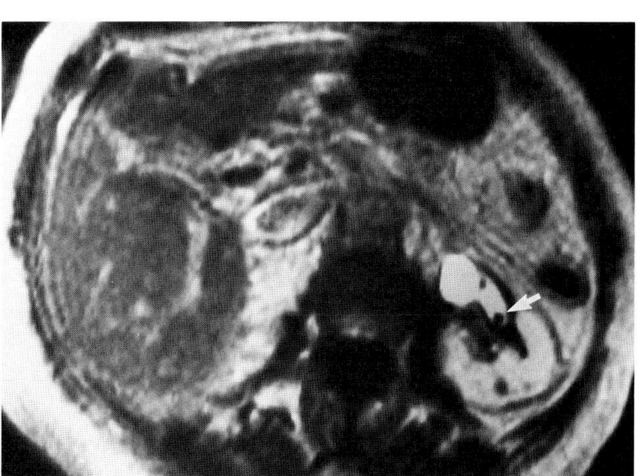 B

FIG. 25. Small renal calculus. One-second (**A**) and 10-minute (**B**) postcontrast FLASH images in a 71-year-old woman with a renal calculus. The signal-void calculus is not apparent in urine (A) or in urine containing concentrated (signal-void) gadolinium. The high SI of dilute gadolinium provides excellent contrast for the signal-void 2-mm calculus (*white arrow*, B).

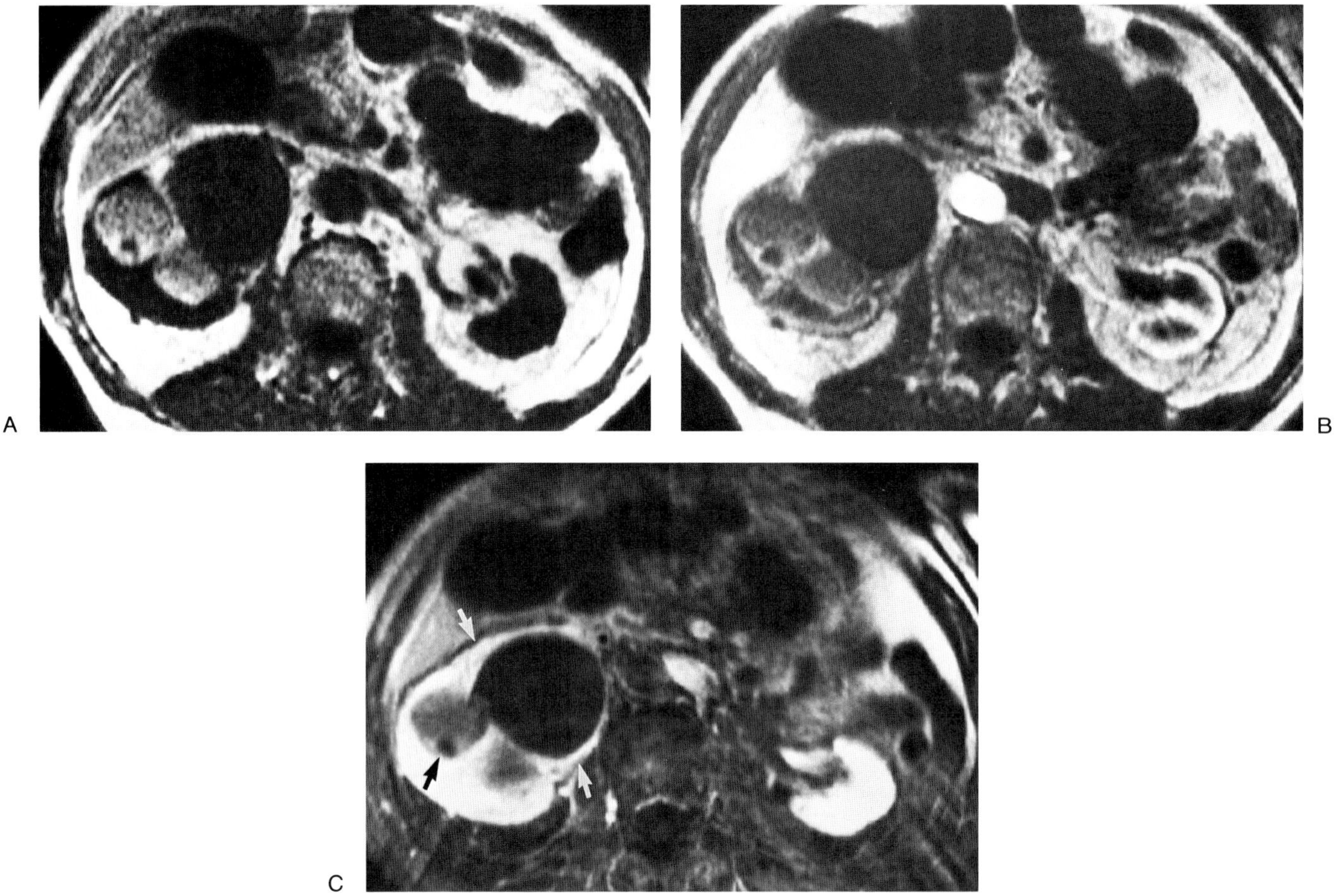

FIG. 26. Blood clot in the renal pelvis. FLASH (**A**), 1-second postcontrast FLASH (**B**), and Gd-DTPA-enhanced T1FS (**C**) images in a 73-year-old man with transitional cell cancer of the renal pelvis and a large intrapelvic blood clot. High SI in dilated renal calyces on the precontrast FLASH image is consistent with blood. A 4.5-cm, oval blood clot in the renal pelvis is low in SI on the FLASH image (A) and does not enhance with contrast (B,C). Cortical perfusion of the involved kidney is diminished in comparison to that of the contralateral kidney during the capillary enhancement phase (B). Thickening of the proximal portion of the renal pelvis on the Gd-DTPA-enhanced T1FS image represents the transitional cell carcinoma (*white arrows,* C). A 1-cm blood clot or calculus is observed in a dilated calyx (*black arrow,* C).

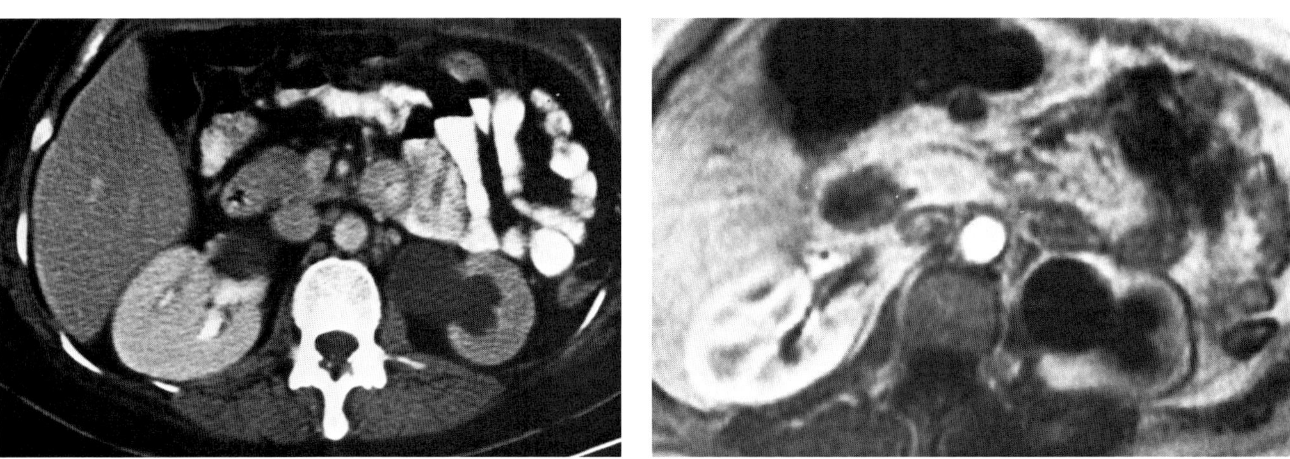

FIG. 27. Chronic renal obstruction. Contrast-enhanced CT (**A**) and 1-second postcontrast FLASH (**B**) images in a 44-year-old woman with chronic ureteric obstruction of the left renal collecting system. The chronically obstructed kidney is smaller, has diminished cortical enhancement and corticomedullary differentiation, and has smooth cortical thinning. These features are also observed in chronic ischemia (see Fig. 28). The distinguishing feature is the presence of a dilated collecting system.

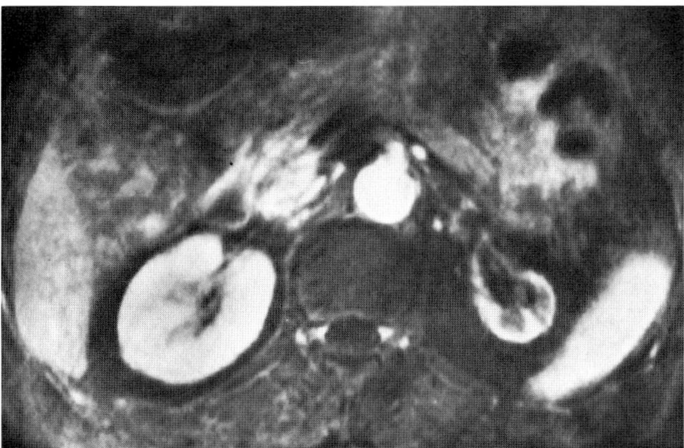

FIG. 28. Chronic ischemia. Gd-DTPA-enhanced T1FS image in a 74-year-old man with atherosclerotic disease of the aorta and left renal artery. The left kidney is chronically ischemic and is reduced in size, with diminished cortical enhancement and smooth cortical thinning. Delayed and persistent corticomedullary differentiation is apparent.

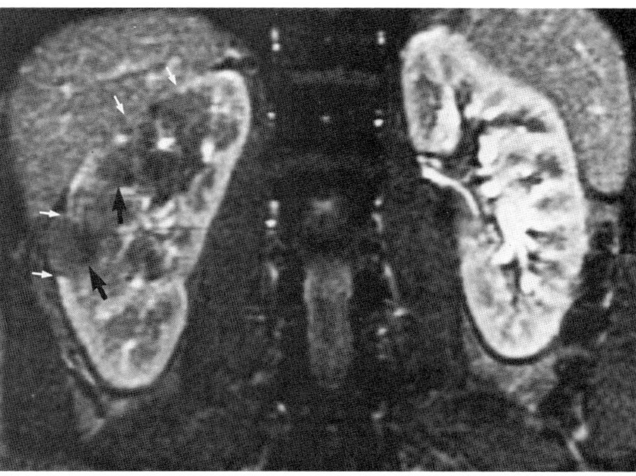

FIG. 30. Reflux nephropathy. Coronal capillary phase gradient echo MR image in a 26-year-old man with reflux nephropathy of the right kidney. Cortical thinning (*small white arrows*) of the upper and middle aspects of the right kidney is associated with calyceal dilatation (*black arrows*).

be achieved by comparing SI increase between the kidneys. Acute ischemia results in a normal or slightly enlarged kidney with diminished contrast enhancement. A chronically ischemic kidney has a smooth boundary, is small, shows diminished contrast enhancement, and has persistence of corticomedullary differentiation (Fig. 28).

Renal emboli are a relatively common occurrence in patients who have a source of emboli, since the kidneys receive approximately 20% of the cardiac output. The most common cause of renal emboli is embolism of mural thrombi in patients with atrial arrhythmias or prior myocardial infarction (53). Renal infarction from embolic events tends to occur between calices and demonstrates well-defined wedge-shaped defects in the renal outline (Fig. 29).

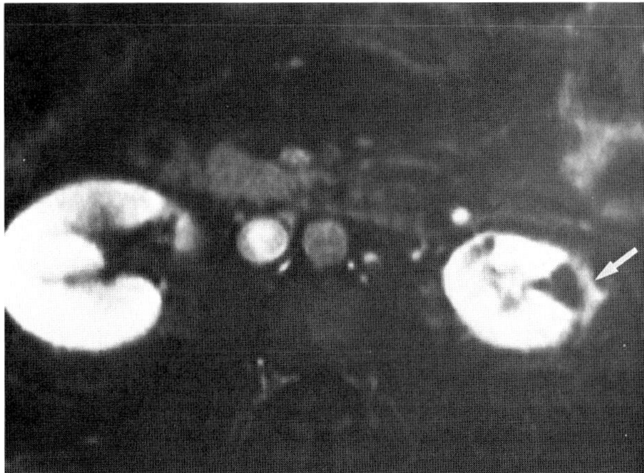

FIG. 29. Embolic renal infarction. Gd-DTPA-enhanced T1FS image in a 54-year-old man with renal infarction secondary to emboli from a left atrial thrombus. A well-defined wedge-shaped defect is present in the lower pole of the left kidney, with a thin rim of enhancement from a vessel in the renal capsule (*white arrow*). This is the typical appearance of embolic infarction.

Reflux Nephropathy and Chronic Pyelonephritis

Renal scarring is a frequent sequela of reflux nephropathy and is typically located in the polar regions adjacent to renal calyces (Fig. 30). Chronic pyelonephritis is characterized by the combination of calyceal dilatation and overlying cortical scarring. Cortical thinning is well demonstrated in images acquired in the capillary phase of enhancement (Fig. 31).

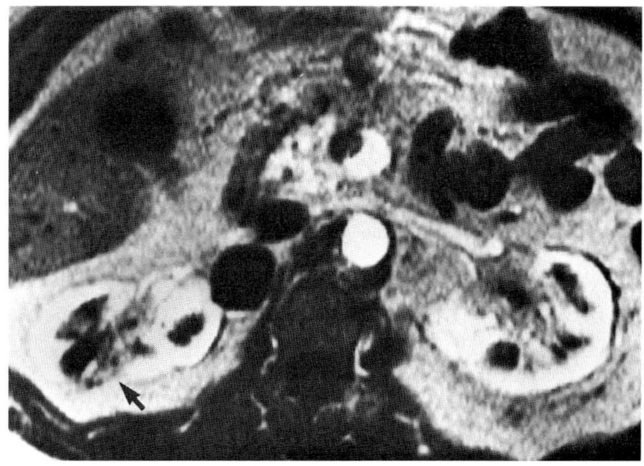

FIG. 31. Renal scarring. One-second postcontrast FLASH image in a 62-year-old man with cortical thinning secondary to scarring (*arrow*).

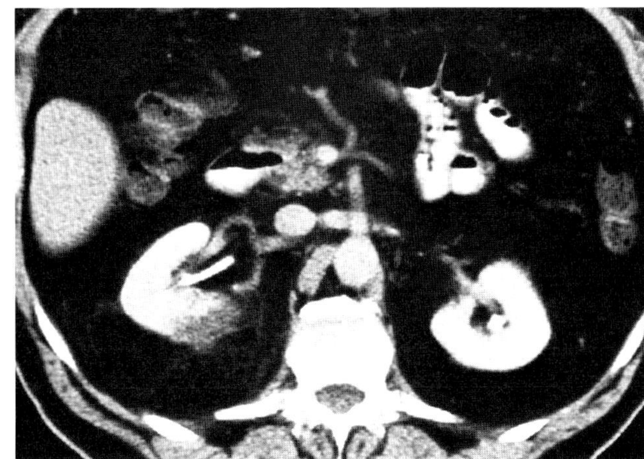

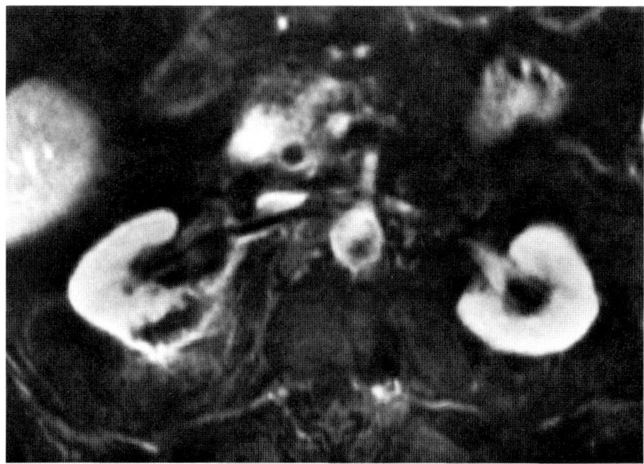

A B

FIG. 32. Renal abscess. Contrast-enhanced CT (**A**) and Gd-DTPA-enhanced T1FS (**B**) images in a 48-year-old man with a renal abscess. An ill-defined mass with reticular densities extending into the perirenal fat is identified arising from the posterior cortex of the right kidney. The signal void in the center of the mass on the Gd-DTPA-enhanced MR image more clearly demonstrates that the mass is an abscess than does the CT image, which shows the center to be of low attenuation.

Infections

Acute Infections

Acute pyelonephritis usually results in enlargement of the infected kidney. The infection is most commonly caused by a gram-negative bacillus as an ascending infection from the lower urinary tract. In general, MRI is not indicated in this condition, which is usually managed on the basis of clinical examination alone.

Abscesses

Fever, shaking, chills, and rigors in the presence of renal infection suggest the development of renal abscess. The clinical presentation may be insidious. Renal abscess usually occurs as a complication of an ascending urinary tract infection; however, hematogenous infections also occur. Hematogenous infection may be seen in tuberculosis, secondary to other sites of infection, or in the setting of intravenous drug use. Hematogenous infections are often due to gram-positive cocci. On MR images renal abscesses appear as irregular mass lesions with a signal-void center (Fig. 32). Based on the findings of imaging, a renal abscess cannot be distinguished from a necrotic tumor; follow-up studies are required to ensure resolution after treatment (54).

Renal tuberculosis is an uncommon form of infection. It is frequently associated with calcification and may result in severe renal destruction.

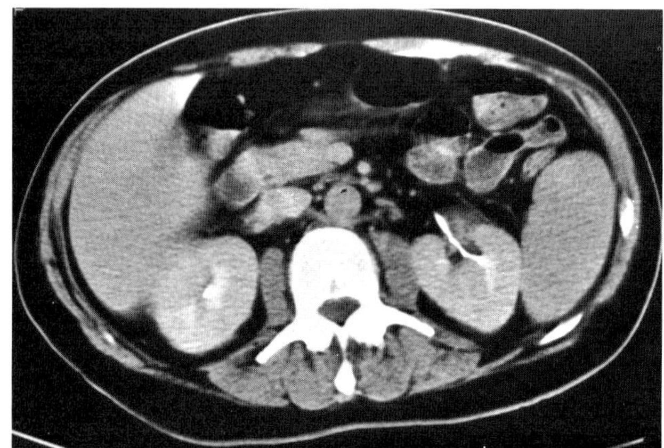

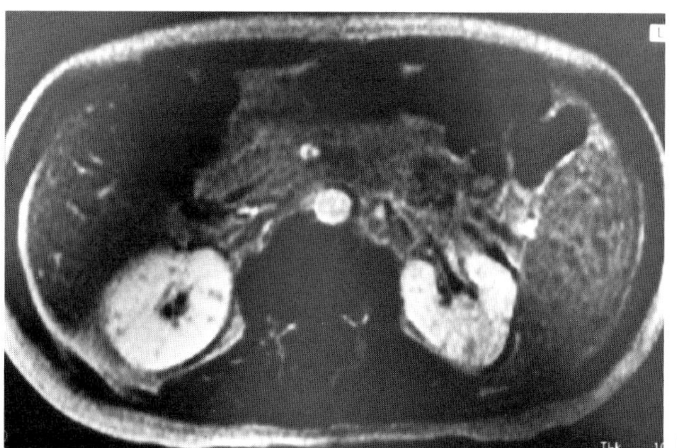

A B

FIG. 33. Renal candidiasis. Contrast-enhanced CT (**A**) and 90-second postcontrast FLASH (**B**) images of a 48-year-old man with hepatosplenic candidiasis. Multiple 1- to 2-mm signal-void lesions in the kidneys on the Gd-DTPA-enhanced FLASH image are compatible with the microabscesses of candidiasis. The CT image acquired 6 days earlier did not identify these lesions. Multiple splenic lesions are also apparent on the FLASH image.

A

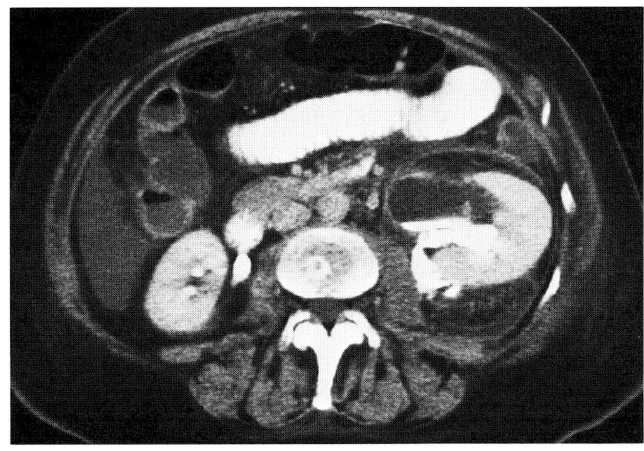

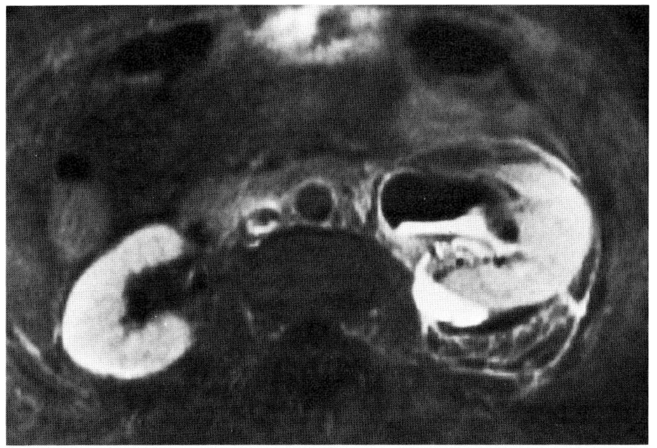

B

FIG. 34. Pyelosinus rupture. Contrast-enhanced CT (**A**) and Gd-DTPA-enhanced T1FS MR (**B**) images in a 65-year-old woman with pyelosinus rupture secondary to ureteral obstruction by ovarian metastases. Contrast agent is identified extravasating from the renal pelvis into the dependent portion of the perirenal space. Thickening of Gerota's fascia and of renorenal septae is apparent.

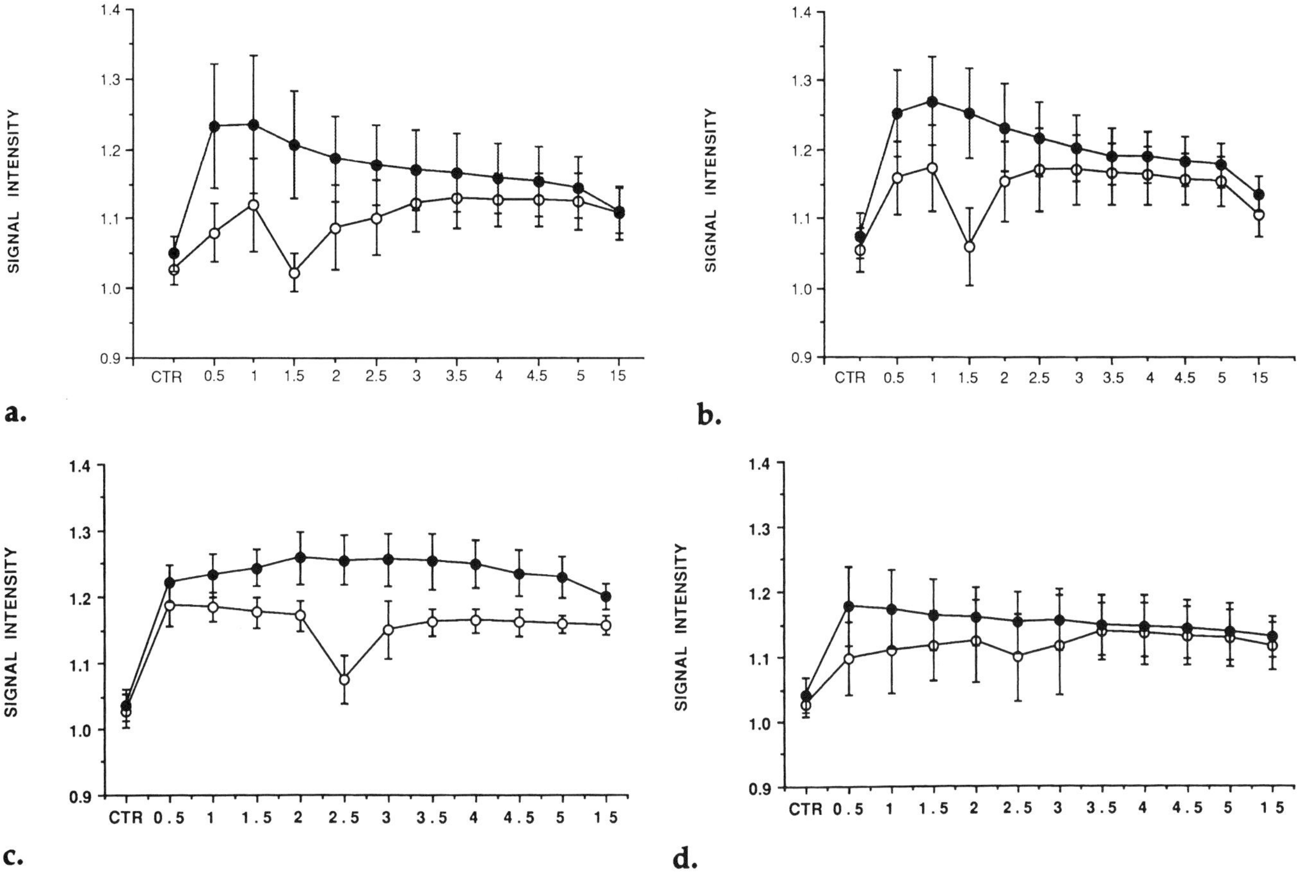

SIGNAL INTENSITY

1.4 1.3 1.2 1.1 1.0 0.9

CTR 0.5 1 1.5 2 2.5 3 3.5 4 4.5 5 15

a.

SIGNAL INTENSITY

1.4 1.3 1.2 1.1 1.0 0.9

CTR 0.5 1 1.5 2 2.5 3 3.5 4 4.5 5 15

b.

SIGNAL INTENSITY

1.4 1.3 1.2 1.1 1.0 0.9

CTR 0.5 1 1.5 2 2.5 3 3.5 4 4.5 5 15

c.

SIGNAL INTENSITY

1.4 1.3 1.2 1.1 1.0 0.9

CTR 0.5 1 1.5 2 2.5 3 3.5 4 4.5 5 15

d.

FIG. 35. Temporal course of SI changes for renal cortex (●) and medulla (○). SI is expressed as a ratio to SI of psoas muscle. *Bars* represent standard deviations (SD). The horizontal axis shows time, expressed in minutes; *CTR,* control (preinjection). **A:** Normal kidneys (n = 14). **B:** Dilated nonobstructed kidneys (n = 8). **C:** Kidneys with acute renal obstruction (n = 6). **D:** Kidneys with chronic renal obstruction (n = 10). Reprinted with permission from ref. 2.

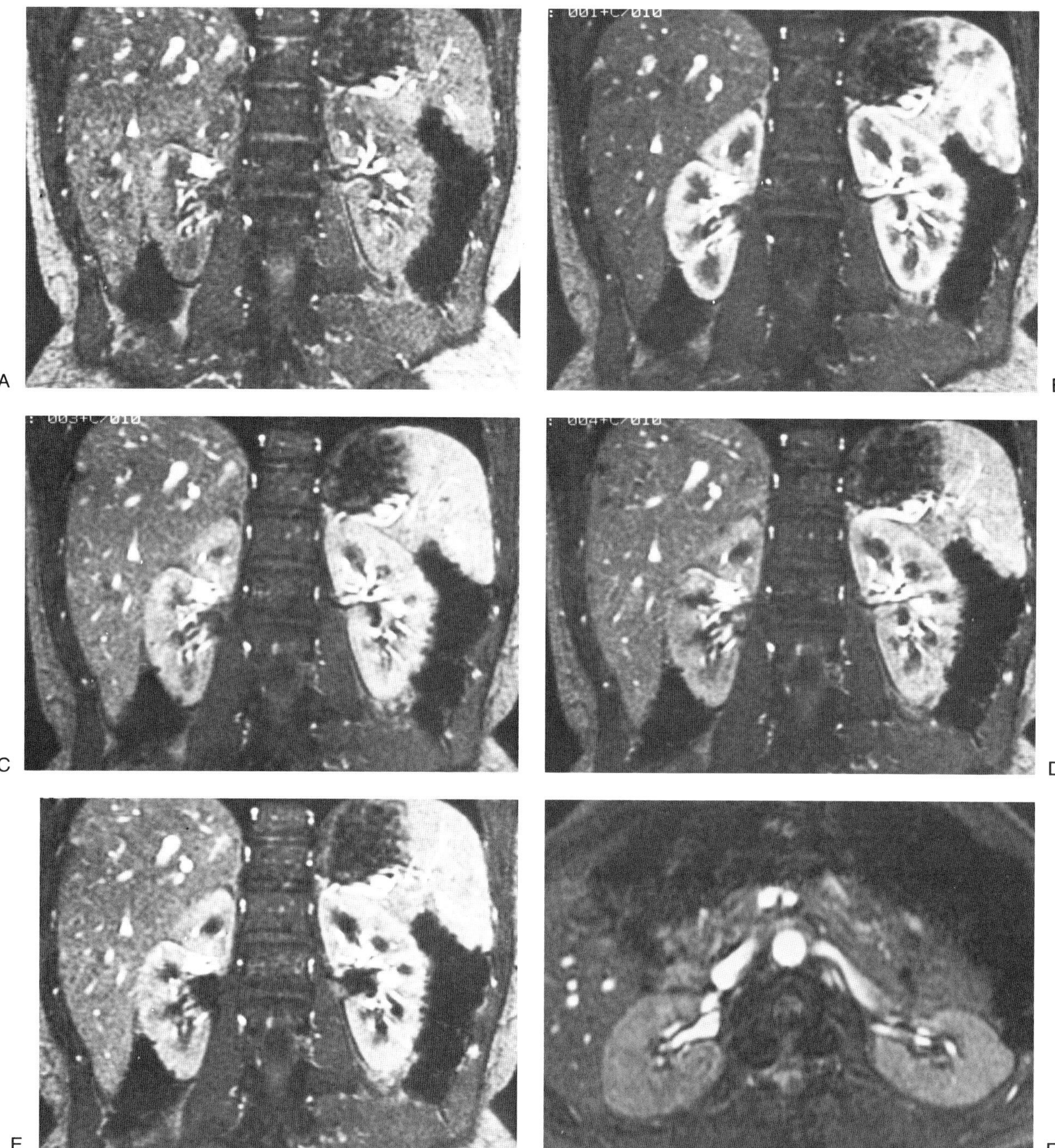

FIG. 36. Normal kidneys. **A:** Precontrast image. Minimal corticomedullary contrast is present. **B:** Cortical enhancement phase. Cortex SI is increased by 17%. Columns of Bertin are well visualized. The corticomedullary boundary is distinct because of differential blood flow. Note the high increase in SI of spleen with serpiginous low-SI bands (normal appearance) and the lower increase in SI of liver. **C:** Early tubular phase. SI of medulla is transiently increased while there is little change in cortical SI. **D:** Ductal phase. SI of medulla is decreased (6% from vascular phase) because of concentration of Gd-DTPA in distal convoluted tubules and collecting ducts. There is minimal decrease in cortical SI (2%). Decreased SI is apparent in the inner medulla and therefore mainly represents concentrated Gd-DTPA in collecting ducts. **E:** Excretory phase. Concentrated (low SI) urine appears in renal collecting systems. **F:** Excretory phase (15 minutes after injection). No corticomedullary contrast is apparent. Urine contains dilute (high-SI) Gd-DTPA (*arrows*) because of rapid clearance of Gd-DTPA from the body. Reprinted with permission from ref. 2.

Xanthogranulomatous Pyelonephritis

Xanthogranulomatous pyelonephritis (XGPN) is an unusual, chronic infection that develops in the presence of chronic obstruction (54). Sixty percent of cases are associated with *Proteus* infection. XGPN usually involves the kidney globally, but focal XGPN has been described (55).

Candidiasis

Renal candidiasis occurs in the context of hepatosplenic candidiasis. These lesions are typically small (2 mm) and well defined (Fig. 33).

Fungus balls may also develop in the collecting system. Diabetes predisposes to this condition.

Hemorrhage

Parenchymal or subcapsular hemorrhage appears as high- or mixed high-SI fluid on MR images. MRI is more sensitive to the presence of hemorrhage in fluid collections than is CT.

JUXTARENAL PROCESSES

Tumor, hemorrhage, abscess, and urine leaks all may occur in a juxtarenal location. Urine extravasation most commonly occurs either as a result of trauma or secondary to pyelosinus rupture due to elevated intracollecting system pressure. Although acute obstruction on the basis of renal calculi is the most common cause of pyelosinus rupture, this can also be due to other causes of obstruction (Fig. 34).

TRAUMA

Renal trauma is a frequent occurrence in abdominal injury. Tomographic imaging is the most accurate method to assess the severity of injury, which is generally classified as mild (contusion), moderate (laceration into the collection system), or severe (disruption of the renal pedicle or complete crush) (56). Dynamic Gd-DTPA-enhanced images demonstrate renal vessels high in SI and are useful to assess their integrity.

MEDICAL RENAL DISEASE

The role of MRI in medical renal disease has not been defined as yet. It may be that MR assessment of parenchymal enhancement or tubular function will be of value. Examination for mass lesions in the presence of decreased renal function is well performed with Gd-DTPA-enhanced MRI.

RENAL FUNCTION

Gd-DTPA-enhanced dynamic serial imaging of the kidneys permits identification of distinct phases of contrast enhancement based on the location of the bulk of the contrast agent. The phases of enhancement can be separated into (a) cortical (or capillary), (b) early tubular, (c) ductal, and (d) excretory enhancement (2). Evalua-

A

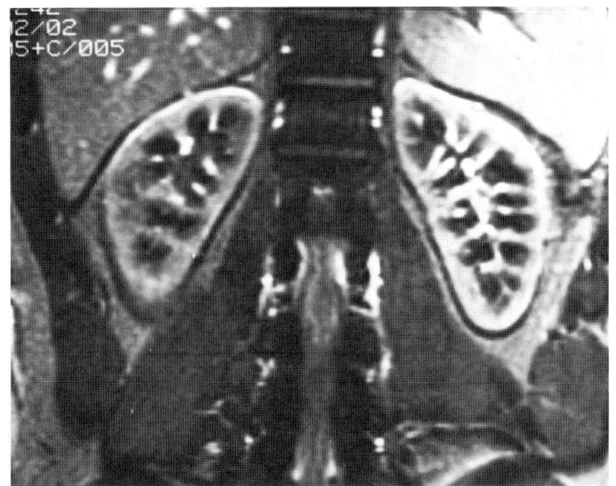

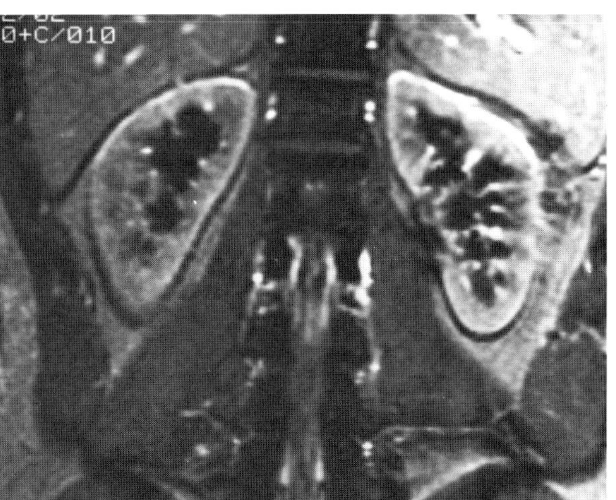

B

FIG. 37. Gradient echo images of subject with a dilated nonobstructed kidney on the left. **A:** Ductal phase. Low SI of medulla appears simultaneously in the dilated nonobstructed right kidney and in the normal left kidney. **B:** Excretory phase. Excretion of concentrated urine appears symmetrical bilaterally. Note susceptibility-induced image distortion of the renal collecting systems due to the high concentration of Gd-DTPA. Reprinted with permission from ref. 2.

tion of the concentrating ability of the kidneys can be made because of the ability of Gd-DTPA to change the SI of the fluid medium in which it is contained based on concentration. The assessment of these phases of enhancement distinguishes among normal kidneys and kidneys with dilated, nonobstructed collecting systems and those with acute and chronic obstruction. It is critical when performing these studies to ensure that the patient is mildly dehydrated to provide the physiological condition for renal concentration. This can be achieved by a 5-hour fast. The change in signal intensity of renal cortex and medulla in the normal kidney is illustrated in quantitative graphic form in Fig. 35A. This corresponds to SI changes illustrated in Fig. 36. Dilated, nonobstructed kidneys have signal intensity changes similar to those of normal kidneys, since renal transit is not abnormal (Fig. 37). Graphically, these SI changes have a similar pattern to those of normal kidneys (Fig. 35B). Acutely obstructed kidneys are enlarged and have increased renal transit time. This corresponds to an appearance of a prolonged, increasing SI nephrogram and the delayed appearance of contrast in the renal ducts and collecting system (Fig. 38). Different quantitative temporal enhancement is appreciated (Fig. 35C). Chronic

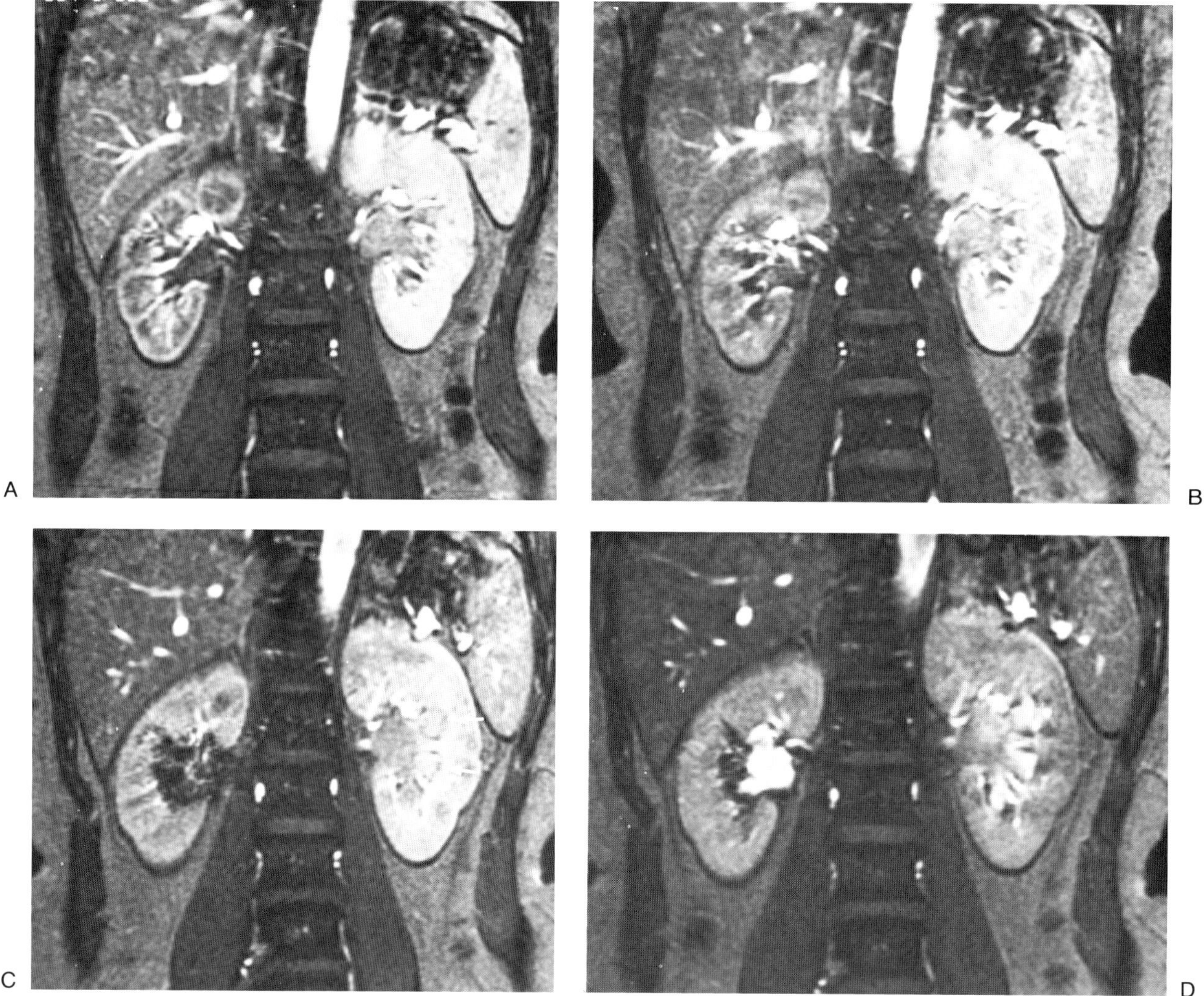

FIG. 38. Gradient echo images of subject with an acutely obstructed kidney on the left and normal kidney on the right. **A:** Cortical enhancement phase. Acutely obstructed left kidney is larger and swollen compared with the right kidney. Obstruction to venous drainage results in an abnormal pattern of contrast enhancement on the obstructed side, with increased parenchymal SI and decreased corticomedullary distinction. **B:** Ductal phase. Tubular concentration is apparent on the normal right side but not on the obstructed left side. Cortical enhancement is persistent on the obstructed side, analogous to the persistent nephrogram on intravenous urogram (IVU) examinations. **C:** Excretory phase. Delayed image obtained at 3.5 minutes shows dilute (high-SI) urine in dilated calyces on the left (*arrows*). Concentrated (low-SI) urine is excreted from the right kidney. **D:** Excretory phase (15 minutes after injection). Dilute urine is excreted on the normal side. Excretion into dilated calyces can be better appreciated. Reprinted with permission from ref. 2.

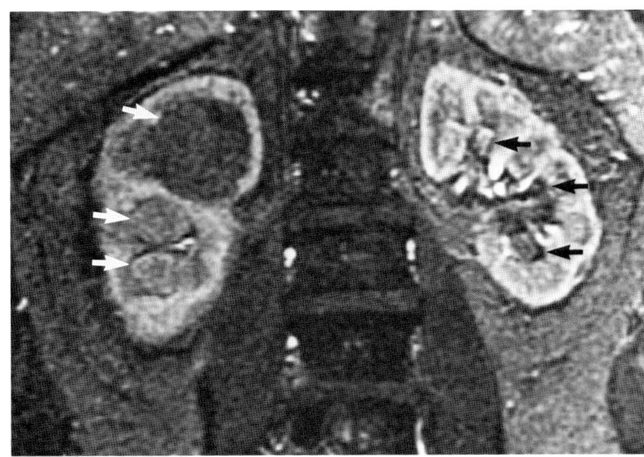

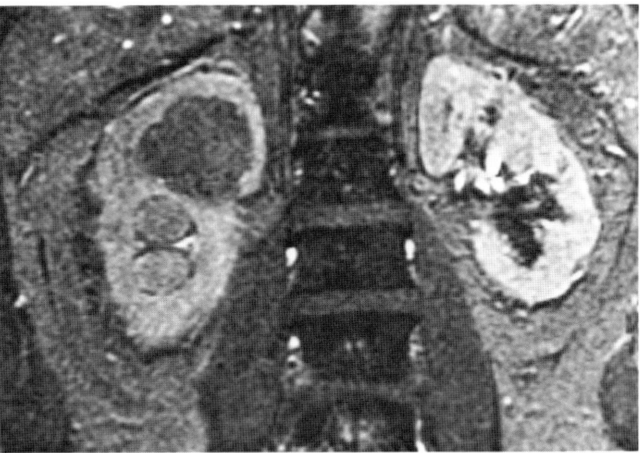

FIG. 39. Gradient echo images of a subject with a chronically obstructed kidney on the right and a dilated nonobstructed kidney on the left. **A:** Cortical enhancement phase. Normal corticomedullary enhancement on the left demonstrates corticomedullary distinction. Cortical enhancement is lower in chronically obstructed kidney on the right, with no distinction between cortex and medulla. Low-SI Gd-DTPA-free urine is present in both collecting systems (*arrows*). **B:** Excretory phase. Concentrated urine is excreted by the dilated nonobstructed left kidney. There is no apparent excretion by the chronically obstructed right kidney, no development of corticomedullary contrast, and no significant changes in parenchymal SI from the cortical enhancement phase. Reprinted with permission from ref. 2.

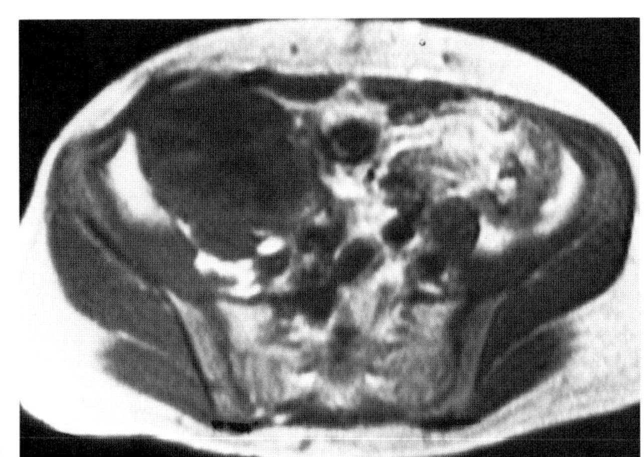

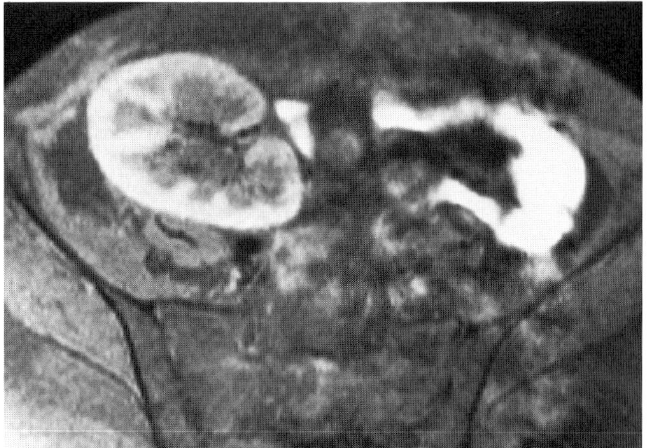

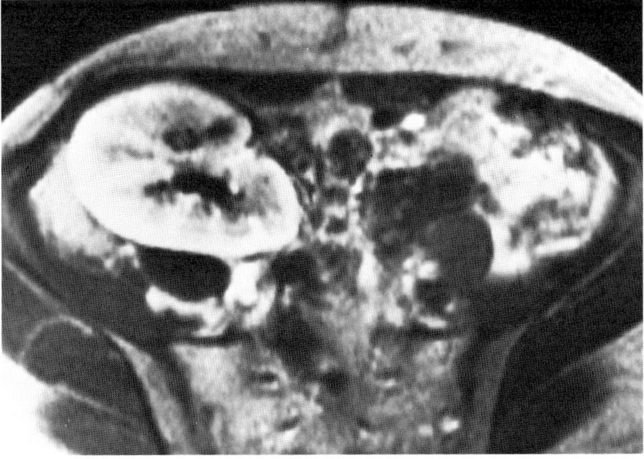

FIG. 40. Functioning renal transplant. FLASH (**A**), T1FS (**B**), and 1-second postcontrast FLASH (**C**) images of a 50-year-old woman with a functioning renal transplant. Normal corticomedullary difference present on the FLASH images (A) is better shown on the T1FS images (B). Corticomedullary difference on the dynamic Gd-DTPA-enhanced images (C) is consistent with a normal pattern of renal blood flow.

obstruction shows diminished cortical enhancement and increased transit time (Fig. 39). SI changes follow a different pattern than those observed in the other groups (Fig. 35D).

RENAL TRANSPLANTS

Loss of renal corticomedullary differentiation is seen in renal allograft undergoing rejection (57). In a study comparing the accuracy of MR, quantitative scintigraphy, and sonography for the detection of renal transplant rejection, the respective sensitivities of these techniques were 97%, 80%, and 70% (58). Unfortunately, the loss of corticomedullary differentiation is nonspecific and is also observed in cyclosporine toxicity and other infiltrative or medical renal diseases. Improved demonstration of corticomedullary difference on fat-suppressed T1-weighted and on dynamic Gd-DTPA-enhanced images requires reassessment of the role of MRI in this context. Normally functioning transplants have good corticomedullary differentiation on T1FS and dynamic Gd-DTPA-enhanced images (Fig. 40). Chronic rejection results in loss of corticomedullary differentiation on T1FS images. The degree of loss of corticomedullary differentiation on dynamic Gd-DTPA-enhanced images may correlate with the severity of rejection (Fig. 41). Assessment of surgical complications such as urinoma formation and renal vascular patency is also achieved with MRI. In addition, MRI permits accurate assessment of the presence of avascular necrosis of bone, which is not uncommon in these patients.

NEW DIRECTIONS

Lymph node-specific contrast agents have been used in animal models (59,60). These agents have the potential to distinguish enlarged hyperplastic from malignant nodes in patients with renal cancer.

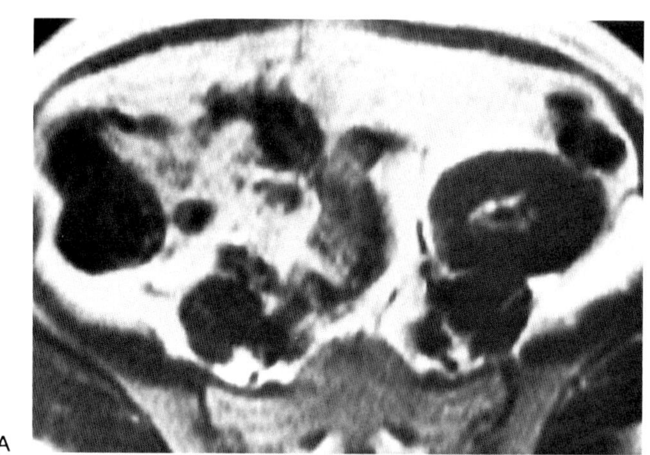
A

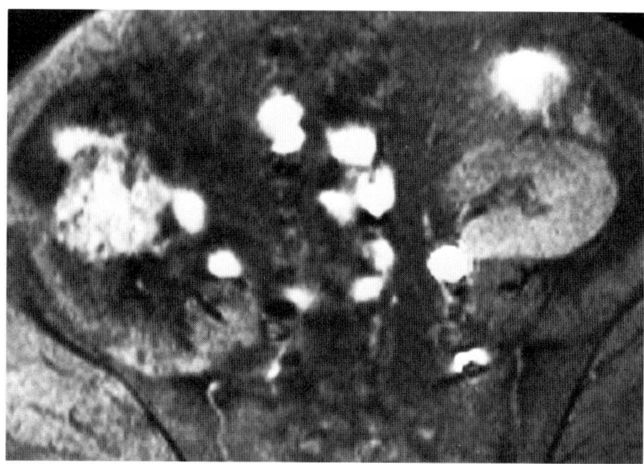
B

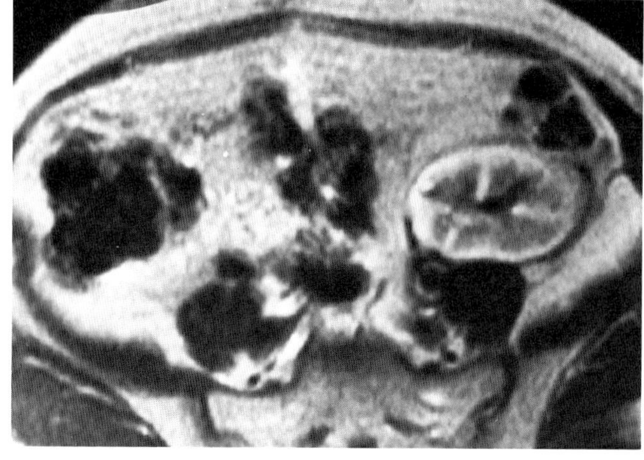
C

FIG. 41. Chronic rejection of renal transplant. FLASH (**A**), T1FS (**B**), and 1-second postcontrast FLASH (**C**) images in a 44-year-old woman with a renal transplant undergoing chronic rejection. Loss of corticomedullary differentiation is present on the precontrast FLASH image (A), with the loss better shown on the T1FS image (B). The presence of corticomedullary differentiation on the capillary phase enhancement image suggests some preservation of a normal pattern of renal blood flow consistent with some persistent renal function.

REFERENCES

1. Barnhart JL, Kuhnert N, Douglas BA, et al. Biodistribution of Gd-CL and Gd-DTPA and their influence on proton magnetic relaxation in rat tissues. *Magn Reson Imaging* 1987;5:221–231.
2. Semelka RC, Hricak H, Tomei E, Floth A, Stoller M: Obstructive nephropathy: evaluation with dynamic Gd-DTPA-enhanced MR imaging. *Radiology* 1990;175:797–803.
3. Choyke PL, Frank JA, Girton ME, et al. Dynamic Gd-DTPA-enhanced MR imaging of the kidney: experimental results. *Radiology* 1989;170:713–720.
4. Kikinis R, von Schulthess GK, Jager P, et al. Normal and hydronephrotic kidney: evaluation of renal function with contrast-enhanced MR imaging. *Radiology* 1987;165:837–842.
5. Semelka RC, Shoenut JP, Kroeker MA, MacMahon RG, Greenberg HM. Renal lesions: controlled comparison between CT and 1.5T MR imaging with nonenhanced and gadolinium-enhanced fat-suppressed spin-echo and breath-hold FLASH techniques. *Radiology* 1992;182:425–430.
6. Dalton D, Neiman H, Grayhack JT. The natural history of simple renal cysts: a preliminary study. *J Urol* 1986;135:905–908.
7. Semelka RC, Hricak H, Stevens SK, Fingold R, Tomei E, Carroll PR. Combined gadolinium-enhanced and fat saturation MR imaging of renal masses. *Radiology* 1991;178:803–809.
8. Lawson TL, McClennan BL, Shirkhoda A. Adult polycystic kidney disease: ultrasonographic and computed tomographic appearance. *J Clin Ultrasound* 1981;6:295–302.
9. Cho C, Friedland GW, Swenson RS. Acquired renal cystic disease and renal neoplasms in hemodialysis patients. *Urol Radiol* 1984;6:153–157.
10. Ishikawa I. Uremic acquired cystic disease of kidney. *Urology* 1985;26:101–107.
11. Levine E, Grantham JJ, Slucher SL, Greathouse JL, Krohn BP. CT of acquired cystic kidney disease and renal tumors in long term dialysis patients. *AJR Am J Roentgenol* 1984;142:125–131.
12. Mitnick JS, Bosniak MA, Mitton S, Raghavendra BN, Subramanyan BR, Genieser NB. Cystic renal disease in tuberous sclerosis. *Radiology* 1983;147:85–87.
13. Gutierrez OH, Burgener FA, Schwartz S. Coincident renal cell carcinoma and renal angiomyolipoma in tuberous sclerosis. *AJR Am J Roentgenol* 1979;132:848–850.
14. Levine E, Lee KR, Weigel JW, Farber B. Computed tomography in the diagnosis of renal carcinoma complicating Hippel Lindau syndrome. *Radiology* 1979;130:703–706.
15. Levine E, Collins DL, Horton WA, Schmenke RN. CT screening of the abdomen in von Hippel-Lindau disease. *AJR Am J Roentgenol* 1982;139:505–510.
16. Bosniak MA. Angiomyolipoma (hamartoma) of the kidney: a preoperative diagnosis is possible in virtually every case. *Urol Radiol* 1981;3:135–142.
17. Totty WG, McClennan BL, Melson GL, Patel R. Relative value of computed tomography and ultrasonography in the assessment of renal angiomyolipoma. *J Comput Assist Tomogr* 1981;5:173–177.
18. Osterling JE, Fishman EK, Goldman SM, Marshall FF. The management of renal angiomyolipoma. *J Urol* 1986;135:1121–1124.
19. Quinn MJ, Hartman DS, Friedman AC, et al. Renal oncocytoma: new observations. *Radiology* 1984;153:49–53.
20. Press GA, McClennan BL, Melson GL, Weyman PJ, Mauro MA, Lee JKT. Papillary renal cell carcinoma: CT and sonographic evaluation. *AJR Am J Roentgenol* 1984;143:1005–1010.
21. Bosniak MA. The small (≤3.0 cm) renal parenchymal tumor: detection, diagnosis, and controversies. *Radiology* 1991;179:307–317.
22. Birnbaum BA, Bosniak MA, Megibow AJ, Lubat E, Gordon RB. Observations on the growth of renal neoplasms. *Radiology* 1990;176:695–701.
23. Levine E, Huntrakoon M, Wetzel LH. Small renal neoplasms: clinical, pathologic, and imaging features. *AJR Am J Roentgenol* 1989;153:69–73.
24. Curry NS, Schabel SI, Betsill WL Jr. Small renal neoplasms: diagnostic imaging, pathological features and clinical course. *Radiology* 1986;158:113–117.
25. Ball DS, Friedman AC, Hartman DS, Radecki PD, Caroline DF. Scar sign of renal oncocytoma: magnetic resonance imaging appearance and lack of specificity. *Urol Radiol* 1986;8:46–48.
26. Boring CC, Squires TS, Tony T. Cancer statistics, 1991. *CA Cancer J Clin* 1991;41:19.
27. Hricak H, Thoeni RF, Carroll PR, Demas BE, Marotti M, Tanagho EA. Detection and staging of renal neoplasms: a reassessment of MR imaging. *Radiology* 1988;166:643–649.
28. Hricak H, Amparo E, Fisher MR, Crooks L, Higgins CB. Abdominal venous system: assessment using MR. *Radiology* 1985;156:415–422.
29. Hricak H, Demas BE, Williams RD, et al. Magnetic resonance imaging in the diagnosis of renal and perirenal neoplasms. *Radiology* 1985;154:709–715.
30. Patel SK, Stack CM, Turner DA. Magnetic resonance imaging in staging of renal cell carcinoma. *Radiographics* 1987;156:415–422.
31. Pritchett TR, Raval JK, Benson RC, et al. Preoperative magnetic resonance imaging of vena caval tumor thrombi: experience with five cases. *J Urol* 1987;138:1220–1222.
32. Fein AB, Lee JKT, Balfe DM, et al. Diagnosis and staging of renal cell carcinoma: a comparison of MR imaging and CT. *AJR Am J Roentgenol* 1987;148:749–753.
33. Eilenberg SS, Lee JKT, Brown JJ, Mirowitz SA, Tartar VM. Renal masses: evaluation with gradient-echo Gd-DTPA-enhanced dynamic MR imaging. *Radiology* 1990;176:333–338.
34. Zeman RK, Cronan JJ, Rosenfield AT, Lynch JH, Jaffe MH, Clark LR. Renal cell carcinoma: dynamic thin-section CT assessment of vascular invasion and tumor vascularity. *Radiology* 1988;167:393–396.
35. Roubidoux MA, Dunnick NR, Sostman HD, Leder RA. Renal carcinoma: detection of venous extension with gradient echo MR imaging. *Radiology* 1992;182:269–272.
36. Studer UE, Scherz S, Scheidegger J, et al. Enlargement of regional lymph nodes in renal cell carcinoma is often not due to metastases. *J Urol* 1990;144:243–245.
37. Semelka RC, Shoenut JP, Magro CM, Kroeker MA, MacMahon R, Greenberg HM. Renal cancer staging: Comparison of contrast-enhanced CT and Gadolinium-enhanced fat suppressed spin echo and breath hold gradient echo MRI. *JMRI* 1992 (*in press*).
38. Goldstein HA, Kashanian FK, Blumetti RF, Holyoak WL, Hugo FP, Blumenfield DM. Safety assessment of gadopentatate dimeglumine in U.S. clinical trials. *Radiology* 1990;174:17–23.
39. Krestin GP, Schuhmann-Giamjsieri G, Haustein J, et al. Functional dynamic MRI, pharmacokinetics and safety of Gd-DTPA in patients with impaired renal function. *Eur Radiol* 1992;2:16–23.
40. Rofsky NM, Weinreb JC, Bosniak MA, Libes RB, Birnbaum BA. Renal lesion characterization with gadolinium-enhanced MR imaging: efficacy and safety in patients with renal insufficiency. *Radiology* 1991;180:85–89.
41. Thompson IM, Peek M. Improvement in survival of patients with renal cell carcinoma: the role of the serendipitous detected tumor. *J Urol* 1988;140:487–490.
42. Smith SJ, Bosniak MA, Megibow AJ, Hulnick DH, Horii SC, Raghavendra BN. Renal cell carcinoma: earlier detection and increased detection. *Radiology* 1989;170:699–703.
43. Johnson DE, Voneschenbach A, Sternberg J. Bilateral renal cell carcinoma. *J Urol* 1978;119:23–24.
44. Carini M, Selli C, Barbanti G, Lapini A, Turini D, Constantine A. Conservative surgical treatment of renal cell carcinoma: clinical experience and reappraisal of indications. *J Urol* 1988;140:725–731.
45. Zincke H, Sen SE. Experience and extra-corporeal surgery and autotransplantation for renal cell and transitional cell cancer of the kidney. *J Urol* 1988;140:25–27.
46. Pronet J, Tessler A, Brown J, Golimbu M, Bosniak M, Morales P. Partial nephrectomy for renal cell carcinoma: indications, results and implications. *J Urol* 1991;145:472–476.
47. Kasper TE, Osborne RW Jr, Semerdjian HS, Miller HC. Urologic abdominal masses in infants and children. *J Urol* 1976;116:629–633.
48. Hartman DS, Davis CJ Jr, Goldman SM, Friedman AC, Fritzsche P. Renal lymphoma: radiologic-pathologic correlation of 21 cases. *Radiology* 1982;144:759–766.
49. Heiken JP, McClennan BL, Gold RP. Renal lymphoma. *Semin Ultrasound CT MR* 1986;7:58–66.

50. Cholankeril JV, Freundlich R, Ketyer S, Spirito AL, Napolitano J. Computed tomography in urothelial tumors of renal pelvis and related filling defects. *J Comput Assist Tomogr* 1986;10:263–272.
51. Baron RL, McClennan BL, Lee JKT, Lawson T. Transitional cell carcinoma of the pelvis and ureter—CT evaluation. *Radiology* 1982;144:125–130.
52. Elliot JS. Urinary calculus disease. *Surg Clin North Am* 1965; 45:1393–1404.
53. Lessman RK, Johnson SF, Coburn JW, et al. Renal artery embolism: clinical features and long-term follow-up of 17 cases. *Ann Intern Med* 1978;89:477–481.
54. Bova JG, Potter JL, Arevalos E, Hopens T, Goldstein HM, Radwin HM. Renal and perirenal infection: the role of computerized tomography. *J Urol* 1985;133:375–378.
55. Goldman SM, Hartman DS, Fishman EK, Finizio JP, Gatewood OM, Siegelman SS. CT of xanthogranulomatous pyelonephritis: radiologic-pathologic correlation. *AJR Am J Roentgenol* 1984;142:963–969.
56. Bretan PN, McAninch JW, Federle MP, Jeffrey RB. Computerized tomographic staging of renal trauma: 85 consecutive cases. *J Urol* 1986;136:561–565.
57. McCreath GT, McMillan N, Patterson J, et al. Magnetic resonance imaging of renal transplants: initial experience. *Br J Radiol* 1988;61:113–118.
58. Hricak H, Terrier F, Marotti M, et al. Post-transplant renal rejection: comparison of quantitative scintigraphy, ultrasonography and magnetic resonance imaging. *Radiology* 1987;162:685–688.
59. Weissleder R, Elizondo G, Josephson L, et al. Experimental lymph node metastases: enhanced detection with MR lymphography. *Radiology* 1989;171:835–839.
60. Hamm B, Taupitz M, Hussman P, Wagner S, Wolf K-J. MR lymphography with iron oxide particles: dose-response studies and pulse sequences optimization in rabbits. *AJR Am J Roentgenol* 1992;158:183–190.

CHAPTER 9

The Gastrointestinal Tract

J. Patrick Shoenut, Richard C. Semelka, Richard Silverman, Clifford S. Yaffe, and Allan B. Micflikier

Magnetic resonance imaging has had limited effect on the diagnosis of gastrointestinal disease until quite recently. This has been due to the long imaging times of conventional sequences that resulted in increased phase artifact and the lack of suitable oral contrast agents. The inherent strengths of MRI, which include high contrast resolution, high sensitivity for intravenous contrast, and safety, have recently resulted in better-defined clinical applications for MRI of bowel disease. MRI seems to have particular utility in distinguishing Crohn's disease from ulcerative colitis, defining the pathological extent of inflammatory bowel disease, and accurately staging malignant neoplasms of the gastrointestinal tract preoperatively.

THE ESOPHAGUS

Normal Anatomy

The esophagus is composed of three layers, an inner circular and outer longitudinal layer of muscle and a squamous epithelial lining. The lack of a serosal surface accounts for the rapid spread of tumor into mediastinal fat. The esophagus lies posterior to the trachea in the neck and the thoracic inlet is posterior and slightly to the left. The esophagus traverses the diaphragm through the esophageal hiatus and lies immediately anterior to the aorta at this level. The normal thickness of the esophagus is approximately 3 mm; on tomographic images it is usually collapsed, although a small amount of air in the lumen is not uncommon (Fig. 1).

MR Technique

Successful imaging of the esophagus necessitates the use of cardiac gating or saturation of the heart to diminish cardiac phase artifact, which is particularly problematic throughout the middle and lower esophagus. Gd-DTPA-enhanced fat-suppressed sequences are ideal in demonstrating the esophageal anatomy.

Mass Lesions

Benign Tumors

Leiomyomas are the most common benign tumors of the esophagus and arise from the circular smooth muscle layer. These lesions generally are found in the distal esophagus and may be single or multiple (1,2). They present as small, oval masses and may be pedunculated (Fig. 2).

Duplication Cysts

Duplication cysts of the esophagus are small, fluid-filled, oval lesions that are usually located in the lower esophagus.

Varices

Varices develop along the lower esophagus, the stomach, and other locations with portosystemic communica-

J. P. Shoenut: University of Manitoba and Department of Medicine, Saint Boniface General Hospital, Winnipeg, Manitoba R2H 2A6.

R. C. Semelka: Department of Radiology and Magnetic Resonance Services, University of North Carolina at Chapel Hill, Chapel Hill, North Carolina 27599.

R. Silverman and C.S. Yaffe: Department of Surgery, University of Manitoba, Winnipeg, Manitoba R2H 2A6.

A. B. Micflikier: Department of Medicine, University of Manitoba, Winnipeg, Manitoba R2H 2A6.

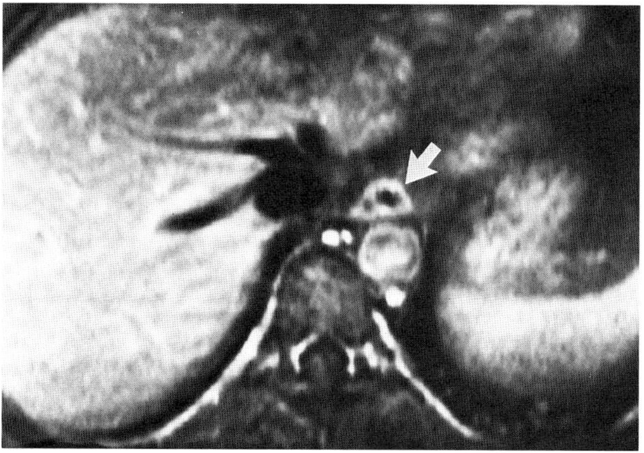

FIG. 1. Normal esophagus. Gd-DTPA-enhanced T1FS image of the normal esophagus. The esophagus (*arrow*) is thin walled and contains a small amount of air. Moderate mural enhancement is present.

tions in patients with portal hypertension. Varices can be demonstrated as signal-void tubular structures on spin echo images, high-SI structures on cine MR techniques, or enhancing tubular structures on dynamic Gd-DTPA-enhanced images (Fig. 3).

Malignant Disease

Squamous cell carcinoma is the most common malignant lesion of the esophagus, accounting for approximately 98% of all primary malignant neoplasms. The etiology is not clear but the incidence seems greater with increased consumption of alcohol and tobacco (3). The lesion is more common in male patients (3:1) and blacks (4). Primary adenocarcinoma of the esophagus arises from columnar cells or Barrett's epithelium (5,6). White males seem to be most at risk. Adenocarcinoma accounts for most of the malignant neoplasms reported in the distal esophagus (Fig. 4). This lesion may invade the esophagus from the proximal stomach, causing pseudoachalasia (7). As with CT, the role of MRI in staging esophageal carcinoma is uncertain. This is primarily because of the early spread of tumor to mediastinal fat, which may be undetectable on imaging studies, and the frequent tumor involvement of normal-sized lymph nodes. There is, however, a definite role for the detection of liver metastases. Invasion of the tracheobronchial tree and descending aorta is also well shown. Tumors that most commonly metastasize to the esophagus include breast and lung cancer and melanoma (Fig. 5).

Inflammatory Disease

The most common esophageal disorder requiring medical attention is reflux esophagitis; 20% of the North American population experience heartburn, and many seek medical help (8,9). Achalasia is a primary disorder of the esophagus. The features include the failure of the lower esophageal sphincter (LES) to relax completely and nonperistaltic, simultaneous esophageal contractions. Palliation of this condition will sometimes lead to problems associated with reflux (10–13). A dilated, slightly thick-walled esophagus with increased mural enhancement may be observed on MR images (Fig. 6). Scleroderma may manifest in the esophagus. As a result of this connective tissue disorder, the esophagus and stomach function as a common cavity. The nonfunctioning lower esophageal sphincter in these patients may permit substantial reflux (14). Inflammatory changes of the lower esophagus appear as high-SI changes of the esophageal wall on Gd-DTPA-enhanced MR images.

Infectious Disease

The herpes simplex virus and *Candida albicans* are the two most common infectious organisms to involve

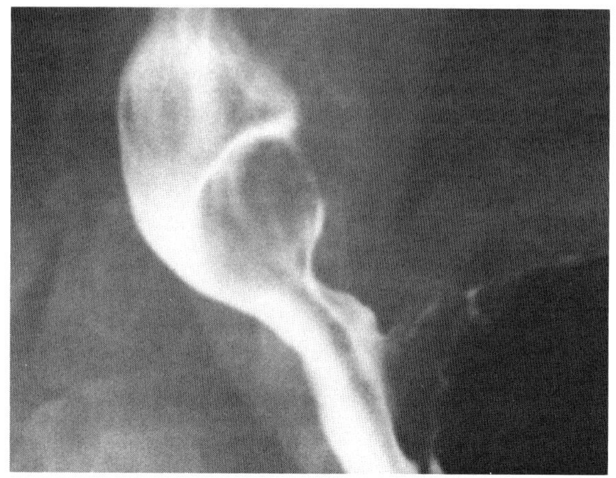

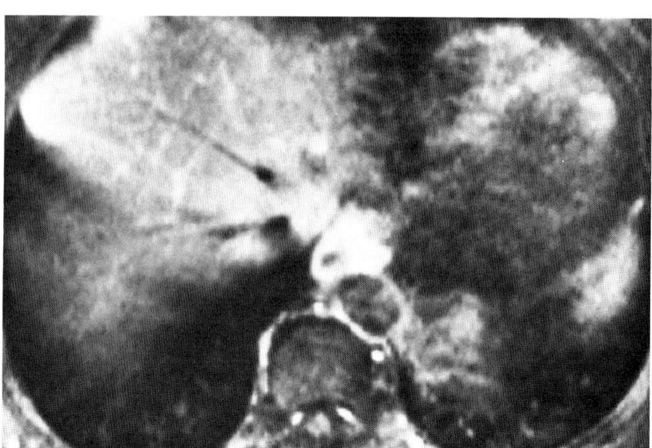

FIG. 2. Leiomyoma. Barium swallow (**A**) and Gd-DTPA-enhanced T1FS (**B**) images in a 52-year-old woman demonstrate a 2-cm leiomyoma arising from the left aspect of the wall of the distal esophagus.

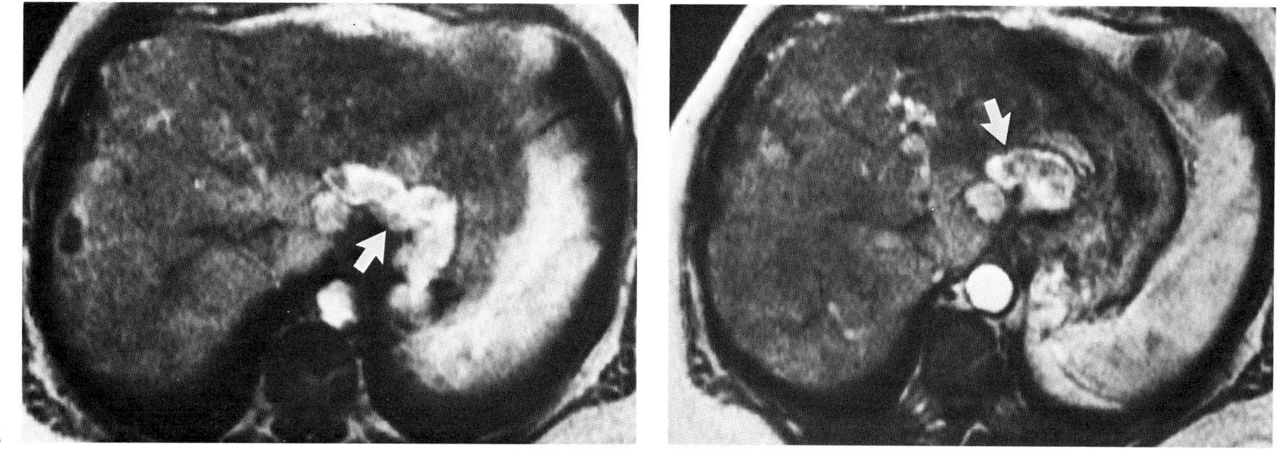

FIG. 3. Gastroesophageal varices. One-second postcontrast FLASH images in a 54-year-old woman with hepatic cirrhosis and portal hypertension. Tubular high-SI structures are identified along the lesser curvature of the stomach (*arrow,* **A**) extending to the lower esophagus (*arrow,* **B**), consistent with gastroesophageal varices.

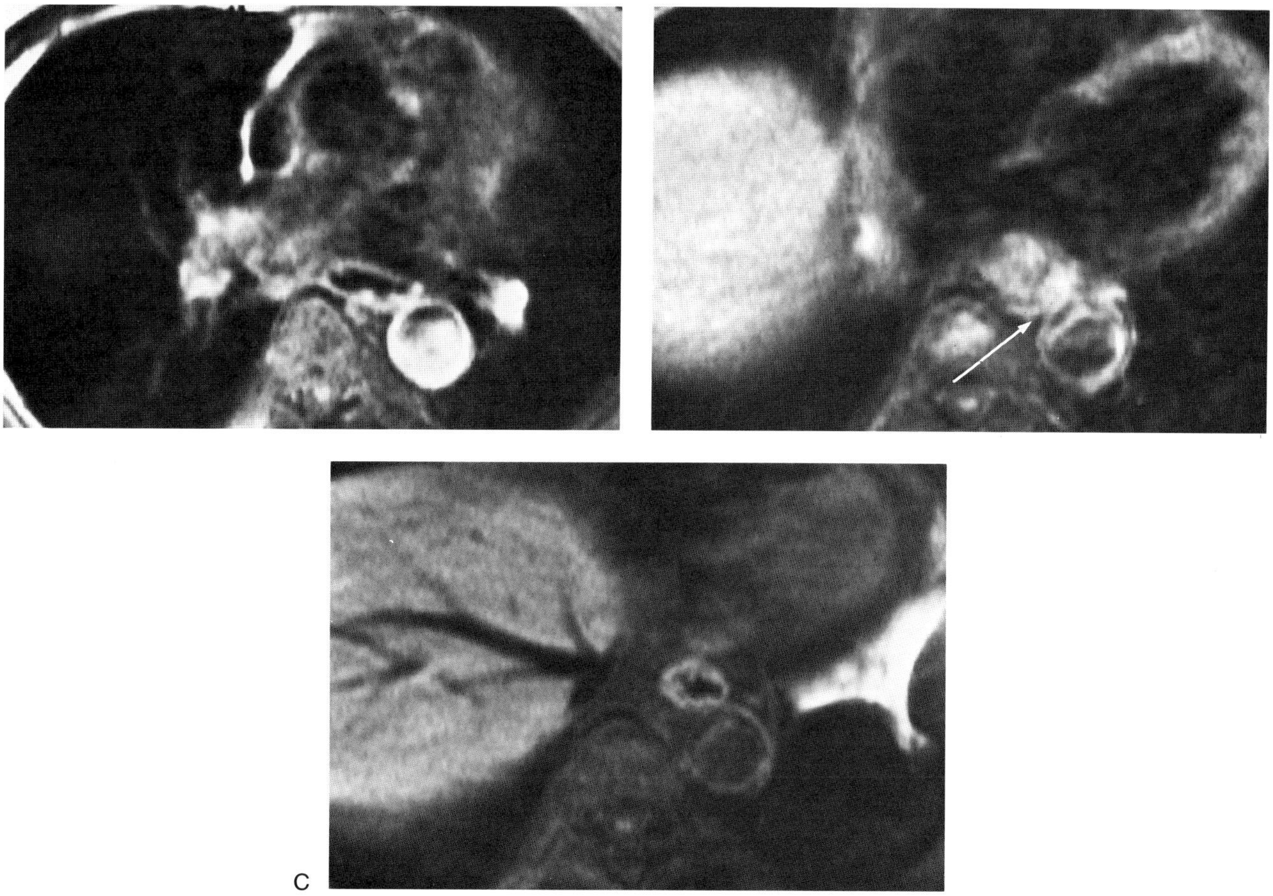

FIG. 4. Adenocarcinoma of the esophagus. Fat-suppressed MR sections from cranial to caudal locations through the lower thorax in a 64-year-old man with adenocarcinoma of the lower esophagus. At the level of the midthorax, the esophagus has a thin, normal-appearing wall (**A**). More inferiorly, at the level of the mitral valve (**B**), a 2.5-cm solid tumor is identified in the esophagus, which has a $<90^\circ$ interface with the descending thoracic aorta (*arrow*). Immediately above the gastroesophageal (GE) junction (**C**), the esophagus possesses a normal appearance. A 2.5-cm cancer with no local invasion was found at surgery, confirming the imaging findings.

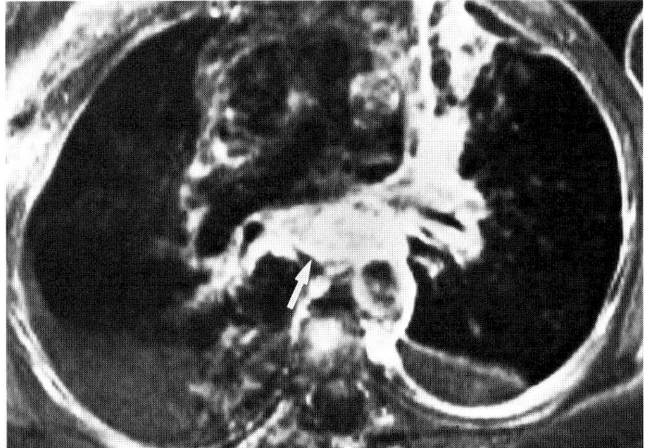

FIG. 5. Breast cancer metastases to the esophagus. Gd-DTPA-enhanced T1FS image in a 57-year-old woman with extensive metastatic disease to the mediastinum. Enhancing tumor encases the esophagus (*arrow*) and extends along the left hilum and left mediastinum to the anterior chest wall. The tumor caused high-grade obstruction of the esophagus.

the esophagus. Tuberculosis of the esophagus is very rare (15).

THE STOMACH

Normal Anatomy

The stomach is an expansion of the digestive tract which disrupts food by mechanical and chemical means. The anatomical components of the stomach include the cardia, fundus, body, antrum, and pylorus. The curved shape of the stomach permits anatomical description of the lesser and greater curvature.

MR Technique

Optimal examination of the stomach has not been defined using MRI but, as with CT, delineation of the wall is better demonstrated by gastric distension. This is best achieved by administering a substantial volume of fluid. Air is a poor distending agent, since it may cause magnetic susceptibility artifact. Gastric mucosa enhances the most intensely of all bowel mucosa with Gd-DTPA and is well shown on immediate post-Gd-DTPA-enhanced MR images. Gd-DTPA-enhanced fat-suppressed MR images are useful in demonstrating gastric abnormalities and possess high contrast resolution (Fig. 7).

Mass Lesions

Benign Tumors

Gastric polyps are benign lesions that occur most commonly in older patients. The majority are classified as hyperplastic polyps, whereas 20% are found to be adenomatous. Of the latter group, approximately one-third contain a focus of adenocarcinoma (16). Polyps smaller than 2 cm are usually benign. Anemia, when present, may be due to chronic blood loss or associated deficiencies in iron or vitamin B_{12} absorption. Leiomyomas are the most common benign nonepithelial tumors of the stomach, arising from the smooth muscle of the gastric wall. Other gastric lesions include duplication cysts and pancreatic rests. Gastric diverticula are uncommon pulsion diverticula usually found near the gastroesophageal junction (17). Infrequently they may occur in the gastric antrum. Symptoms suggestive of peptic ulcer disease may be present, and the radiologic appearances must be differentiated from ulcer disease.

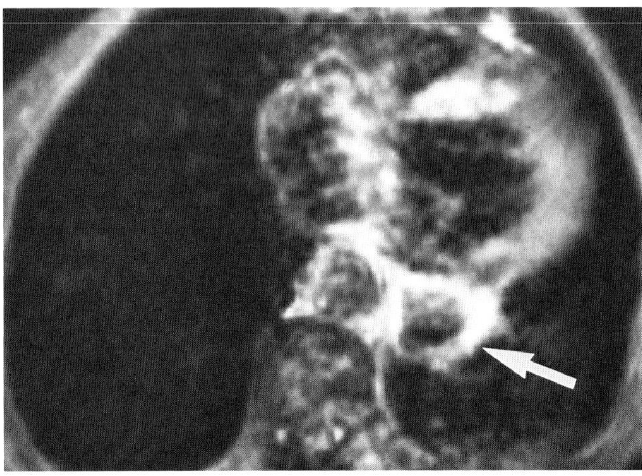

FIG. 6. Achalasia. A dilated, slightly thick-walled esophagus with increased mural enhancement (*arrow*) in an 80-year-old woman with achalasia is observed on the Gd-DTPA-enhanced T1FS image.

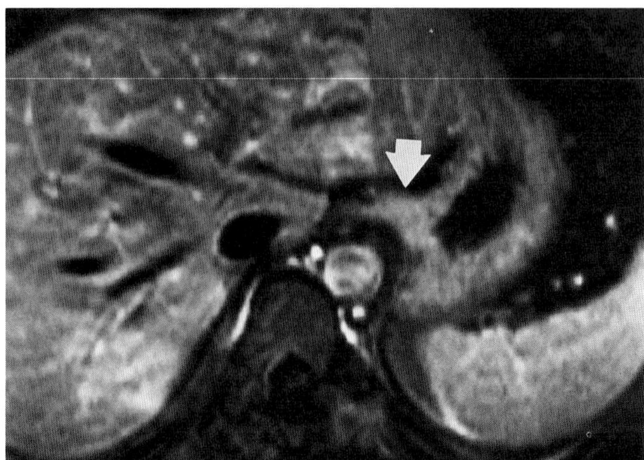

FIG. 7. Normal stomach. The normal gastric wall enhances in a moderate fashion on Gd-DTPA-enhanced T1FS images. In the collapsed state normal wall may usually be distinguished from disease processes because of the good contrast resolution of this technique. The image is obtained at the level of the GE junction (*arrow*).

Varices

Varices may be observed in patients with portal hypertension or splenic vein thrombosis. Splenic vein thrombosis causes enlargement of short gastric veins along the greater curvature in the absence of lesser curvature varices.

Malignant Tumors

Adenocarcinomas

Although the incidence of gastric carcinoma is now substantially lower than it was several decades ago, 25,000 cases are diagnosed each year in the United States. The incidence varies in different countries, with maximum rates of 70 per 100,000 males in Japan (18,19). The male to female disease ratio is approximately 2:1. These lesions are almost always adenocarcinomas and are morphologically categorized as ulcerating, polypoid, superficial spreading, or linitis plastica. Gastric cancer spreads by (a) hematogenous metastasis to lung and liver, (b) direct extension to contiguous structures, (c) lymph node metastasis, and (d) intraperitoneal seeding. The overall prognosis is poor.

The majority of carcinomas arise in the antrum and body of the stomach. Symptoms tend to be vague, with dyspepsia and anorexia preceding weight loss. Later symptoms of vomiting and hematemesis may occur in association with a palpable epigastric mass and anemia.

MRI is sensitive in the detection of the peritoneal spread of disease because of high contrast resolution of enhancing tumor deposits in a background of suppressed fat on Gd-DTPA-enhanced fat-suppressed images. The role of CT or MRI in the staging of gastric cancer is uncertain at present; however, demonstration of tumor bulk and detection of liver metastases are reliably performed by both techniques (Fig. 8). Although MRI cannot detect microscopic lymph node involvement, the detection of enlarged adenopathy is comparable to that of CT (Fig. 9).

Leiomyosarcomas

Leiomyosarcomas frequently have a large extragastric tumor bulk that assists in differentiating this entity from either adenocarcinoma or lymphoma. Central necrosis is common. Liver metastases and extension to adjacent viscera are the most common forms of tumor extension.

Lymphomas

The stomach is the segment of the gastrointestinal tract most frequently involved with lymphoma. Non-Hodgkin's lymphoma is the most common type (20). Typically, substantial wall thickening is present; however, gastric distensibility is maintained so that obstruction is unusual (Fig. 10). Mesenteric and retroperitoneal lymphadenopathy also suggest the diagnosis. Hodgkin's disease tends to be a more desmoplastic lesion, and gastric luminal narrowing is frequently present.

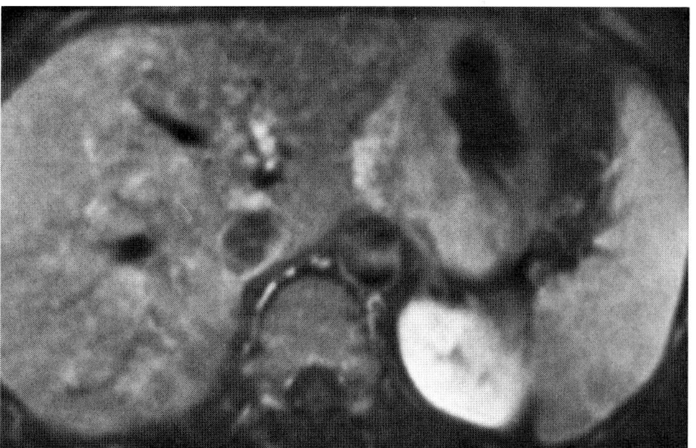

FIG. 8. Adenocarcinoma of the stomach. Gd-DTPA-enhanced T1FS image in a 37-year-old man. A large tumor arises from the cardia of the stomach. No invasion of adjacent organs was demonstrated on the MR images, and this was confirmed at surgery.

Metastases

Metastases to the stomach occur by direct extension or hematogenous or lymphatic spread. Breast cancer metastases are noteworthy in that submucosal involvement of the stomach can occur with an appearance indistinguishable from scirrhous carcinoma.

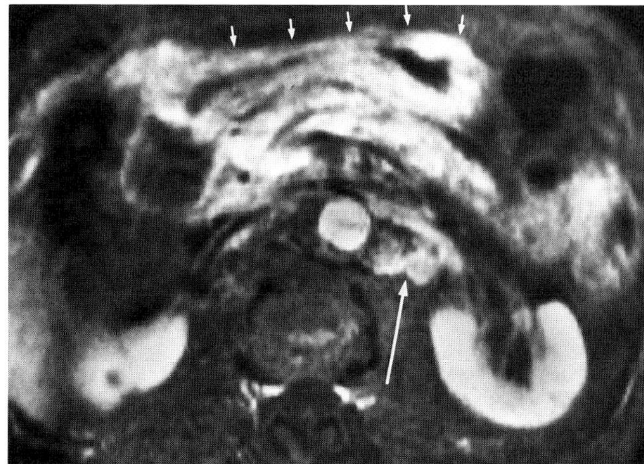

FIG. 9. Adenocarcinoma of the stomach. Gd-DTPA-enhanced T1FS image in a 72-year-old man with gastric cancer involving the body and antrum of the stomach in a circumferential fashion (*small arrows*). Associated lymphadenopathy in a left paraaortic location is present (*large arrow*).

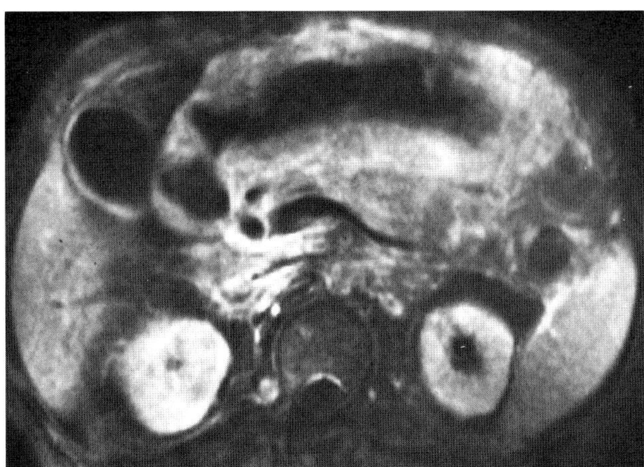

FIG. 10. Non-Hodgkin's lymphoma of the stomach. Gd-DTPA-enhanced T1FS image in a 74-year-old man with non-Hodgkin's lymphoma of the stomach. Substantial circumferential thickening of the gastric wall is present. Extensive retroperitoneal adenopathy is also identified (better seen on other tomographic sections) and is suggestive of the diagnosis.

Inflammation—Gastric Ulcers

Benign gastric ulcer has its peak incidence in middle age and is usually located on the lesser curvature of the stomach. Three types are described. Type I ulcers occur in patients with normal or low gastric acid output. These are associated with antral gastritis and the presence of *Helicobacter* pylori in gastric aspirate cultures. Type II ulcers are associated with duodenal ulcers and are frequently prepyloric in location. Type III ulcers typically are formed in the antrum and are associated with the use of nonsteroidal antiinflammatory medications.

A variety of other inflammatory conditions involve the stomach, including Crohn's disease, tuberculosis, and sarcoidosis. Crohn's disease involving the stomach is uncommon, with less than 5% of patients being affected (21). Marked hypertrophy of the gastric rugae may be seen in Zollinger-Ellison syndrome or Menetrier disease.

THE SMALL INTESTINE

Normal Anatomy

The adult small intestine measures 15 to 18 feet from the ligament of Treitz to the ileocecal valve. The duodenum begins at the pylorus and extends in a C-shaped curve around the head of the pancreas to meet the jejunum at the duodenojejunal flexure. The pancreatic and common bile ducts enter the second portion of the duodenum on the posteromedial side. In comparison to jejunum, the ileum has a narrower lumen with fewer mucosal folds and a greater number of mesenteric vascular arcades. MRI has been limited in assessing the small bowel because of the lack of a suitable oral contrast agent. The oral formulation of Gd-DTPA has been shown to produce a relatively uniform high SI throughout all segments of small bowel (22). Alternatively, negative contrast agents, either ferrous (iron oxide) (23) or diamagnetic perfluoroctylbromide (PFOB) (24), produce relatively uniform low SI throughout the small bowel. In the absence of oral contrast agent, however, fat-suppressed spin echo alone or in combination with intravenous Gd-DTPA adequately demonstrates small bowel. Normal small bowel on fat-suppressed images has a feathery appearance because of the presence of valvulae conniventes and, after intravenous Gd-DTPA, enhances in a moderately uniform fashion (Fig. 11). The wall thickness of normal small bowel should not exceed 3 to 4 mm.

MR Technique

Fat-suppressed spin echo and Gd-DTPA-enhanced fat-suppressed spin echo have been effective in studying small bowel. A critical element in successful MR examination is having the patient fast for at least 5 hours to reduce gut motility. The role and type of oral contrast agent have not been defined; however, a negative agent may be useful in combination with intravenous Gd-DTPA or when examining for adenopathy. A positive agent would be useful in examining for small bowel fistula or in trying to distinguish bowel from abscess.

Congenital Abnormalities

Rotational abnormalities of small bowel are not infrequent. The most common form, nonrotation, is readily apparent on tomographic images by demonstration of the lack of passage of the third and fourth parts of the duodenum anterior to the aorta. Duplication cysts are small and located distally in the small bowel along the mesenteric wall.

A Meckel's diverticulum is a remnant of the omphalomesenteric duct and occurs within 25 cm of the ileocecal valve (25). These diverticula frequently contain gastric mucosa and thus may be recognized on MR images because gastric mucosa enhances to a greater extent than does the mucosa of adjacent small or large bowel (Fig. 12).

Mass Lesions

Small intestinal neoplasms are most commonly found in the terminal ileum. These tumors account for less than 5% of all gastrointestinal tract neoplasms.

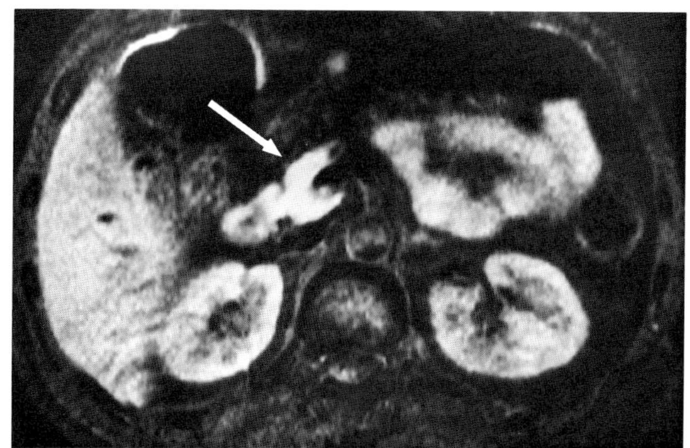

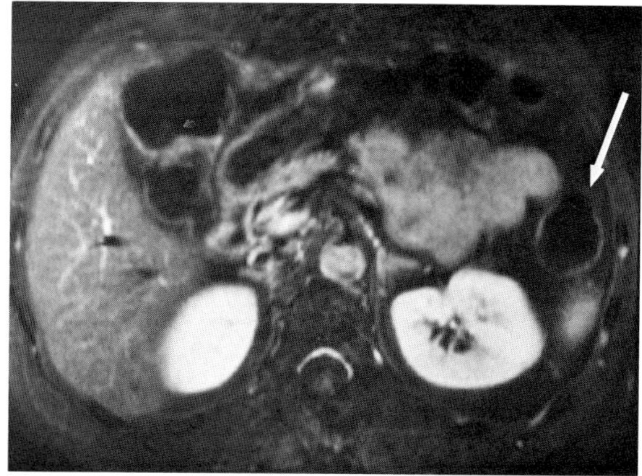

FIG. 11. Normal bowel. T1FS (**A**) and Gd-DTPA-enhanced T1FS (**B**) MR images. On the precontrast image jejunum has a typical feathery appearance, which readily distinguishes jejunum from the more homogeneous high SI of pancreas (*arrow*). After intravenous contrast administration, jejunum and other bowel segments enhance to a minor extent, which can be appreciated in the normal descending colon (*arrow*). Reprinted with permission from ref. 62.

Benign Tumors

Small bowel lesions are rare; these are equally divided between benign and malignant types (26). Small intestinal adenomas are rare in comparison to colonic polyps. They are usually asymptomatic, although symptoms may arise as a result of bleeding or obstruction associated with intussusception. Hamartoma polyps may occur as solitary lesions or be multiple, often in association with Peutz-Jeghers syndrome. Multiple adenomatous polyps, particularly of the duodenum, may occur in familial adenomatous polyposis syndromes. Juvenile polyps are considered to be a form of hamartomatous polyp which may occur in the small bowel as well as the colon. Other small bowel benign tumors include leiomyomas (Fig. 13), lipomas, neurofibromas, and fibromas.

Varices

Duodenal varices may exist in patients with or without portal vein obstruction. These have life-threatening potential but have been treated successfully by sclerotherapy (27,28).

Malignant Tumors

Adenocarcinomas

Adenocarcinomas account for 50% of malignant small bowel tumors (29,30). Primary small intestinal adenocarcinomas arise most commonly in the duodenum and proximal jejunum. These tumors are frequently asymptomatic for prolonged periods, and metastases are present in up to 80% of cases at the time of surgical resection. Tumor bulk, invasion of adjacent structures, and hepatic metastases are well shown on MR images (Fig. 14).

Carcinoid Tumors

Carcinoid is the most common primary neoplasm in the small intestine. Carcinoid tumors are of neuroendocrine origin. The appendix is a common site (31), where the tumor is virtually always benign. The most frequent location of malignant carcinoid tumors is the rectum,

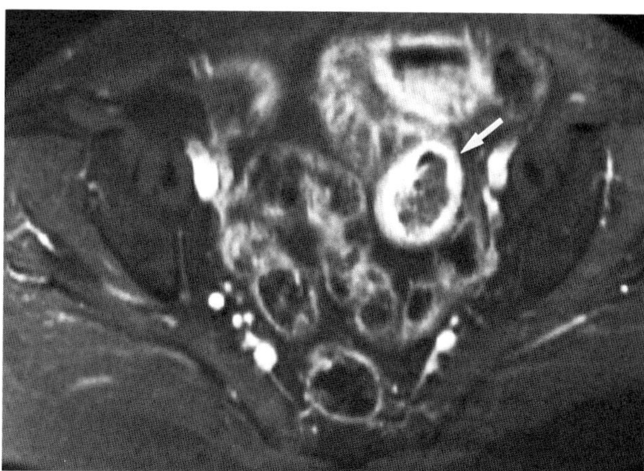

FIG. 12. Meckel's diverticulum. Gd-DTPA-enhanced T1FS image in a 66-year-old woman with a Meckel's diverticulum who presented with lower GI bleeding. The wall of the diverticulum (*arrow*) enhances to a greater extent than neighboring colon, permitting detection. The presence of gastric mucosa probably accounts for the increased contrast enhancement.

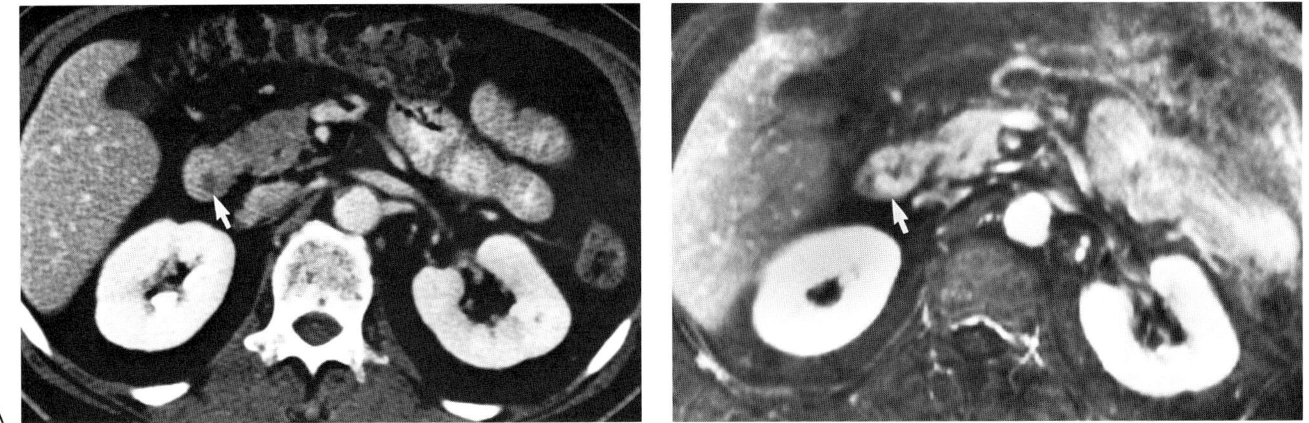

FIG. 13. Leiomyoma. CT (**A**) and contrast-enhanced T1FS (**B**) images in a 66-year-old man with a leiomyoma of the second part of the duodenum. The tumor appears as a filling defect on the contrast-enhanced CT images (*arrow*, A) while tumor enhancement is appreciated on the contrast enhanced MR image (*arrow*, B).

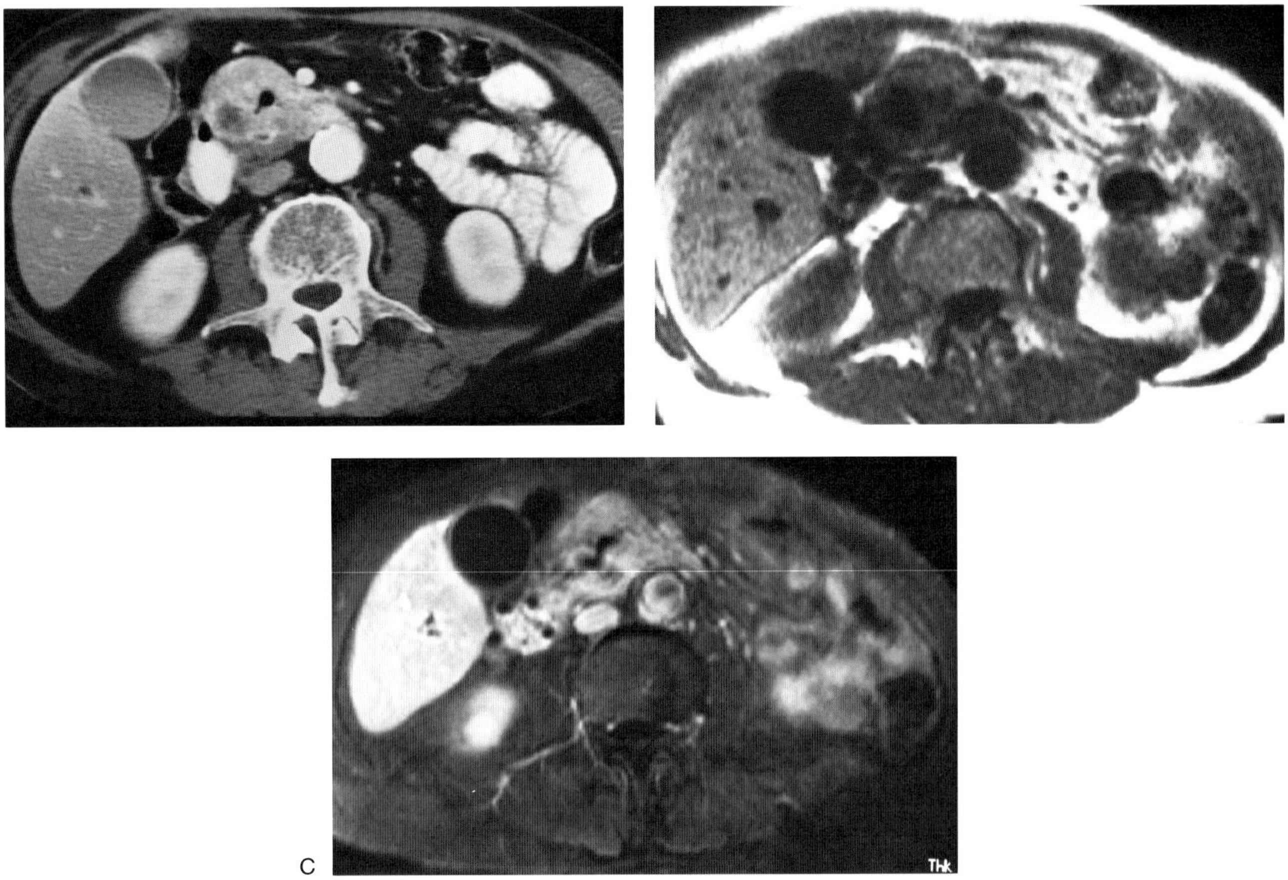

FIG. 14. Duodenal cancer. Dynamic contrast-enhanced CT (**A**), FLASH (**B**), and postcontrast T1FS (**C**) images in a 62-year-old man with duodenal cancer. Tumor size and extent are well demonstrated on the CT and postcontrast T1FS images. Reprinted with permission from ref. 62.

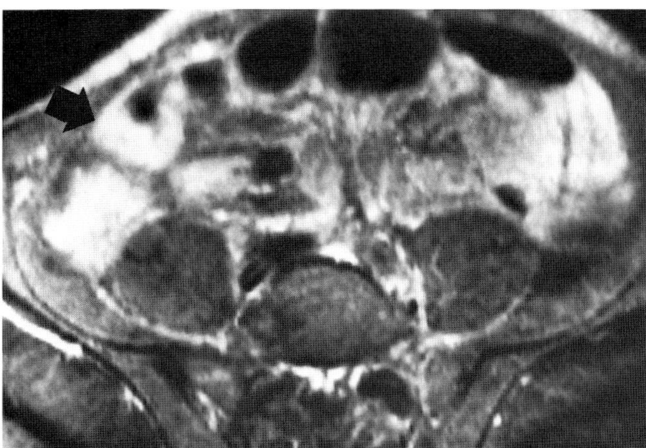

FIG. 15. Carcinoid tumor. Gd-DTPA-enhanced T1FS image in a 48-year-old man with carcinoid tumor. Asymmetrical thickening of the wall of a distal loop of ileum is present, consistent with the primary tumor (*arrow*).

followed by the distal ileum. The primary malignant tumor frequently is small and is not detected on tomographic images. On occasion, asymmetrical thickening of the bowel wall with moderate enhancement may be appreciated (Fig. 15). Desmoplastic fibrotic tissue in the root of the mesentery is characteristic of the tumor. Liver metastases are frequently hypervascular and possess a distinct ring enhancement pattern on dynamic Gd-DTPA-enhanced FLASH images (Fig. 16).

Lymphomas

Primary small intestinal lymphoma arises from mural lymphoid tissue, most commonly in the terminal ileum. The most frequent cell types to involve the small bowel are diffuse histiocytic and poorly differentiated lymphocytic lymphoma (32). These tumors may remain well localized as polypoid or ulcerating lesions, or they may diffusely infiltrate a long segment of intestine. Multiple lesions are found in 20% of cases. Secondary intestinal involvement may be seen in up to 50% of cases of advanced lymphoma arising outside the abdominal cavity. Thickening of bowel wall is appreciated on MR images, and contrast enhancement is usually moderate (Fig. 17). The frequent presence of lymph nodes in the mesentery suggests the diagnosis. Splenic involvement and retroperitoneal metastases are also features suggestive of the diagnosis.

Leiomyosarcomas

Leiomyosarcomas are the most common small bowel sarcomas. They are found most frequently in the ileum and least often in the duodenum (33). Leiomyosarcomas tend to be vascular and undergo central necrosis. A large exophytic component of the tumor is common (Fig. 18).

Metastases

Small bowel metastases occur most frequently via peritoneal seeding or by direct extension along the mesentery and are seen in ovarian, gastric, and pancreatic cancer. Hematogenous metastases occur less commonly and are seen in patients with lung or breast cancer or melanoma. Hematogenous metastases are found on the antimesenteric surface of the bowel wall.

Inflammation

Crohn's disease is the most common inflammatory condition to affect the small bowel in North America.

A

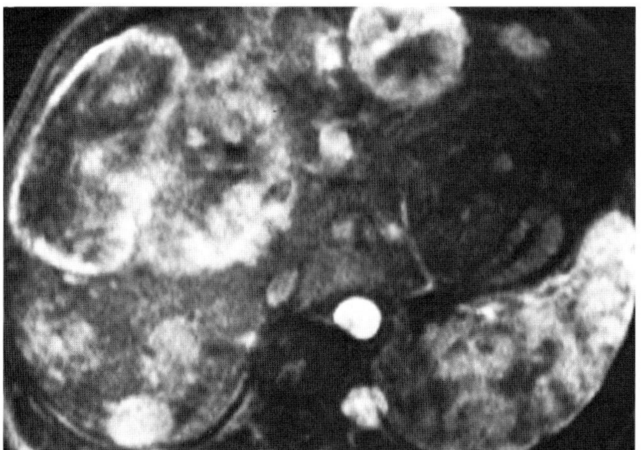

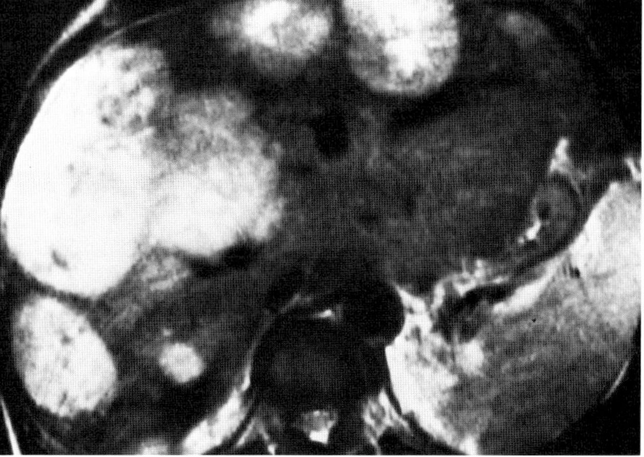

B

FIG. 16. Carcinoid liver metastases. One-second postcontrast FLASH (**A**) and T2-weighted (512 × 512) RARE (**B**) images in a 48-year-old man with carcinoid tumor. Vascular metastases from carcinoid tumor have a typical ring enhancement pattern on immediate postcontrast images (A). These lesions also are high in SI on T2-weighted images (B), which is typical for vascular metastases.

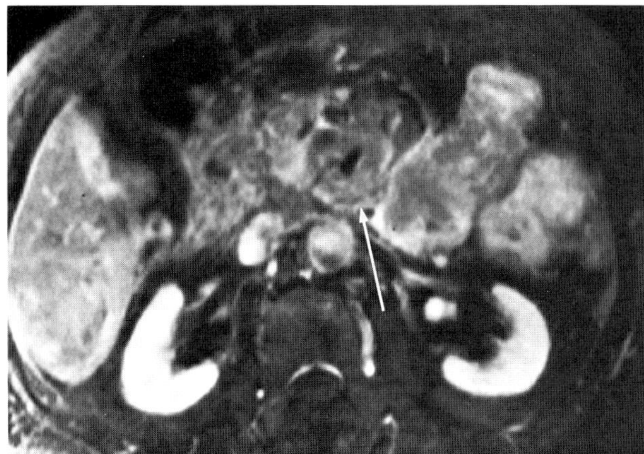

FIG. 17. Lymphoma of small bowel. Gd-DTPA-enhanced T1FS image in a 52-year-old man with non-Hodgkin's lymphoma. Abnormal thickened loops of jejunum are present with heterogeneous enhancement. Wall thickness of >1 cm is common in lymphoma (*arrow*).

Identification of the site of involvement and the extent of bowel disease is important for the assessment of response to medical management over time and to indicate when surgery may be advisable (34,35). Approximately 30% of Crohn's patients have exclusively small bowel disease, and the majority of that is confined to the distal ileum (36,37). Forty percent of patients with Crohn's disease will have involvement of the distal ileum and proximal colon. Five percent will manifest primary Crohn's disease in the jejunum or duodenum. Twenty to thirty percent will have isolated colon involvement (38). Gd-DTPA-enhanced fat-suppressed MR images are very sensitive in the detection of Crohn's disease. MR findings include full-thickness wall involvement, circumferential involvement of segments interspersed with segments of asymmetrical involvement, skip lesions, and inflammatory stranding in the mesentery. Mesenteric stranding is due to dilated vasa recta and sinus tracts. Associated findings include the presence of inflammatory nodes and abscesses. The length of diseased bowel, the bowel wall thickness, and the signal intensity increase from precontrast to postcontrast fat-suppressed images have been shown to correlate with disease activity (Table 1)(39). The following criteria are those we use on MR images to determine mild, moderate, and severe bowel inflammation. Mild disease is determined by the presence of two of the following findings: involvement of <5 cm of bowel, wall thickening of <5 mm, and contrast enhancement of <50% (Fig. 19). The appreciation of bowel wall >4 mm thick is necessary to suggest the presence of mild IBD as small bowel in patients with no bowel symptoms occasionally shows substantial enhancement without wall thickening. Moderate disease is determined by the presence of wall thickening of 0.5 to 1.0 cm and contrast enhancement of <100% (Fig. 20). Wall thickening of >1 cm and contrast enhancement of >100% is consistent with severe disease (Fig. 21). The typical appearance of Crohn's disease on Gd-DTPA-enhanced MR images is a thickened, high-SI segment of distal ileum which is often associated with asymmetrical involvement of the cecum (Fig. 22). Segments of fixed, stenotic bowel can result in dilated proximal small bowel (Fig. 23).

Reflux Ileitis

Reflux or backwash ileitis is a condition associated with severe IBD of the right side of the colon causing a

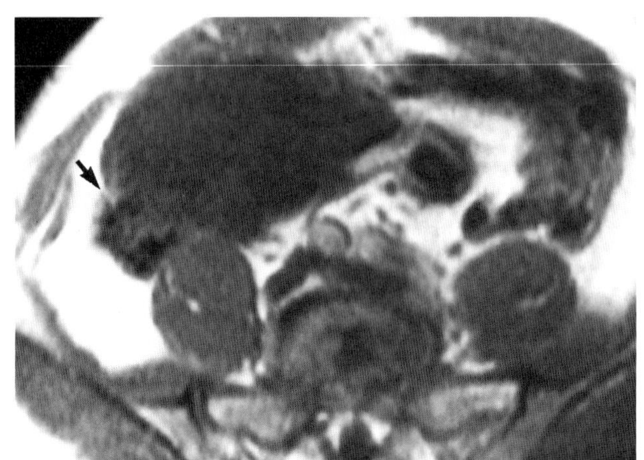

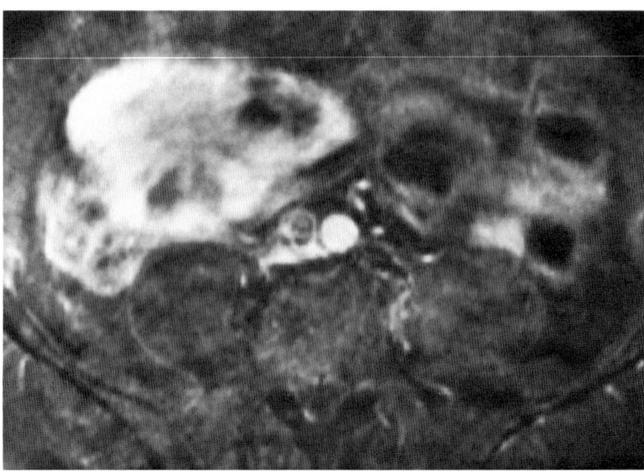

FIG. 18. Leiomyosarcoma. FLASH (**A**) and contrast-enhanced T1FS (**B**) MR images in a 75-year-old man with leiomyosarcoma arising from small bowel. A large tumor is present in the lower right abdomen which invades and/or arises from adjacent bowel (*arrow*, A). The exophytic nature of the tumor is reflected by the lack of substantial bowel obstruction despite the tumor's large size. Following contrast administration the tumor enhances heterogenously and central necrotic regions are demonstrated (B).

TABLE 1. *Comparison of MRI and surgical/pathological findings*

Patient	Inflammation		Length of involvement (cm)		Bowel wall thickness (cm)	
	MR	Surgery	MR	Surgery	MR	Surgery
1	S	S	>10.0	70.0	>1.0	1.0
2	S	S	>10.0	20.0	>1.0	1.2
3	S	S	>10.0	36.0	>1.0	0.7
4	S	S	>10.0	10.0	>1.0	>1.0
5	S	S	10.0	12.0	>1.0	0.8
6	S	S	>10.0 (skip lesions)	94.0 (skip lesions)	1.0	1.0
7	S	S	>10.0	48.0	>1.0	1.4
8	M	S	>10.0	35.0 (skip lesions)	<1.0	0.7
9	M	M	10.0	68.0	<1.0	<1.0
10	S	M	>10.0	97.0	1.0	0.5

S, severe; M, moderate.

patulous ileocecal valve and reflux of colon contents into the terminal ileum. This is most commonly observed in the context of full colon involvement with ulcerative colitis. The lumen of the ileum is moderately dilated and the wall is inflamed (Fig. 24).

Infection

Acute inflammation may be due to a variety of bacterial or viral pathogens. Bowel diseases caused by *Yersinia enterocolitica* infection include acute gastroenteritis, terminal ileitis, mesenteric lymphadenitis, and colitis (40). *Yersinia* ileitis is most common in young adults, and preoperative differentiation from appendicitis may not be possible. The imaging features of *Yersinia* enterocolitis may resemble those of Crohn's disease. Tuberculosis of the intestine caused by the bovine strain of the tuberculosis mycobacteria is rare in North America. Secondary intestinal tuberculosis (TB) due to swallowing the human pathogen occurs in 1% of patients with pulmonary TB. The terminal ileum is most commonly involved, and symptoms result from acute inflammation or late fibrotic stenosis (41). *Mycobacterium avium intracellulare* is a pathogen that can affect bowel. The infection is increasing in frequency because of the association with human immunodeficiency virus infection. *Campylobacter jejuni* may produce diarrhea, severe gastroenteritis, or a colitis that may resemble idiopathic ulcerative colitis (42). *Giardia lamblia* and *Strongyloides stercoralis* are protozoa that typically involve proximal small bowel.

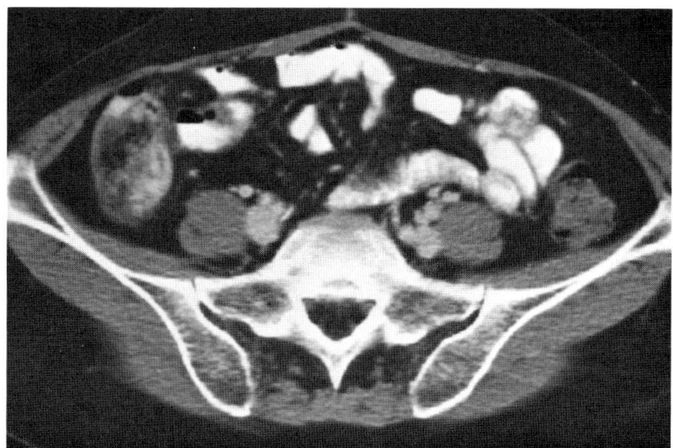
A

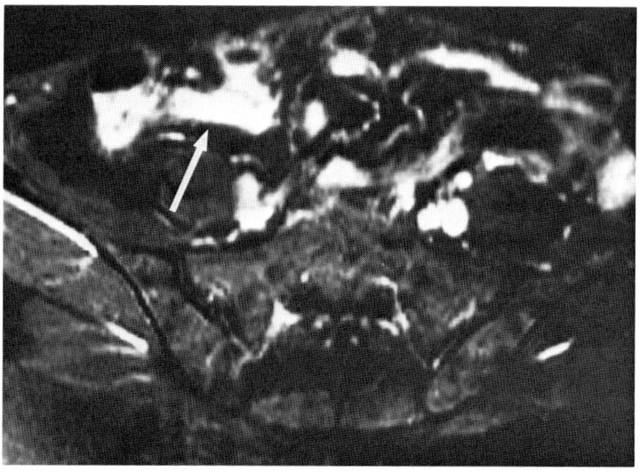
B

FIG. 19. Mild bowel inflammation. Contrast-enhanced CT (**A**) and postcontrast T1FS (**B**) images in a 38-year-old woman with Crohn's disease of the terminal ileum. The CT study demonstrates normal wall thickness of the terminal ileum; on the postcontrast T1FS image, however, enhancement of the distal 4 cm of terminal ileum was identified (*white arrow*), which was compatible with mild inflammatory disease found at endoscopy. High-SI bowel content is present in multiple bowel loops. The extension of high SI to the serosal surface in the diseased terminal ileum is consistent with bowel wall inflammation and distinguishes this entity from high-SI bowel content. Reprinted with permission from ref. 62.

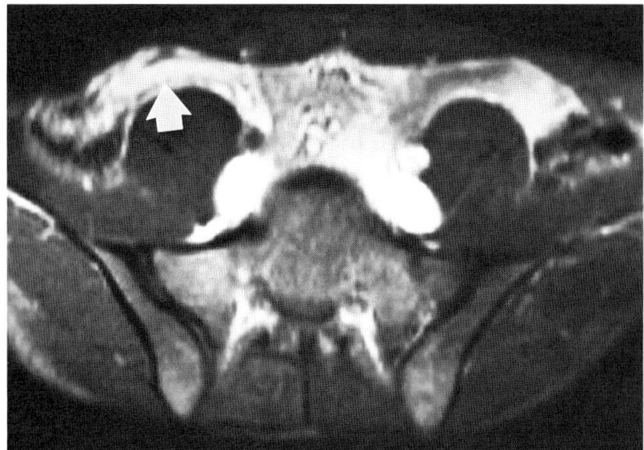

FIG. 20. Moderate Crohn's disease. Gd-DTPA-enhanced T1FS image in an 18-year-old man with Crohn's disease. Inflammatory disease of the terminal ileum is shown (*arrow*), with a wall thickness of 8 mm, 7 cm of diseased bowel, and 92% contrast enhancement. These features are consistent with moderate disease.

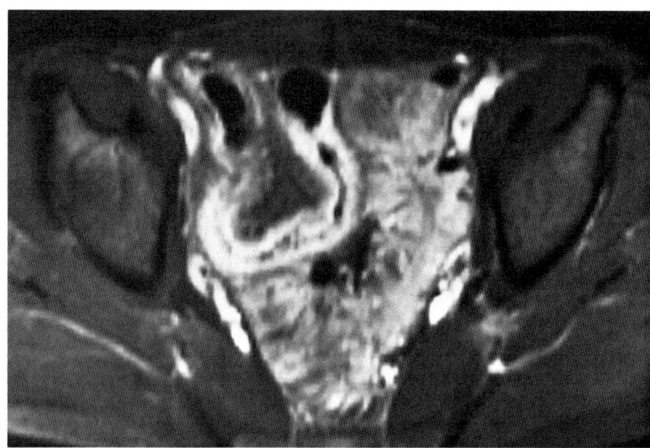

FIG. 21. Severe Crohn's disease. Gd-DTPA-enhanced T1FS image in a 24-year-old man with Crohn's disease. A long segment of IBD is shown with a wall thickness of 1 cm, 15 cm of diseased bowel, and 138% contrast enhancement. These are features consistent with severe disease.

A B C D

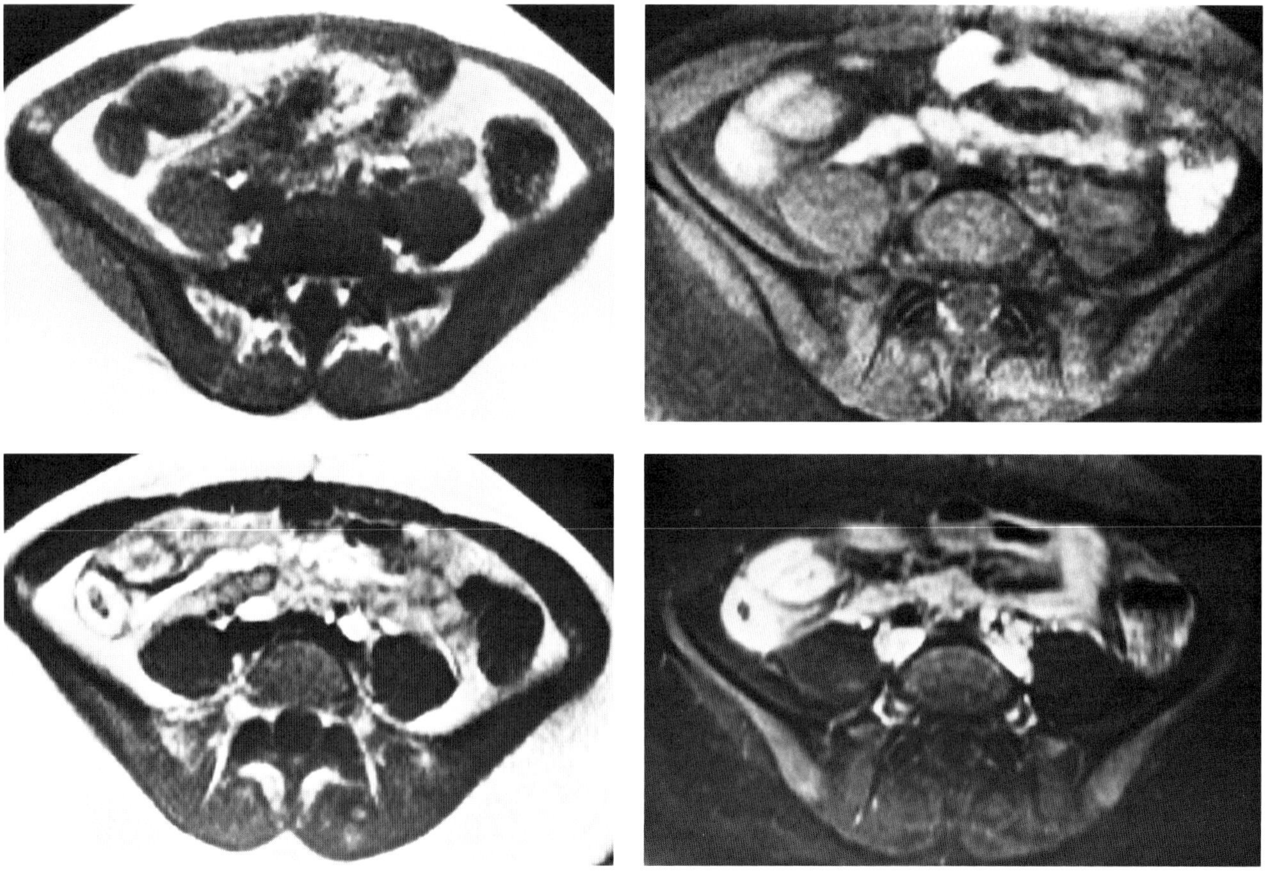

FIG. 22. Crohn's disease with severe inflammatory changes. Precontrast FLASH (**A**), precontrast T1FS (**B**), 1-second postcontrast FLASH (**C**), and postcontrast T1FS (**D**) images in a 23-year-old woman with Crohn's disease. Increased thickness of the terminal ileum and ascending colon is apparent, and these areas enhance substantially (>100%) after contrast administration. Enhancement of bowel on the 1-second postcontrast FLASH image is apparent, and this finding is identified only in cases of severe inflammation. Bowel content, which is high in SI on the precontrast T1FS image, is low in SI on the postcontrast T1FS image. Reprinted with permission from ref. 62.

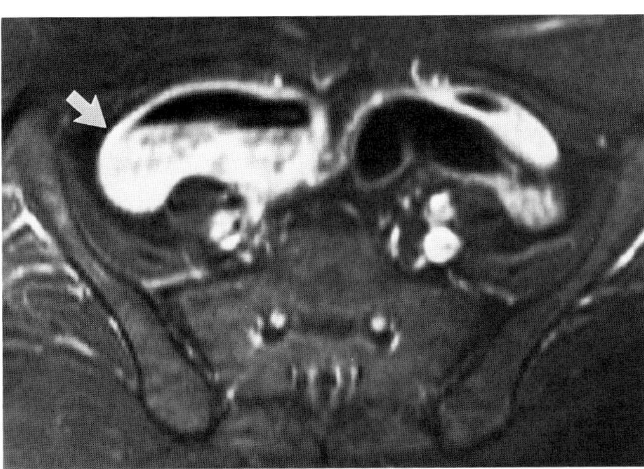

FIG. 23. Crohn's disease with dilated stagnant bowel loops. Gd-DTPA-enhanced T1FS image in a 28-year-old woman with Crohn's disease and severe stenosis of the terminal ileum and ascending colon. A large, relatively stagnant loop of ileum proximal to the stenotic bowel contains a substantial volume of debris (*arrow*).

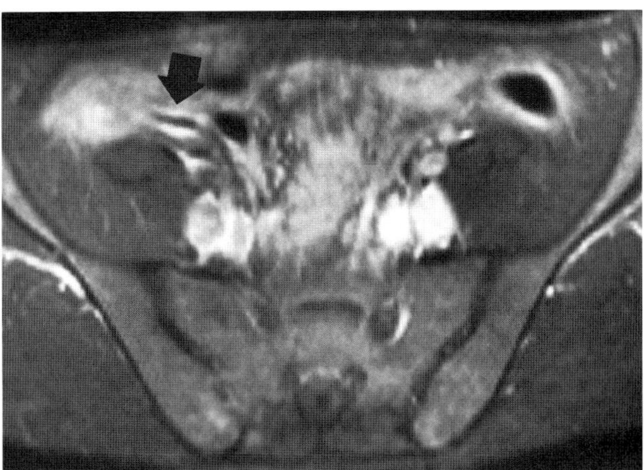

FIG. 24. Reflux ileitis. Gd-DTPA-enhanced T1FS image in a 26-year-old man with full colon involvement with ulcerative colitis. Mild dilatation and increased mural enhancement of the terminal ileum (*arrow*) is consistent with reflux ileitis.

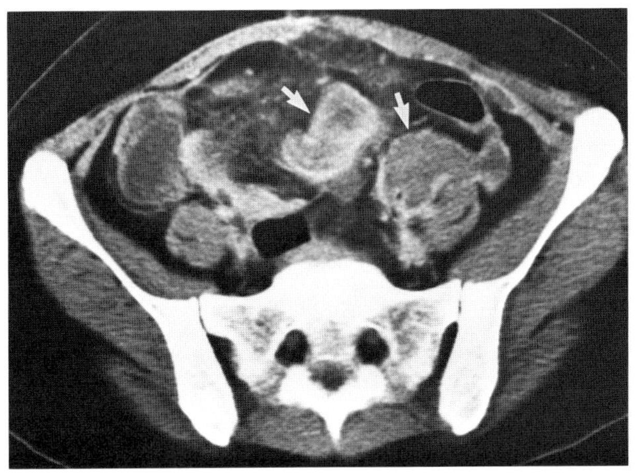

A

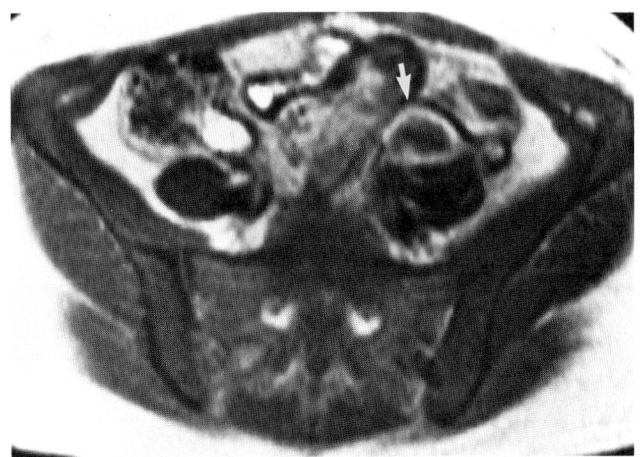

B

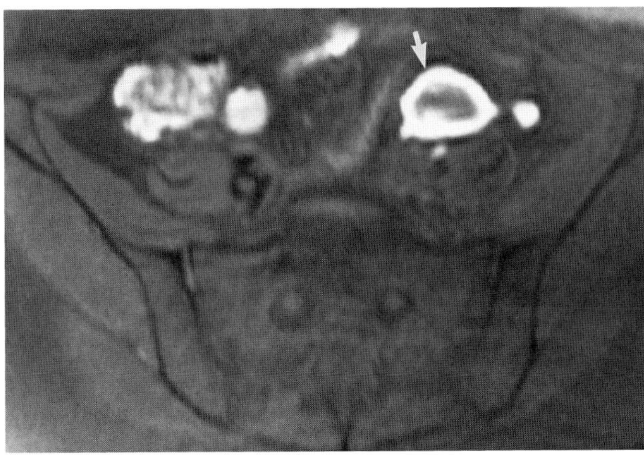

C

FIG. 25. Submucosal hemorrhage. CT (**A**), FLASH (**B**), and T1FS (**C**) images in a 26-year-old woman with submucosal hemorrhage. One week after hysterectomy this woman developed abdominal pain and lower GI bleeding, and peristalsis remained diminished after surgery. The CT image demonstrated abnormal thickening of the wall of small bowel loops (*arrows,* A). Increased SI of the bowel wall on the FLASH images becomes more conspicuous after fat suppression (*arrow,* B, C). This finding is consistent with submucosal hemorrhage. The patient had undergone vigorous small bowel retraction during the hysterectomy.

Submucosal Fluid

Submucosal edema can result from a number of causes including congestive heart failure, hypoalbuminemia, vasculitis (such as polyarteritis nodosa), radiation changes, and lymphangiectasia. A specific role for MRI in assessing submucosal disease is in the detection of submucosal hemorrhage. MRI is more sensitive than CT in the detection of blood and can better evaluate the presence of submucosal hemorrhage secondary to trauma or medication (Fig. 25).

THE COLON

Normal Anatomy

The ascending and descending colon is located in the anterior pararenal space. The transverse colon is located anteriorly in the peritoneal cavity suspended by the transverse mesocolon, which originates from the peritoneal covering of the anterior surface of the pancreas. The superior surface of the transverse colon is connected to the greater curvature of the stomach by the gastrocolic ligament. The sigmoid colon is mobile, suspended on a mesentery, and the rectum is retroperitoneal. Normal bowel wall thickness does not exceed 4 mm. The colonic luminal diameter is greatest in the cecum, which gradually narrows distally to the level of the rectal ampulla, where it again dilates. Normal sigmoid colon is illustrated in Fig. 26.

MR Technique

The technique and considerations for studying the colon are the same as for the small bowel. Intravenous glucagon has been used to improve the image quality of the rectum. Endorectal coil imaging of the rectum improves the signal to noise ratio and has met with success in the evaluation of rectal cancer.

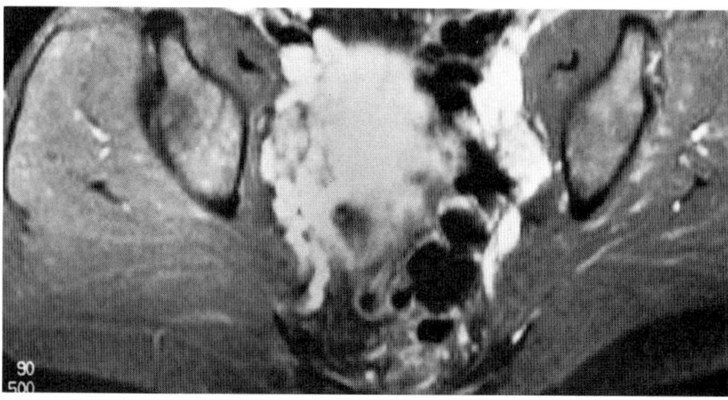

FIG. 26. Normal colon. Gd-DTPA-enhanced T1FS image of normal sigmoid colon. The colon is thin walled and enhances <30%.

Mass Lesions

Benign Tumors

A polyp is a descriptive term denoting a demarcated projection above the epithelial surface of the bowel lumen. Polyps may vary in size from diminutive 1- to 2-mm polyps to large lesions several centimeters in diameter (43). The most common polyp of the large intestine is the hyperplastic polyp. This lesion is usually less than 5 mm and results from a nonneoplastic alteration in cell growth and maturation (44). Juvenile polyps are retention polyps most frequently found in children under 10 years of age. They occur in approximately 1% of asymptomatic children (45) and may result in bleeding, anal protrusion, or transient intussusception with abdominal pain.

Adenomatous polyps are the most common true neoplasms of the colon. They are morphologically categorized as tubular, tubulovillous, or villous. The characteristic dysplastic changes in these polyps consist of distortion of cellular morphology and nuclear changes of hyperchromatism and increased mitotic activity. Adenomas are commonly observed in geographic areas with a high incidence of colorectal carcinoma. The synchronous occurrence of adenomatous polyps and carcinoma is not uncommon (46). Polyps increase in frequency with age and are found with equal frequency in males and females. They are usually asymptomatic, although larger lesions may result in gastrointestinal tract bleed-

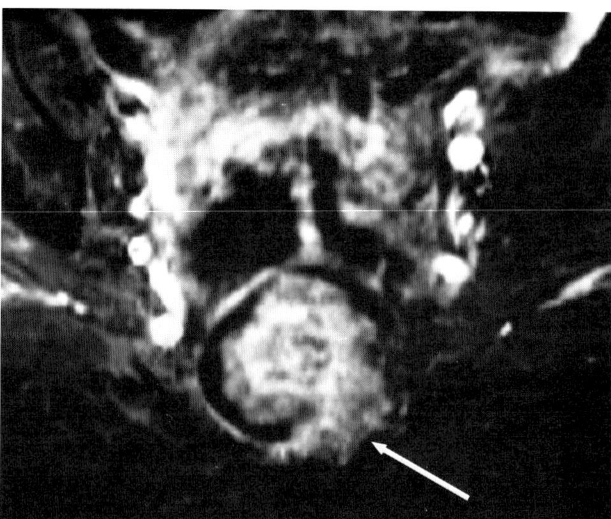

FIG. 27. Rectal villous adenoma. Gd-DTPA-enhanced T1FS image demonstrates a large, polypoid, heterogeneously enhancing tumor mass in a 56-year-old woman. The MR image suggests that the tumor has invaded the full thickness of the bowel wall with extension into perirectal fat (*white arrow*). Histopathological findings showed that the tumor was confined within the muscularis mucosa. Reprinted with permission from ref. 52.

ing, mucous diarrhea, or, rarely, obstructive symptoms. Villous adenomas often have a frondlike or cauliflower appearance and may be quite large. There is a greater tendency for villous adenomas than for other types of polyps to undergo malignant degeneration (Fig. 27).

Lipoma is the commonest intramural lesion of the colon but is a rare entity (0.2% to 0.3% on autopsy series) (46). Approximately 90% are submucosal and 10% are subserosal. Most are asymptomatic, although symptoms of changes in bowel habit or bleeding have been reported in patients with large lesions. The most common locations for colonic lipomas are the cecum, ascending colon, and sigmoid colon. The MR appearance of lipomas with T1-weighted and fat-suppressed T1-weighted images is pathognomonic. Lesions are high in SI on T1-weighted images and diminish in SI on fat-suppressed images (Fig. 28). Other benign colonic tumors include fibromas, leiomyomas, and neurofibromas. Leiomyomas occur uncommonly in the colon. Myxomas may arise from the appendix.

Varices

Rectal varices may develop in patients with portal hypertension. The incidence of hemorrhoids is not increased in these patients (47).

Malignant Tumors

Adenocarcinomas

Colorectal carcinoma is the second most common visceral cancer in North America. The estimated incidence in the United States in 1988 was 147,000 new cases (48). The 5-year survival is less than 50% (49). The incidence

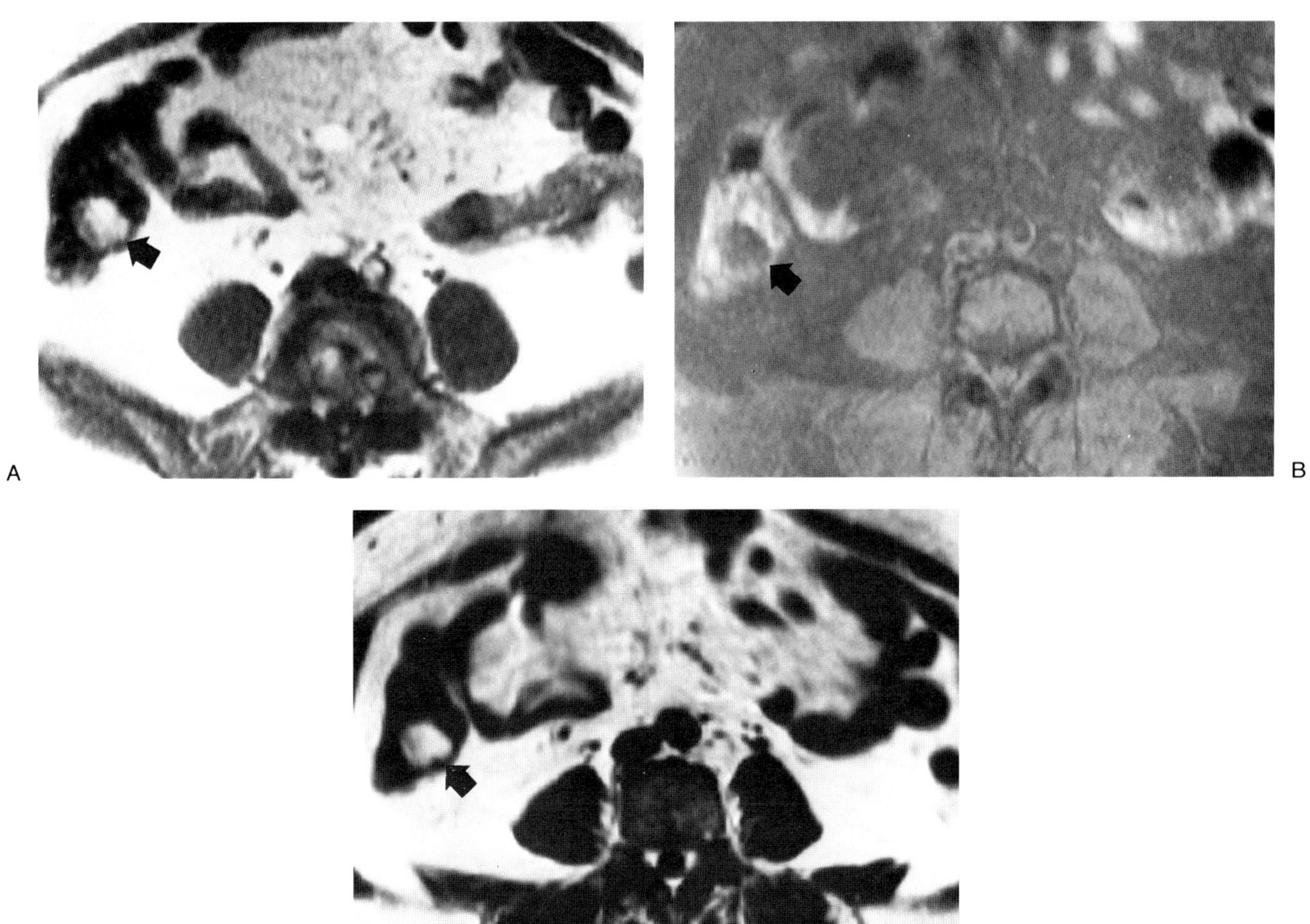

FIG. 28. Cecal lipoma. FLASH (**A**), T1FS (**B**), and water-suppressed spin echo (**C**) MR images in a 71-year-old woman. The FLASH image (A) demonstrates a well-defined high-SI mass in the cecum. The T1FS image (B) demonstrates attenuation of the signal intensity consistent with a fatty lesion. The water-suppressed spin echo image (C) shows that the mass does not attenuate, confirming the fatty nature of the lesion (*arrow* points to lipoma). Reprinted with permission from ref. 52.

increases with increasing age. Sporadic cancers are increased in first degree family relatives of patients with known colorectal cancers. Several congenital syndromes predispose to the development of these malignant neoplasms, including familial adenomatous polyposis syndromes and Lynch syndromes. Patients with chronic ulcerative colitis, Crohn's colitis, and previous ureterosigmoidostomies are also at increased risk. The rectum and sigmoid colon are the most frequent sites of occurrence; however, over the last few decades, right-sided cancers have increased in frequency (50,51). The classic clinical signs of colorectal cancer include alterations in bowel habit, rectal bleeding (either overt or occult), rectal or abdominal pain, and weight loss.

Adenocarcinoma of the colon is the most common malignant tumor of the gastrointestinal tract. Tumors are irregular soft tissue masses that can be polypoid, asymmetrical, or circumferential. Occasionally, the tumor may contain air and simulate diverticulitis (Fig. 29). Tomographic imaging is best used to demonstrate the exophytic extent of tumor and the presence of liver metastases (Fig. 30). Currently, MR is limited by the inability to determine the depth of tumor penetration of the wall and the inability to distinguish hyperplastic from neoplastic lymph nodes. Detection of nodal involvement is difficult, as involved nodes are frequently small. An attractive feature of MRI is the ability to image directly in the sagittal plane, which best demonstrates the length of disease in tumors involving the rectosigmoid colon (Fig. 31)(52). MRI is probably superior to CT in determining the intraperitoneal extent of tumor seeding due to the high soft tissue contrast on Gd-DTPA-enhanced MR images (Fig. 32).

One of the most widely used applications of MRI is in

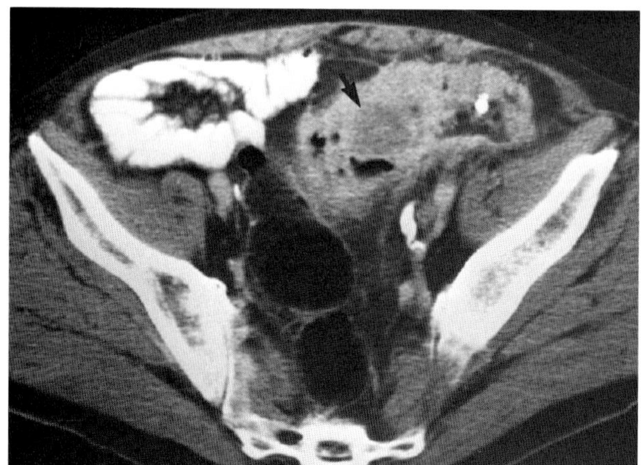

A

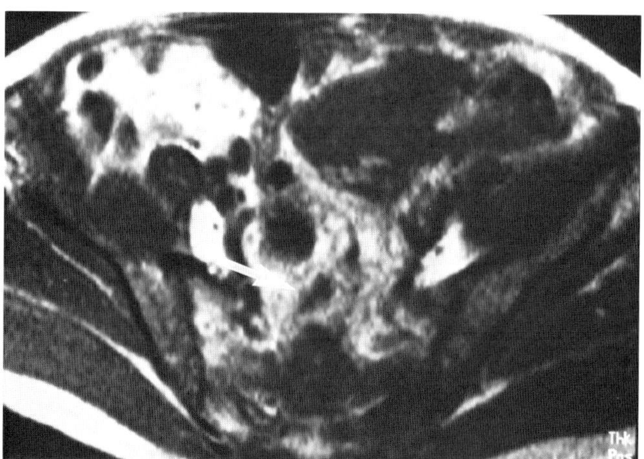

B

C

FIG. 29. Colon cancer simulating diverticulitis. CT (**A**), FLASH (**B**), and Gd-DTPA-enhanced T1FS (**C**) images in a 62-year-old man who presented with fever and bowel symptoms. The CT image demonstrates a large mass lesion containing air and a low-attenuation center (*arrow,* A), which were interpreted as consistent with diverticulitis with a diverticular abscess. The FLASH image demonstrates a large mass arising from the sigmoid colon with extensive inflammatory stranding in the pericolonic fat (*arrow,* B). On the Gd-DTPA-enhanced T1FS image, the low-attenuation center identified on the CT image is shown to enhance in a diminished fashion (*arrow,* C), which is not consistent with an abscess but is compatible with solid hypovascular tumor. At surgery a colon cancer with surrounding inflammatory changes was identified.

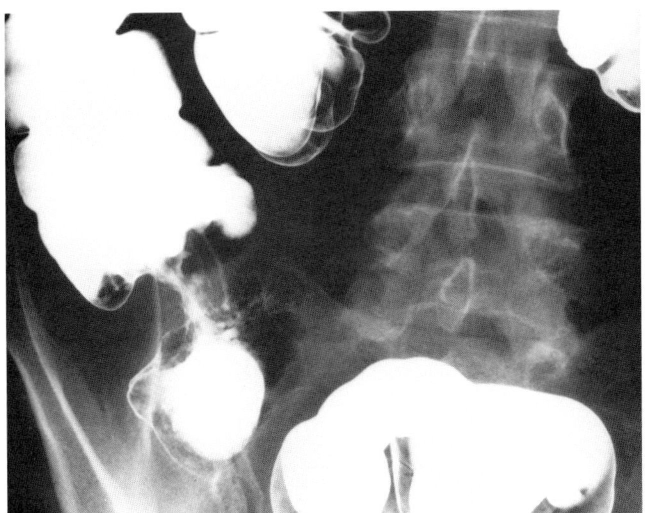

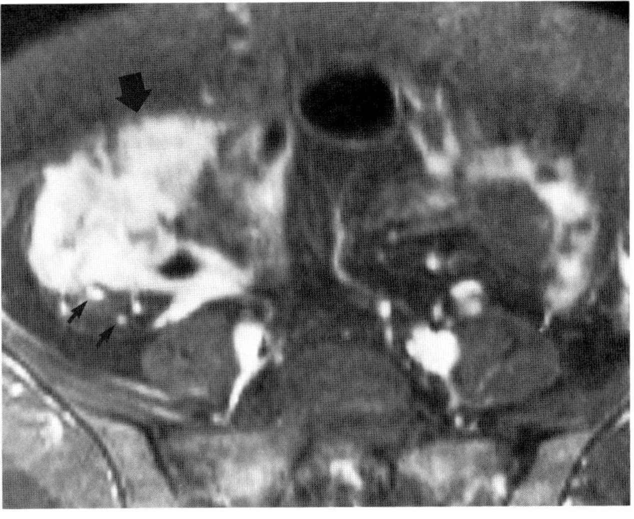

FIG. 30. Cecal adenocarcinoma. Barium enema (**A**) and Gd-DTPA-enhanced T1FS MR (**B**) images in a 48-year-old woman with cecal cancer. The barium enema image (A) demonstrates a circumferential adenocarcinoma of the cecum with a classic "apple core" appearance. Local extension of the tumor cannot be determined on the barium study. The Gd-DTPA-enhanced T1FS image (B) demonstrates a large heterogeneous adenocarcinoma with direct extension to the anterior abdominal wall (*large arrow*). Multiple small lymph nodes were also identified (*small arrows*). These nodes were histologically malignant. Reprinted with permission from ref. 52.

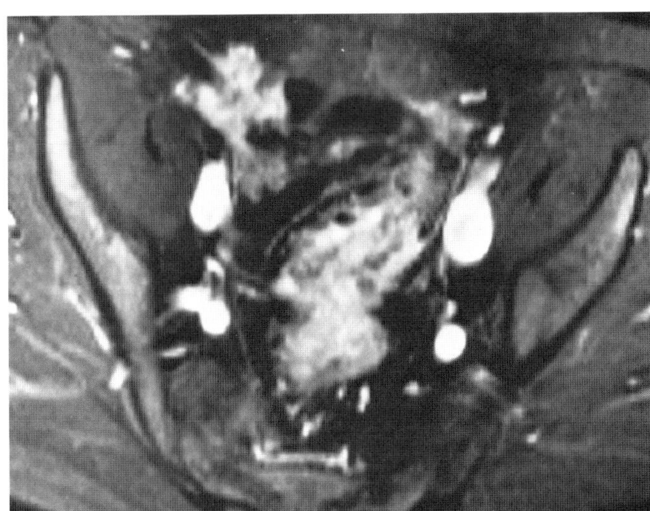

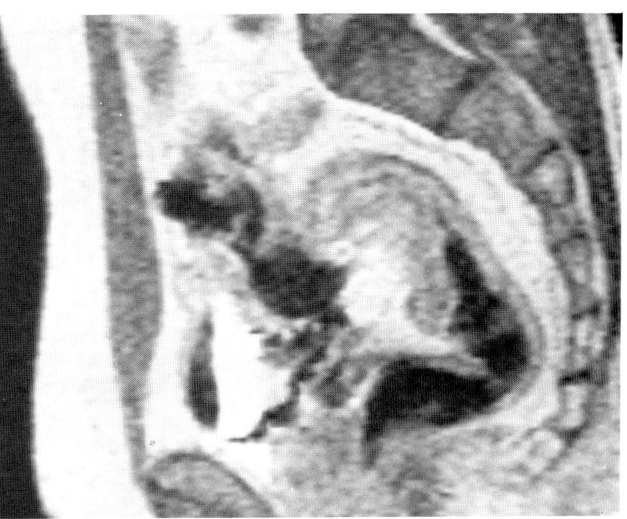

FIG. 31. Sigmoid adenocarcinoma. Gd-DTPA-enhanced T1FS (**A**) and 10-minute postcontrast sagittal FLASH (**B**) MR images in a 34-year-old man with colon cancer. The Gd-DTPA-enhanced T1FS image (A) demonstrates a large adenocarcinoma involving the sigmoid colon. Full-thickness invasion of the wall is apparent. The Gd-DTPA-enhanced sagittal FLASH image (B) demonstrates the longitudinal length of the tumor. Reprinted with permission from ref. 52.

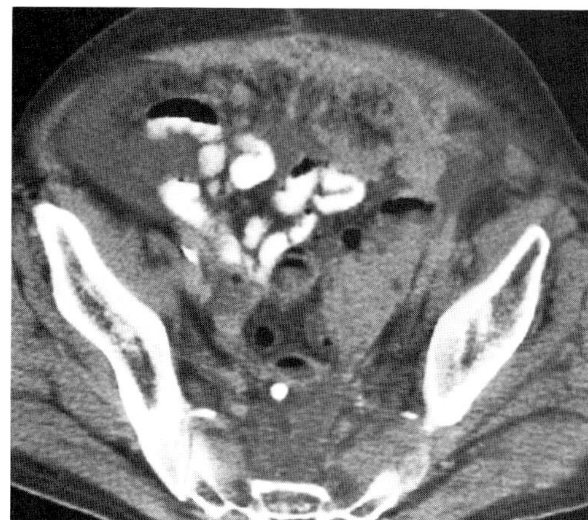

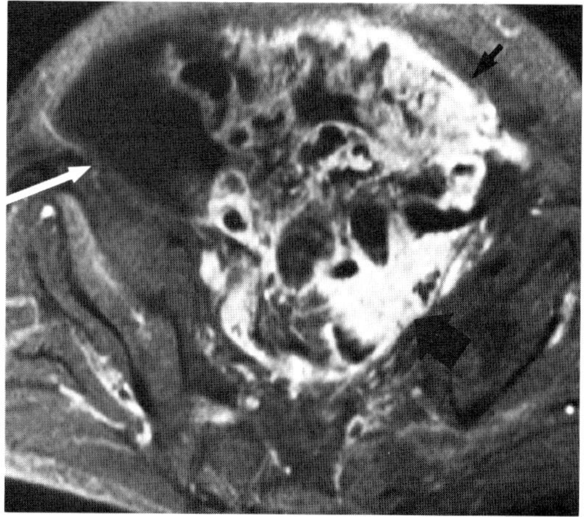

FIG. 32. Colon cancer. Contrast-enhanced CT (**A**) and postcontrast T1FS (**B**) images in a 72-year-old man with advanced adenocarcinoma of the sigmoid colon. Both techniques demonstrate ascites (*white arrow,* B), peritoneal tumor extension (*small black arrow,* B), and the primary tumor (*large arrow,* B). Slightly greater contrast resolution is apparent on the MR image. Reprinted with permission from ref. 62.

the evaluation of recurrent rectal cancer. The rectum is relatively fixed and reasonably free of ghosting artifact and has been well assessed by MRI. Comparisons of CT, MRI, and transrectal ultrasound (TRUS) have been made to determine the most effective imaging technique for preoperative staging and recurrence follow-up. MR and TRUS are superior to CT (53,54). Waizer et al. demonstrated that MR is more specific in the detection of recurrent rectal cancer than is TRUS. Although both techniques had difficulty in distinguishing between fibrous tissue and recurrent cancer, MR correctly diagnosed 10 of 12 lesions (83.2%) compared with TRUS, which correctly diagnosed 5 of 12 (41.6%) (55). In addition, the ability of MR to image directly in the sagittal plane permits evaluation of the rectum in the best anatomical display. Seminal vesicles are clearly shown and invasion of bone is demonstrated better than on CT images. Uncomplicated postradiation fibrosis is low in SI on T2-weighted images and does not enhance substantially with gadolinium approximately 1 year after surgery (Fig. 33). Recurrent cancer tends to be relatively high in SI on T2-weighted images. Differentiation between recurrent tumors and postsurgical changes is not absolute, and overlap in appearance persists, particularly

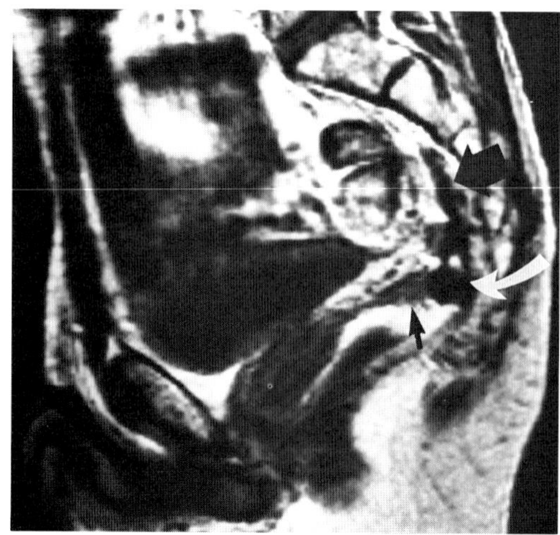

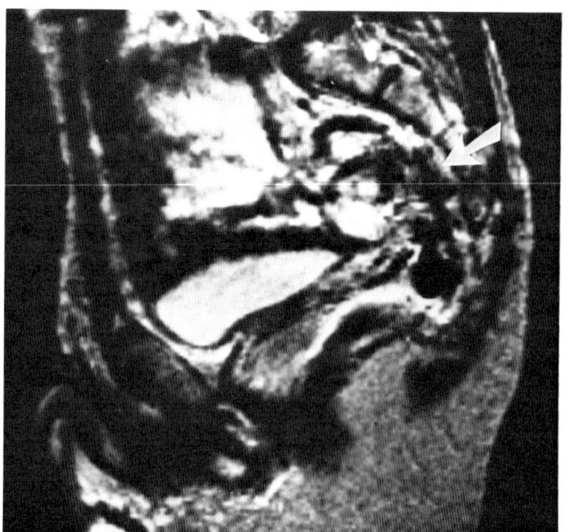

FIG. 33. Postsurgical scarring in the rectal bed. Proton density (2000/15) (**A**) and T2-weighted (2000/70) (**B**) spin echo images in a 56-year-old man 2 years after abdominoperineal resection for rectal cancer. The anatomy is most clearly shown on the proton density image, which demonstrates seminal vesicles (*short black arrow, A*), magnetic-susceptible artifact (*curved white arrow, A*), and postsurgical fibrosis (*large black arrow, A*) in the rectal bed. The presence of these three findings made distinction from recurrent disease difficult on transverse CT images. The linear fibrotic tissue, which was low in SI on the proton density images, remains low in SI on the T2-weighted image (*large white arrow, B*), consistent with postsurgical fibrosis.

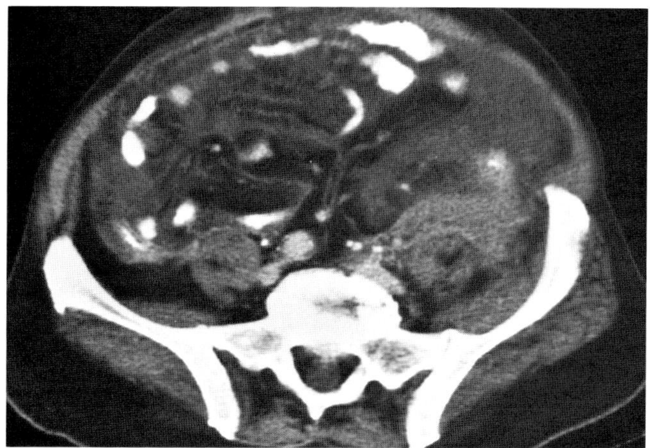

A

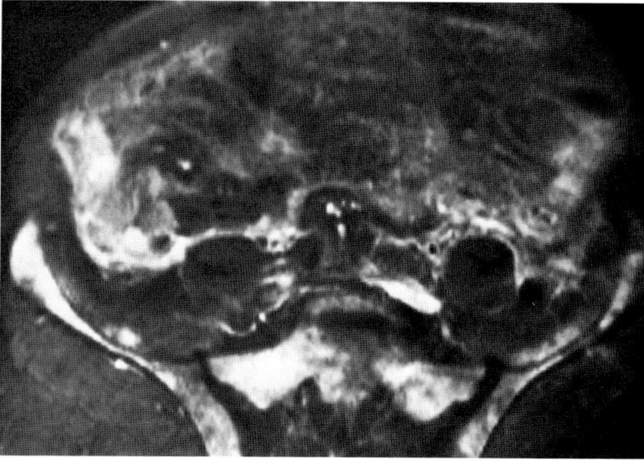

B

FIG. 34. Burkitt's lymphoma. Contrast-enhanced CT (**A**) and Gd-DTPA-enhanced T1FS (**B**) images in a 52-year-old man with Burkitt's lymphoma. The CT image demonstrates increased soft tissue in the left pericolic gutter, thickening of the descending colon, and stranding in the mesentery. Similar findings are identified on the MR image, with extensive linear stranding through the mesentery, and in both pericolic gutters. In addition, a patchy appearance of the bone marrow of the pelvis is appreciated on the MR image, consistent with marrow involvement. This was confirmed by bone marrow biopsy.

when surgery has been performed less than 1 year before the MR study. Occasionally, recurrent tumor can be low in SI because of desmoplastic changes in the lesion. Fibrosis may be high in SI and enhance with gadolinium in certain settings including imaging within 1 year of surgery, infection, and inflammation. Morphological criteria remain important in the assessment of recurrent disease. Presacral pain is an ominous symptom independent of the appearance of presacral tissue.

Lymphomas

Lymphoma can involve the colon, usually as part of widespread disease (Fig. 34). Primary lymphomas of the colon are rare; most are non-Hodgkin's. Human immunodeficiency virus infection is associated with colonic lymphoma (Fig. 35). These tumors account for 10% to 20% of primary gastrointestinal lymphomas. The cecum is the most common site, followed by the rectum. The fifth to seventh decades are the most common ages. These lesions may develop in patients with longstanding ulcerative colitis (56–58).

Other Malignant Tumors

Carcinoid tumors are most frequently diagnosed in the rectum; a 32-year retrospective report (59) found that 94 of 170 carcinoid tumors (55%) were primary rectal lesions. Twenty-eight patients with lesions smaller than 2 cm were treated by local excision with no recurrence; however, only 1 of 10 patients with metastatic rectal carcinoid tumors larger than 4 cm survived for 5 years. Melanoma can be a primary tumor of the colon. This lesion is rare (0.25% to 1.2% of cancers of the anal canal) (60). The prognosis for patients with this cancer is very poor. The lesion can have a characteristic high SI on T1-weighted images and demonstrates ring enhancement, as observed in melanoma lesions in the liver (Fig. 36).

Metastases

The rectum and colon are not infrequently involved in tumor extension from other primary cancers. Cancer

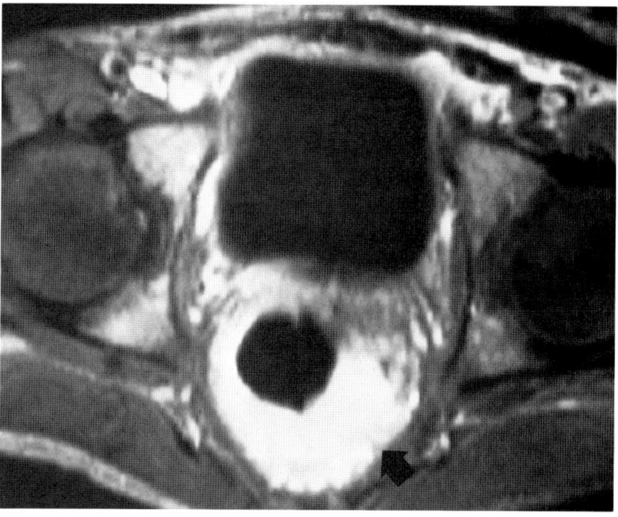

FIG. 35. Rectal lymphoma. Gd-DTPA-enhanced T1FS image in a human immunodeficiency virus (HIV)-positive 26-year-old man demonstrates an enhancing tumor mass surrounding the rectum (*arrow*). Reprinted with permission from ref. 52.

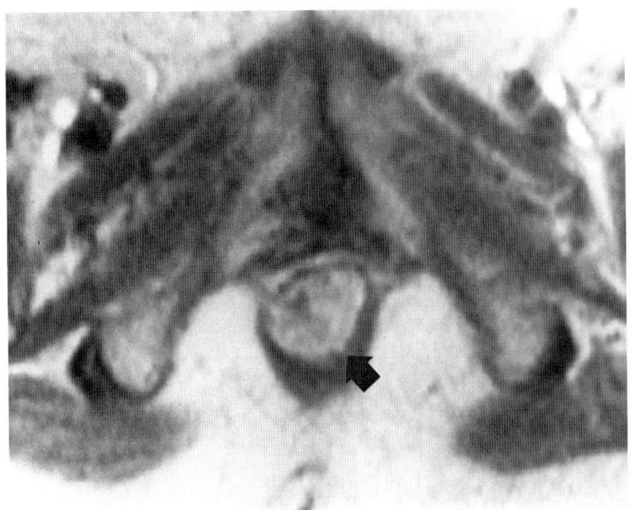

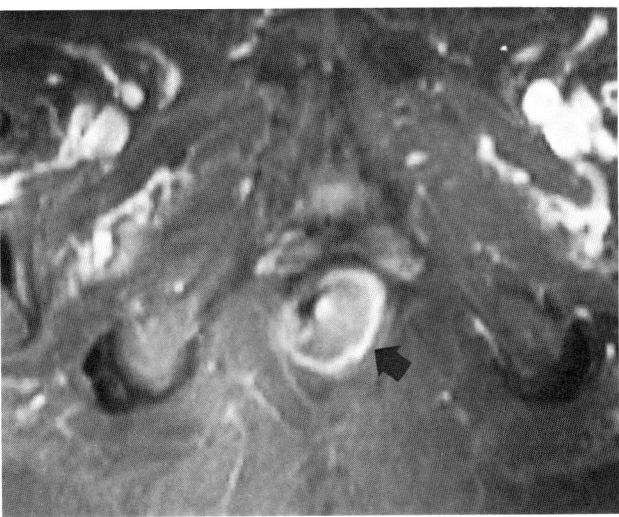

A B

FIG. 36. Anorectal malignant melanoma. FLASH (**A**) and Gd-DTPA-enhanced T1FS (**B**) MR images in a 48-year-old woman. The FLASH image (A) demonstrates a high-SI mass that does not extend beyond the rectal wall (*arrow*). The Gd-DTPA-enhanced T1FS image (B) demonstrates that the mass has an enhancing rim (*arrow*). Reprinted with permission from ref. 52.

of the cervix and ovary are the two most common malignant neoplasms to involve the colon secondarily. These most commonly occur through direct tumor extension. High contrast resolution and the multiplanar imaging capability of MRI permit accurate evaluation of invasion of the colon (Fig. 37).

Inflammation

Ulcerative colitis (UC) and Crohn's colitis are the two most common chronic inflammatory conditions of the colon. Ulcerative colitis usually begins in the rectum and left colon; its proximal course is variable but may include the entire colon. The incidence of UC is greatest in the second, third, and fourth decades of life and is somewhat more frequent among female patients (1.3:1.0). UC is predominately a disease of whites, with a higher incidence among Jews (61). The etiology is unknown, but investigations have focused on infectious agents and genetic, psychosomatic, and immunological mechanisms. UC is variable in presentation, but symptoms are usually indolent and include rectal bleeding and diarrhea. Patients with UC are at greater risk for developing cancer than is the general population.

The two characteristic MR features of ulcerative colitis are (a) colon involvement progressing from the rectum in a retrograde fashion to involve a variable extent

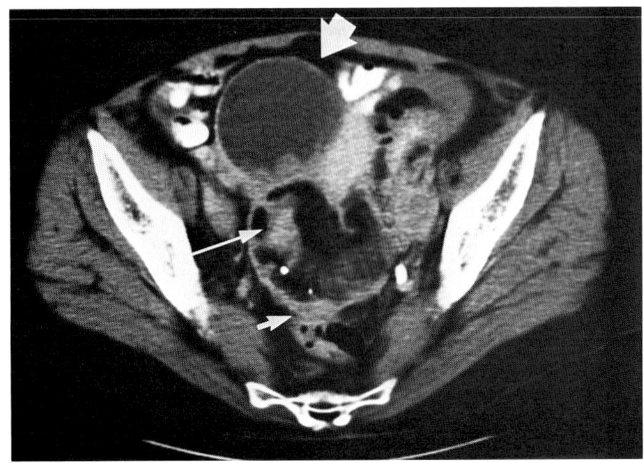

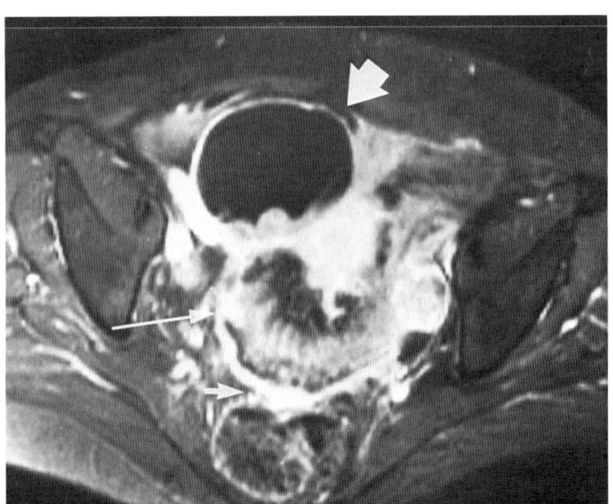

A B

FIG. 37. Ovarian cancer extension to sigmoid colon. Contrast-enhanced CT (**A**) and Gd-DTPA-enhanced T1FS (**B**) images in a 64-year-old woman with ovarian cancer. A mixed cystic/solid ovarian cancer is apparent (*large arrow*). The aggressive local invasion of the tumor is well shown, with encasement of the sigmoid colon (*long arrow*) and invasion of the anterior wall of the rectum (*small arrow*).

of colon and (b) submucosal sparing. Prominent vasa recta are frequently present. Patients who present acutely with toxic colon may have a thick colon wall with substantial enhancement and minimal submucosal sparing (Fig. 38). Patients who present after years of indolent symptoms tend to have more prominent submucosal low SI from submucosal edema and lymphangiectasia (Fig. 39).

Crohn's disease (CD) is transmural and predominately a disease of young people in the second and third decades of life. Males are affected more frequently than females (1.41:1.00), and the incidence of colon involvement in the general population is approximately 2 to 3 per 100,000. Jews are 5 times more likely to have CD than is the general population (62). The etiology is unknown, but investigators have included genetic factors, transmissible infectious agents, and autoimmune phenomena. The presentation of CD is variable and may include intestinal obstruction, intraabdominal fistula, low-grade fever, nonbloody diarrhea, weight loss, moderate anemia, and toxic colon. The distribution of non-small bowel CD includes 27% in the colon and 4% exclusively anorectal.

MRI can generally distinguish UC and CD based on morphological criteria (Table 1). On MR images, the characteristic feature of Crohn's disease is full-thickness enhancement (Fig. 40). Additional features include asymmetrical involvement, relative sparing of the rectum, fistulous tracts, and skip lesions. Associated involvement of the terminal ileum with the typical MR features is definitive for the diagnosis. Patients with a short history who present with toxic colon may not have substantial wall thickening; however, the diseased bowel is usually long and contrast enhancement exceeds 100% (Fig. 41).

Until recently, MRI has had a limited role in the diagnosis, assessment, and treatment response of patients with IBD. This has been due to ghosting artifact, gut peristalsis, and poor resolution. Most studies have used oral contrast agents of high or low signal intensity to

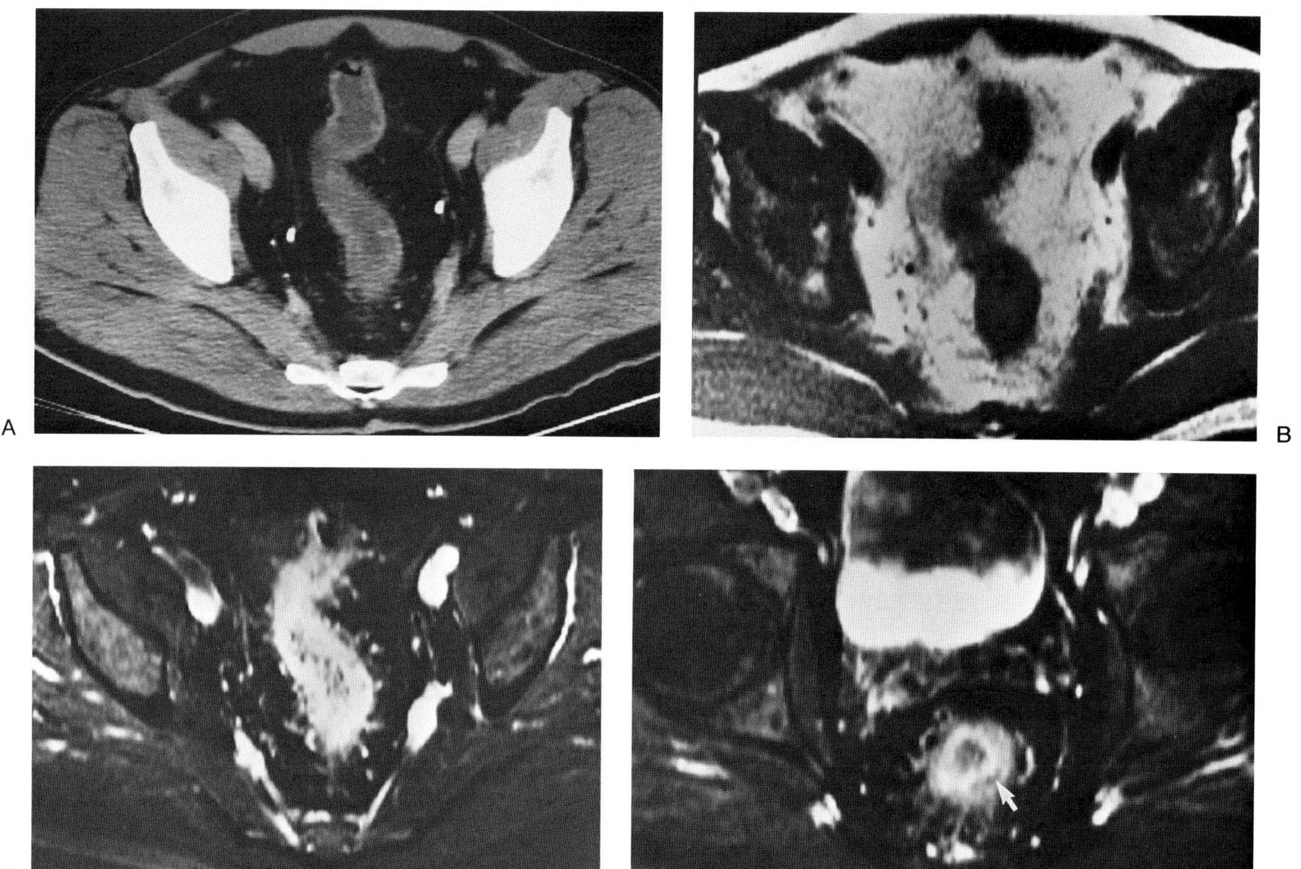

FIG. 38. Ulcerative colitis with severe inflammatory changes. Contrast-enhanced CT (**A**), precontrast FLASH (**B**), and postcontrast T1FS (**C,D**) images in a 57-year-old man with ulcerative colitis. The contrast-enhanced CT and precontrast FLASH images show irregular low-SI strands related to a thick-walled sigmoid colon. The postcontrast T1FS image shows marked enhancement (>100%) of the colon wall, with surrounding reticular strands. These enhancing strands presumably represent a prominent vasa recta and granulation tissue. A similar appearance is apparent in the rectum (D). Submucosal sparing is apparent (*arrow,* D). Reprinted with permission from ref. 62.

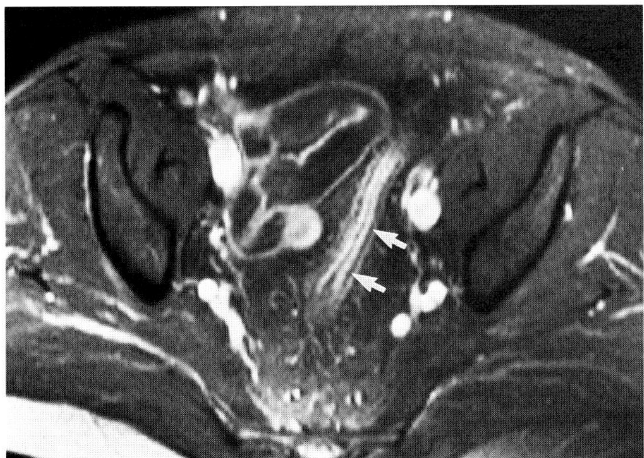

FIG. 39. Chronic ulcerative colitis. Gd-DTPA-enhanced T1FS image in a 52-year-old man with indolent colonic symptoms for >10 years. Substantial submucosal low SI is present (*arrow*), reflecting submucosal edema and lymphangiectasia.

delineate the bowel from surrounding tissue (23–25,63). A recent report has shown promising results for the MR investigation of IBD using T1-weighted spin echo with fat suppression and Gd-DTPA enhancement (64). MR was shown to be comparable to CT in the demonstration of bowel wall thickness and superior in contrast enhancement.

Pouchitis

Patients with UC undergoing colectomy are candidates for the construction of an ileal reservoir (pouch) to simulate a colon and ileorectal anastomosis. Patients with Crohn's disease have a high complication rate after pouch construction (65). Pouchitis occurs in 7% to 42% of patients with ileal pouch anal anastomosis (66). Increased wall thickness and inflammatory changes around the pouch are imaging findings (Fig. 42).

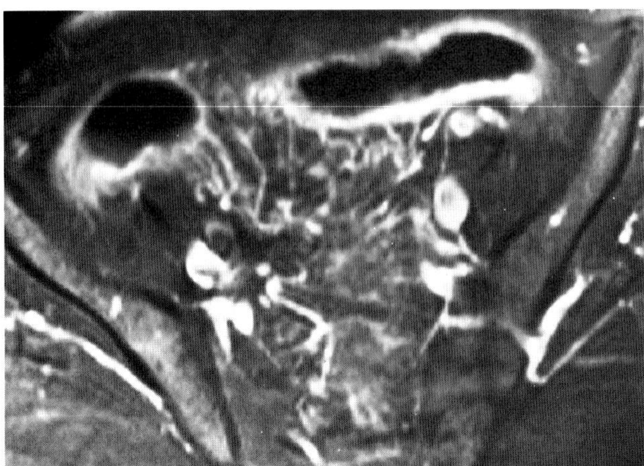

FIG. 40. Crohn's colitis. Gd-DTPA-enhanced T1FS image in a 69-year-old man with Crohn's colitis. Full-thickness mural involvement is present and is characteristic of the disease. Involvement of the sigmoid colon and the ascending colon with relative sparing of the rectum are also present in a distribution consistent with Crohn's disease. Prominent vasa recta are identified.

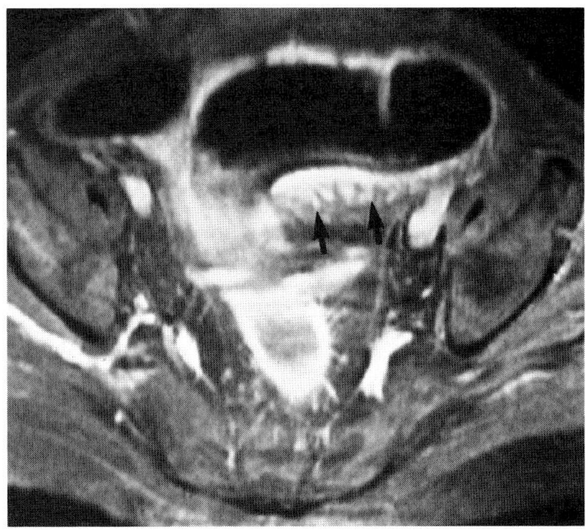

FIG. 41. Crohn's disease. Gd-DTPA-enhanced T1FS MR image in a 57-year-old man with toxic megacolon. The bowel wall thickness is 1 cm, and the bowel wall enhances 70%. Transmural enhancement of the bowel wall is present, with no submucosal sparing demonstrated. Prominent vasa recta are apparent (*arrows*). Reprinted with permission from ref. 39.

Infection

Appendicitis

Appendicitis and appendical abscess are well shown on MR images because of the high sensitivity of MR to

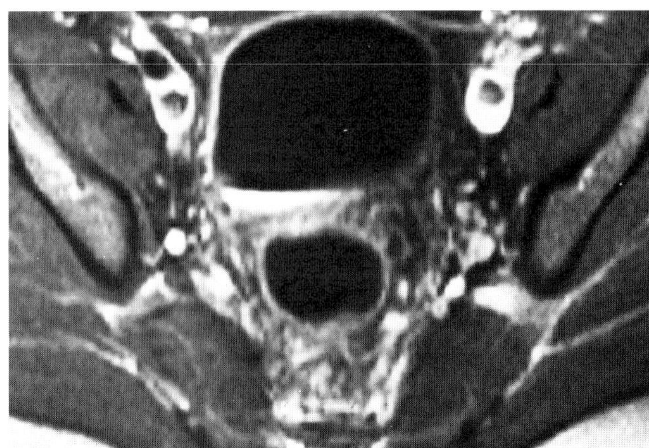

FIG. 42. Pouchitis. Gd-DTPA-enhanced T1FS image in an 18-year-old man with an ileal pouch reconstruction after colectomy for ulcerative colitis. Prominent inflammatory stranding surrounding the pouch is present, with focal increased wall thickness anteriorly. These features are in keeping with pouchitis.

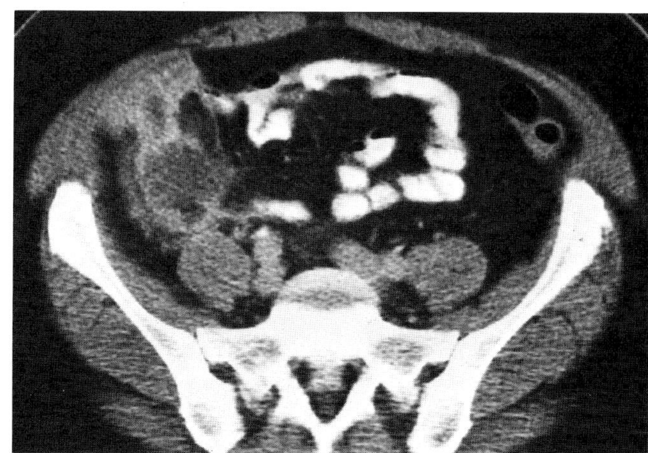

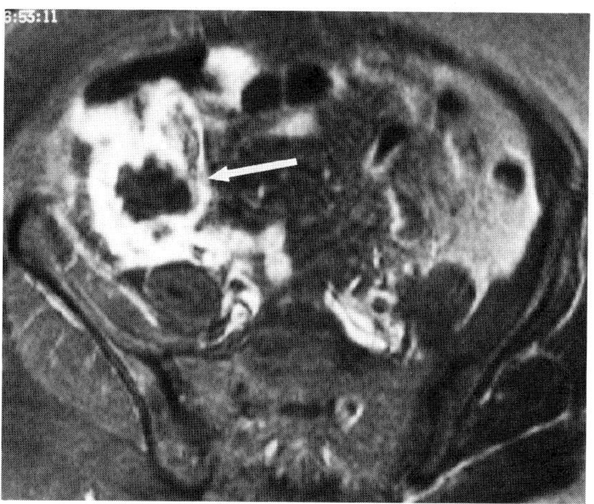

A B

FIG. 43. Appendiceal abscess. Contrast-enhanced CT (**A**) and post-Gd-DTPA T1FS (**B**) images in a 66-year-old woman with an appendiceal abscess. Both CT and T1FS images show thickening of the base of the cecum and the terminal ileum, with an amorphous, rounded mass related to the inferior surface of the cecum. The higher contrast resolution on the MR image shows that the center of the mass is signal void, compatible with an appendiceal abscess (*arrow*). Reprinted with permission from ref. 62.

Gd-DTPA. An appendical abscess appears as a signal-void cavity, and inflammatory changes of distal ileum are frequently present (Fig. 43).

Diverticulitis

Diverticulitis is an inflammatory condition usually affecting the left colon. Diverticula are usually but not invariably seen. Abscess collections are demonstrated as loculated, signal-void lesions with a defined wall (Fig. 44). In the context of diverticulitis, examination for fistulous tracts may be assisted by the use of a positive oral contrast agent.

Infectious Colitis

Pseudomembranous colitis is an infection associated with antibiotic use. The infecting organism is *Clostridium difficile* (67). The severity can vary from mild to life threatening. Enhancement of bowel wall is demonstrated on MR images (Fig. 45).

Neutropenic colitis is seen in the context of malignant disease, frequently leukemia. The right side of the colon is most typically involved. Other infectious agents include *Shigella, Salmonella, Escherichia coli,* amebiasis, and cholera.

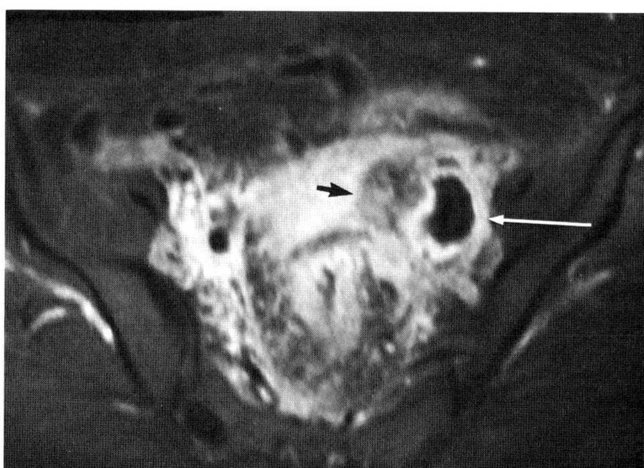

FIG. 44. Diverticulitis. Gd-DTPA-enhanced T1FS image in a 44-year-old woman with diverticulitis. A signal-void fluid collection with an enhancing wall (*thin arrow*) is present adjacent to a thick-walled sigmoid colon (*small black arrow*). Multiple inflammatory strands throughout the pelvis radiate from the thick-walled colon.

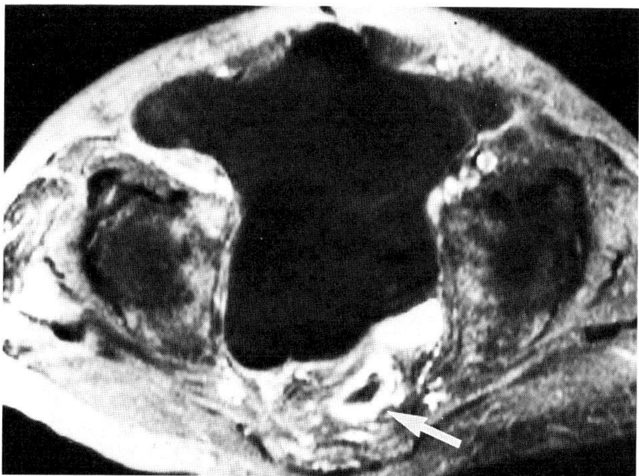

FIG. 45. Pseudomembranous colitis. Gd-DTPA-enhanced T1FS image in a 63-year-old man who had been on a prolonged course of oral antibiotics. The rectum and sigmoid colon are thick walled and show transmural increased SI (*arrow*). This appearance is nonspecific for severe bowel inflammation, consistent with pseudomembranous colitis. A large volume of ascites is present.

Ischemia and Radiation

Submucosal edema is a feature of ischemic and radiation enteritis. The clinical history and distribution of changes are clues to the diagnosis. Ischemia tends to occur in watershed segments of bowel, typically the splenic flexure. Radiation changes occur in segments of bowel that are relatively fixed and within the radiation portal, such as the rectum.

NEW DIRECTIONS

Contrast Agents

Many reports have described improvement in imaging the bowel with either a positive or a negative oral contrast agent. The ideal agent has not been agreed upon.

MR Techniques

Surface coil imaging with either a phased array coil or an endorectal coil has been shown in early reports substantially to improve imaging of the rectum (68). Dynamic MR studies using echo planar imaging (69) may provide useful information on gut motility without the patient discomfort of perfused systems. T1-weighted spin echo techniques and Gd-DTPA have been used to acquire images to study gastric emptying (70). These techniques allow anatomical information to be gathered in a more physiological setting without patient discomfort.

REFERENCES

1. American Joint Committee: Clinical staging systems for cancer of the esophagus. *Cancer* 1975;25:50–57.
2. Habey K, Winnfield AL. Multiple leiomyomas of the esophagus. *Am J Dig Dis* 1974;19:678–680.
3. Wienbeck M, Berges W. Oesophageal lesions in the alcoholic. *Clin Gastroenterol* 1981;10:375–388.
4. Maram ES, Kurland LT, Ludwig J, Brian DD. Esophageal carcinoma in Olmsted County, Minnesota, 1935–1971. *Mayo Clin Proc* 1977;52:24–27.
5. Iascone C, DeMeester TR, Little AG, Skinner DB. Barrett's esophagus: functional assessment, proposed pathogenesis and surgical therapy. *Arch Surg* 1983;118:543–549.
6. Streitz JM, Ellis FH, Gibb SP, Balogh K, Watkins E. Adenocarcinoma in Barrett's esophagus: a clinicopathologic study of 65 cases. *Ann Surg* 1991;213:122–125.
7. Kahrihas PJ, Kishk SM, Helm JF, Dodds WJ, Harig JM, Hogan WJ. Comparison of pseudoachalasia and achalasia. *Am J Med* 1987;82:439–446.
8. Nebel OT, Fornes MF, Castell DO. Symptomatic gastro- esophageal reflux: incidence and precipitating factors. *Am J Dig Dis* 1976;21:953–956.
9. Behar J, Sheahan MB, Biancani P, Spiro HM, Storer EH. Medical and surgical management of reflux esophagitis. *N Engl J Med* 1975;293:263–268.
10. Thomson D, Shoenut JP, Trenholm BG, Teskey JM. Reflux patterns following limited myotomy without fundoplication for achalasia. *Ann Thorac Surg* 1987;43:550–553.
11. Shoenut JP, Trenholm BG, Micflikier AB, Teskey JM. Reflux patterns in patients with achalasia without operation. *Ann Thorac Surg* 1988;45:303–305.
12. Sauer L, Pellegrini CA, Way LW. The treatment of achalasia: a current perspective. *Arch Surg* 1989;124:929–932.
13. Shoenut, Wieler JA, Micflikier AB, Teskey JM. Esophageal reflux before and after isolated myotomy for achalasia. *Surgery* 1990;108:876–879.
14. Murphy JR, McNally P, Peller P, Shay SS. Prolonged clearance is the primary abnormal reflux parameter in patients with progressive systemic sclerosis and esophagitis. *Dig Dis Sci* 1992;37: 833–841.
15. Dow C. Oesophageal tuberculosis. Gut 1981;22:234–236.
16. Nakamura T, Nakano G. Histopathological classification and malignant change in gastric polyps. *J Clin Pathol* 1985;38:754–764.
17. Palmer ED. Gastric diverticula, with special reference to subjective manifestations. *Gastroenterology* 1958;35:406–408.
18. Haenszel W, Kurihara M. Studies of Japanese migrants: 1. Mortality from cancer and other disease among Japanese in the United States. *J Natl Cancer Inst* 1968;40:43–68.
19. Coggon D, Acheson ED. The geography of cancer of the stomach. *Br Med Bull* 1984;40:335–341.
20. Freeman C, Berg JW, Cutler SJ. Occurrence and prognosis of extranodal lymphomas. *Cancer* 1972;29:252–260.
21. Danzi JT, Farmer RG, Sullivan BH, Rankin GB. Endoscopic features of gastroduodenal Crohn's disease. *Gastroenterology* 1976; 70:9–13.
22. Kaminsky S, Laniado M, Gogoll M, et al. Gadopentatate dimeglumine as a bowel contrast agent: safety and efficacy. *Radiology* 1991;178:503–508.
23. Hahn PF, Stark DD, Lewis JM, et al. First clinical trial of a new superparamagnetic iron oxide for use as an oral gastrointestinal contrast agent in MR imaging. *Radiology* 1990;175:695–700.
24. Mattrey RF, Hajek P, Gylys-Morin VM, et al. Perfluoro- chemicals as gastrointestinal contrast agents for MR imaging: preliminary studies in rats and humans. *AJR Am J Roentgenol* 1987; 148:1259–1263.
25. MacKey WC, Dineen P. A fifty year experience with Meckel's diverticulum. *Surg Gynecol Obstet* 1983;156:56–64.
26. Gupta S, Gupta S. Primary tumors of the small bowel: a clinicopathological study of 58 cases. *J Surg Oncol* 1982;20:161–167.
27. Sauerbruch T, Weinzierl M, Dietrich HP, Antes G, Eisenberg J, Paumgartner G. Sclerotherapy on a bleeding duodenal varix. *Endoscopy* 1982;14:187–189.
28. Kirkpatrick JR, Shoenut JP, Micflikier AB. Successful injection sclerotherapy for a bleeding duodenal varix in intrahepatic portal obstruction. *Gastrointest Endosc* 1985;31:259–260.
29. Silberman H, Crichlow RW, Caplan HS. Neoplasms of the small bowel. *Ann Surg* 1974;180:157–161.
30. Freund H, Lavi A, Pfeffermann R, Durst AL. Primary neoplasms of the small bowel. *Am J Surg* 1978;135:757–759.
31. MacDonald RA. A study of 356 carcinoids of the gastrointestinal tract. *Am J Med* 1956;21:867–878.
32. Al-Mondhiry H. Primary lymphomas of the intestine: East-west contrast. *Am J Hematol* 1986;22:89–105.
33. Martin RG. Malignant tumors of the small intestine. *Surg Clin North Am* 1986;66:779–785.
34. Farmer RG, Hawk WA, Turnbull RB. Clinical patterns in Crohn's disease: A statistical study of 615 cases. *Gastroenterology* 1975;68:627–635.
35. Farmer RG, Hawk WA, Turnbull RB. Indications for surgery in Crohn's disease: an analysis of 500 cases. *Gastroenterology* 1976;71:245–250.
36. Crohn BB, Ginsberg L, Oppenheimer GD. Regional ileitis: a pathological and clinical entity. *JAMA* 1932;99:1323–1329.
37. Farmer RG, Hawk WA, Turnbull RB. Clinical patterns in Crohn's disease: a statistical study of 615 cases. *Gastroenterology* 1975;68:627–635.
38. Goldstein F. *Small Bowel Disease: Sulfasalazine Use in Current Management of Inflammatory Bowel Disease,* ed, Bayless TM. BC Decker, Toronto, 1989.
39. Shoenut JP, Semelka RC, Silverman R, Yaffe CS, Micflikier AB. Magnetic resonance imaging in inflammatory bowel disease. *J Clin Gastroenterol* (*in press*).

40. Gutmann LT. *Yersinia enterocilitica* and *Yersinia pseudotuberculosis*. In: Gorbach SL (ed). *Infectious Diarrhea*. Blackwell Scientific, Boston, 1986, p 65.
41. Bentley G, Webster JH. Gastrointestinal tuberculosis: a 10-year review. *Br J Surg* 1967;54:90–96.
42. Lambert ME, Schofield PF, Ironside AG, Mandal BK. Campylobacter colitis. *Br Med J* 1979;1:857–859.
43. Hayashi T, Yatani R, Apostol J, et al. Pathogenesis of hyperplastic polyps of the colon: a hypothesis based on ultrasound and *in vitro* kinetics. *Gastroenterology* 1974;66:347–356.
44. Gelb AM, Minkowitz S, Tresser M. Rectal and colonic polyps occurring in young people. *NY State J Med* 1962;513–518.
45. Morson BC, Dawson IMP. Nonepithelial tumors. In: *Gastrointestinal Pathology*. Blackwell Scientific, Oxford, 1979, pp 187–199.
46. Hancock BJ, Vajcner A. Lipomas of the colon: a clinicopathologic review. *Can J Surg* 1988;31:178–181.
47. Bernstein WC. What are hemorrhoids and what is their relationship to the portal venous system? *Dis Colon Rectum* 1983;26: 829–834.
48. Silverberg E, Lubera S. Cancer statistics, 1988. *CA Cancer J Clin* 1988;38:14–15.
49. Begent RHJ. Colorectal cancer. *Br Med J* 1992;305:246–249.
50. Kee F, Wilson RH, Gilliland R, Sloan JM, Rowlands BJ, Moorehead RJ. Changing site distribution of colorectal cancer. *Br Med J* 1992;305:158.
51. Beart RW, Melton J, Maruta M, Dockerty MB, Frydenberg HB, O'Fallon WM. Trends in right- and left-sided colon cancer. *Dis Colon Rectum* 1983;26:393–398.
52. Shoenut JP, Semelka RC, Silverman R, Yaffe CS, Micflikier AB. Magnetic resonance imaging evaluation of the local extent of colorectal mass lesions. *J Clin Gastroenterol* (*in press*).
53. Krestin GP, Steibrich W, Friedmann G. Recurrent rectal cancer: diagnosis with MR versus CT. *Radiology* 1988;168:307–311.
54. Gomberg JS, Friedman AC, Radecki PD, Grumbach K, Caroline DF. MRI differentiation of recurrent colorectal carcinoma from postoperative fibrosis. *Gastrointest Radiol* 1986;11:361–363.
55. Waizer A, Powsner E, Russo I, et al. Prospective comparative study of magnetic resonance imaging versus transrectal ultrasound for preoperative staging and follow-up of rectal cancer. *Dis Colon Rectum* 1991;34:1068–1072.
56. Dragosics B, Bauer P, Radaasziewicz T. Primary gastrointestinal non-Hodgkin's lymphomas. *Cancer* 1985;55:1060–1073.
57. Loehr W, Mujahed Z, Zah FD, Gray G, Thorbjarnarson B. Primary lymphoma of the gastrointestinal tract: a review of 100 cases. *Ann Surg* 1969;170:232–238.
58. Bartolo D, Goepel JR, Parsons MA. Rectal malignant lymphoma in chronic ulcerative colitis. *Gut* 1982;23:164–168.
59. Jetmore AB, Ray JE, Gathright BJ, McMullen KM, Hicks TC, Timmcke AE. Rectal carcinoids: the most frequent carcinoid tumor. *Dis Colon Rectum* 1992;35:717–725.
60. Pack GT, Oropeza R. A comparative study of melanoma and epidermoid carcinoma of the anal canal. *Dis Colon Rectum* 1967;10:161–176.
61. Acheson ED. The distribution of ulcerative colitis and regional enteritis in United States veterans with particular reference to the Jewish religion. *Gut* 1960;1:291–293.
62. Brahme F, Lindstrom C, Wenckert A. Crohn's disease in a defined population. *Gastroenterology* 1975;69:342–351.
63. Laniado M, Kormesser W, Hamm B, Clauss W, Weinmann HJ, Felix R. MR imaging of the gastrointestinal tract: value of Gd-DTPA. *AJR Am J Roentgenol* 1988;150:817–821
64. Semelka RC, Shoenut JP, Silverman R, Kroeker MA, Yaffe CS, Micflikier AB. Bowel disease: prospective comparison of CT and 1.5T pre- and postcontrast MR imaging with T1-weighted fat-suppressed and breath-hold FLASH sequences. *JMRI* 1991;1: 625–632.
65. Deutsch AA, McLeod RS, Cullen J, Cohen Z. Results of the pelvic-pouch procedure in patients with Crohn's disease. *Dis Colon Rectum* 1991;34:475–477.
66. Rauh SM, Schoetz DR Jr, Roberts PL, Murray JJ, Coller JA, Veidenheimer MC. Pouchitis—is it a wastebasket diagnosis? *Dis Colon Rectum* 1991;34:685–689.
67. Larson H, Price AB, Honour P. *Clostridium difficile* and the etiology of pseudomembranous colitis. *Lancet* 1978;1:1063–1066.
68. Chan TW, Kressel HY, Milestone B, Tomachefski J, Schnall M, Rosato E, Daly J. Rectal carcinoma: staging at MR imaging with endorectal surface coil. *Radiology* 1991;181:461–467.
69. Stehling MK, Evans DF, Lamont G, et al. Gastrointestinal tract: dynamic MR studies with echo-planar imaging. *Radiology* 1989·171:41–46.
70. Schwizer W, Maecke H, Fried M. Measurement of gastric emptying by magnetic resonance imaging in humans. *Gastroenterology* 1992;103:369–376.

CHAPTER 10

The Peritoneal Cavity

Richard C. Semelka and J. Patrick Shoenut

NORMAL ANATOMY

The peritoneal cavity and the abdominal and pelvic organs are covered with peritoneum. Peritoneal folds within the cavity are called ligaments and physically support and provide protection to nutrient vessels. Mesentery are peritoneal folds that connect the small bowel and sigmoid colon to the posterior abdominal wall. The greater omentum extends from the greater curvature of the stomach to lie anterior in the abdomen and reflects back onto the transverse colon. The transverse mesocolon extends from the pancreas to the transverse colon. The lesser omentum or gastrohepatic ligament joins the lesser curvature of the stomach to the liver. The peritoneal cavity is divided into subspaces that communicate with one another. Fluid tends to loculate in these subspaces in inflammatory or neoplastic conditions.

The transverse mesocolon separates the peritoneal cavity into supramesocolic and inframesocolic spaces. The supramesocolic compartment can be further divided into right and left peritoneal spaces. The right peritoneal space includes the right perihepatic space and the lesser sac. These spaces communicate via the epiploic foramen, through which passes the portal vein, common bile duct, and hepatic artery. The right perihepatic space consists of a subphrenic and subhepatic space that is partly separated by the right coronary ligament. The posterior aspect of the right subhepatic space contains a recess between the liver and kidney called the hepatorenal fossa or Morison's pouch. This space commonly accumulates fluid in conditions such as gallbladder inflammation and disease of the second portion of the duodenum, the liver, and the right colon. The lesser sac is a potential space that most commonly becomes distended with fluid in pancreatitis. With the exception of pancreatitis, there is a greater tendency for malignant rather than benign disease to fill both the greater peritoneal cavity and the lesser sac; benign disease affects the greater peritoneal cavity more disproportionately (1,2).

The left peritoneal space can be divided into anterior and posterior perihepatic spaces and anterior and posterior subphrenic spaces. The perihepatic spaces tend to be involved with disease processes affecting the left lobe of the liver and stomach. The anterior subphrenic space tends to be affected additionally by disease of the splenic flexure. The left posterior subphrenic space is most commonly involved in disease of the spleen.

The inframesocolic component is divided into a small right and a larger left infracolic spaces. The right infracolic space is limited inferiorly by the junction of the distal small bowel mesentery with the cecum, whereas the left infracolic space is open to the pelvis.

The paracolic gutters are located lateral to the peritoneal attachment of the ascending and descending colon. The right paracolic gutter is continuous with the right perihepatic space; on the left side, however, the phrenicocolic ligament forms a partial barrier between the paracolic gutter and the left subphrenic space (3). The pelvis is the most dependent location of the peritoneal cavity in both erect and supine positions, and therefore both benign and malignant fluid tends to pool in this location (4,5). The pelvic cavity consists of lateral paravesical spaces and the midline pouch of Douglas (rectovaginal space in women, rectovesical space in men).

The various peritoneal reflections permit passage of intraperitoneal fluid along pathways of least resistance. Flow along the right paracolic gutter is relatively unimpeded, as is flow of fluid into the pelvis (6). Relatively greater resistance to flow occurs along the left paracolic gutter, and flow across the midline is impeded by the falciform ligament (6).

R. C. Semelka: Department of Radiology and Magnetic Resonance Services, University of North Carolina at Chapel Hill, Chapel Hill, North Carolina 27599.

J. P. Shoenut: University of Manitoba and Department of Medicine, Saint Boniface General Hospital, Winnipeg, Manitoba R2H 2A6.

MR TECHNIQUE

T1-weighted sequences are useful to study peritoneal disease because of high contrast resolution between diseased tissue and intraperitoneal fat. Gd-DTPA-enhanced fat-suppressed spin echo is of value to demonstrate peritoneum-based lesions, such as metastatic deposits.

MASS LESIONS

Benign Masses

Benign tumors of the peritoneal cavity are uncommon. The most common entities are mesenteric cysts, desmoid tumors, and mesenteric lipomas (7–11). The most clinically important of these entities is the desmoid tumor, which is most commonly seen in patients with Gardner's syndrome who have undergone bowel resection (9–11). These tumors are extremely fibrous and can vary substantially in size from small to massive tumors. These lesions are low in SI on T1-weighted and T2-weighted images and enhance with Gd-DTPA to a minimal extent (Fig. 1). Sagittal MR images are useful to demonstrate the extent of large desmoid tumors (Fig. 2).

Malignant Tumors

Mesothelioma is a rare primary malignant tumor of the peritoneum. It can occur alone or in combination with pleural mesothelioma (12).

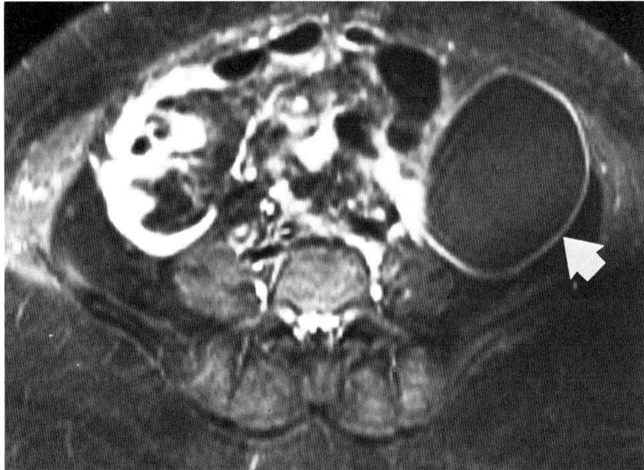

FIG. 1. Desmoid tumor. Gd-DTPA-enhanced T1FS MR image in a 48-year-old woman with Gardner's syndrome and a 6-cm intraabdominal desmoid tumor. The tumor exhibits negligible uptake of gadolinium, consistent with a solid fibrous lesion. Mural enhancement is apparent (*arrow*). This lesion could be confused with a cyst on the basis of this image. On T2-weighted images, these lesions are low in SI, which would distinguish them from cysts that are high in SI.

Metastases

Metastatic tumors that involve the peritoneum most commonly arise from the stomach, colon, ovary, and pancreas (13). Dissemination can occur from direct spread along mesenteric or ligamentous attachments, intraperitoneal seeding, hematogenous emboli, and lymphatic extension (5,14).

Direct Spread

Direct spread along adjacent visceral peritoneal surfaces to involve adjacent structures commonly occurs in tumors that have full-thickness penetration (Fig. 3)(15,16).

Intraperitoneal Seeding

Intraperitoneal seeding of tumor follows pathways of least resistance. The most common locations are the pouch of Douglas, sigmoid mesocolon, right paracolic gutter, and small bowel mesentery near the ileocecal valve (5). Ovarian cancer most frequently spreads in this fashion, followed by colon, stomach, and pancreatic cancer. The technique best suited for detecting small peritoneum-based droplet metastases is the Gd-DTPA-enhanced T1FS sequence (17). The conspicuity of small lesions is much greater than with other MR techniques or with CT (Fig. 4).

The omentum is almost invariably involved with metastases when intraperitoneal metastatic deposits are present. Omental involvement can vary in appearance, including rounded plate-like, ill-defined, and stellate densities (18). Omental metastases typically enhance with Gd-DTPA and possess a lobular contour (Fig. 5).

Pseudomyxoma peritonei are due to diffuse intraperitoneal deposits of malignant mucinous material in the abdomen, usually from an ovarian or appendiceal primary (19–23). The appearance of diffuse intraperitoneal fluid-like material that causes a scalloped margin of the liver is characteristic for this entity (19–23).

Embolic Metastases

Tumor emboli spread via the mesenteric arteries to the antimesenteric border of the bowel (14). The most common neoplasms to spread hematogenously are melanoma and carcinomas of the breast or lung.

Lymphatic Dissemination

Lymphatic dissemination is the primary mode of spread of lymphoma. Both Hodgkin's and non-Hodgkin's lymphoma may involve the abdomen. Mesen-

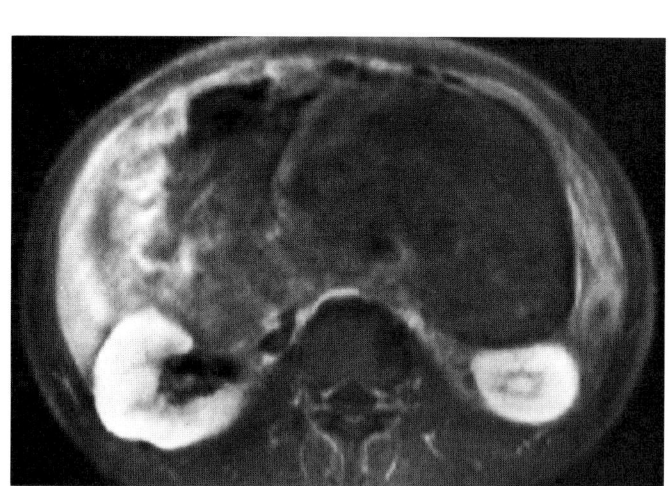

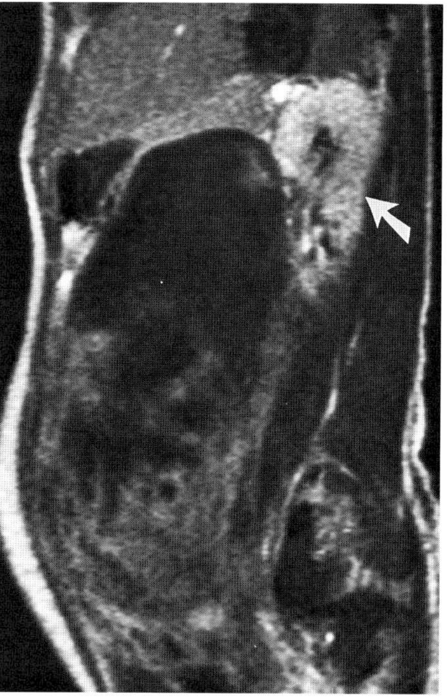

FIG. 2. Desmoid tumor. Gd-DTPA-enhanced transverse T1FS (**A**) and Gd-DTPA-enhanced sagittal FLASH (**B**) images in a 27-year-old woman with Gardner's syndrome and a 20-cm intraabdominal desmoid tumor. Enhancement of the right aspect of the large desmoid tumor is identified, with the remainder of the tumor very hypovascular. A sagittal image acquired to the right of midline demonstrates the longitudinal extent of tumor. Posterior displacement of the right kidney is shown on this image (*arrow*).

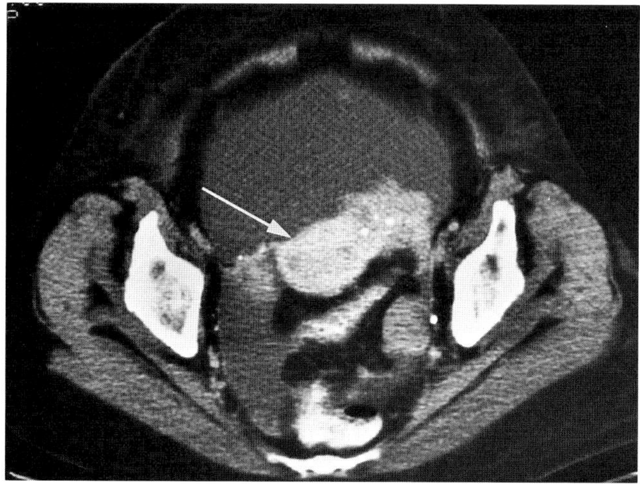

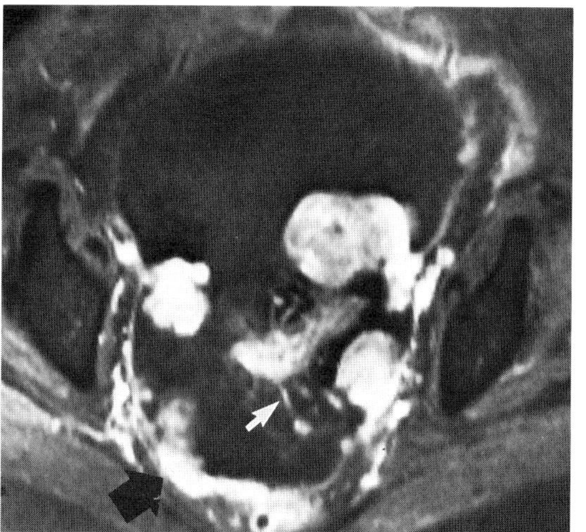

FIG. 3. Relationship of ovarian tumor to adjacent pelvic structures. Contrast-enhanced CT (**A**) and Gd-DTPA-enhanced T1FS MR (**B**) images. Fine tumor strands extending to the sigmoid colon (short white arrow, B) are more conspicuous on the MR image. Extensive peritoneal metastases demonstrate higher contrast on MR images (*large black arrow,* B). Peritoneal disease is better shown on the MR image in part because of a slightly different anatomical section. The MR image is above the level of the uterus (*long white arrow,* A). Bilateral ovarian tumors with peritoneal metastases and involvement of the uterus and sigmoid colon were found at surgery. Reprinted with permission from ref. 17.

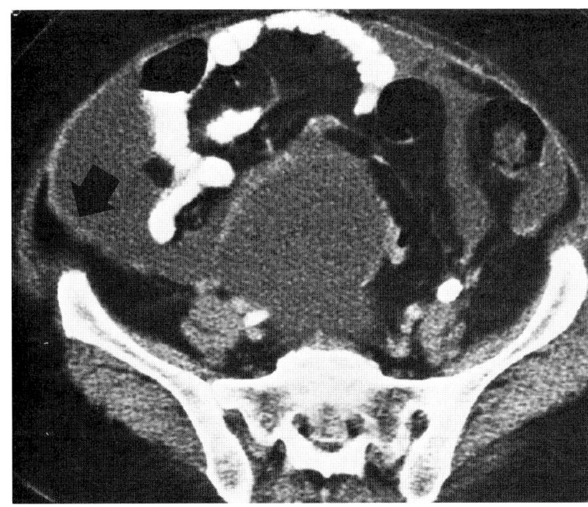

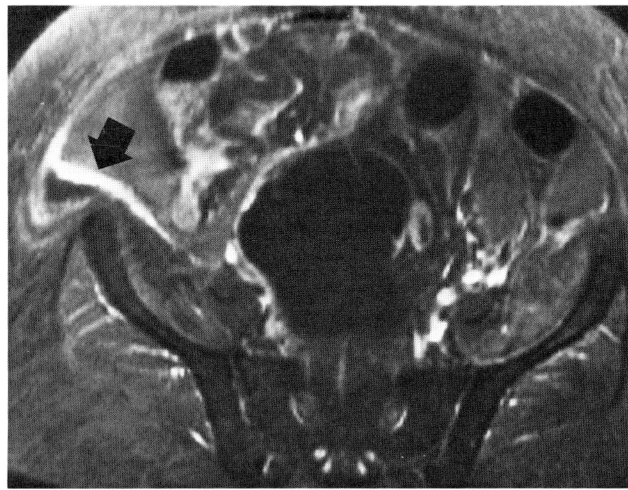

A B

FIG. 4. Peritoneal metastases. Contrast-enhanced CT (**A**) and Gd-DTPA-enhanced T1FS MR (**B**) images. Peritoneal metastases in the right paracolic gutter (*large arrow*) in a 64-year-old woman with ovarian cancer. Peritoneal metastases are well shown on fat-suppressed images because of the uptake of gadolinium and the suppression of background fat and are higher in conspicuity than on CT images. Reprinted with permission from ref. 17.

teric and celiac adenopathy is a frequent occurrence in non-Hodgkin's lymphoma (24–26) (see Chapter 11, Fig. 4) but is rare in Hodgkin's lymphoma. The presence of mesenteric adenopathy on tomographic images suggests the diagnosis of non-Hodgkin's lymphoma.

Mesenteric Lipodystrophy (Fibrosis)

Mesenteric lipodystrophy results from inflammation of adipose tissue, which may involve mesentery, omentum, or retroperitoneum (27). Irregularly thickened strands of soft tissue may be found in the mesentery. These findings are best demonstrated in T1-weighted images, in which fibrous stands are low in SI in a background of high-SI fat (Fig. 6).

Carcinoid Tumors

Carcinoid tumors produce a characteristic appearance of mesenteric involvement. Typically, there is an irregular soft tissue mass in the root of the mesentery, with soft tissue strands radiating from the mass (28,29). Fibrosis is stimulated by the release of 5-hydroxytryptophan and serotonin. Conventional T1-weighted images are best

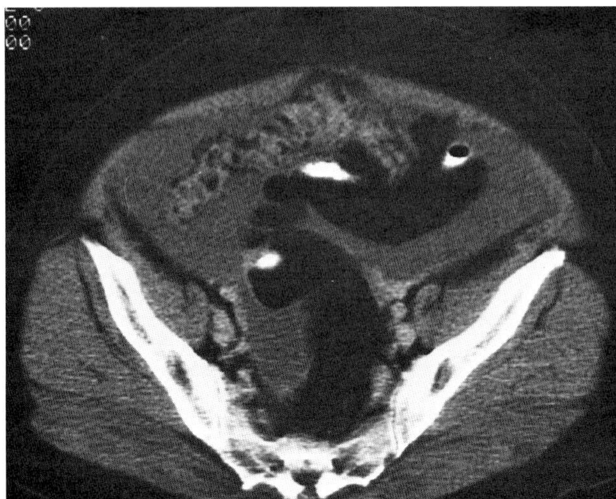

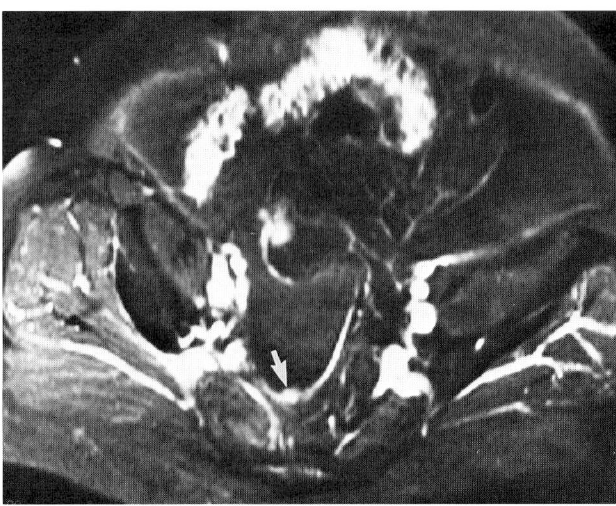

A B

FIG. 5. Omental metastases. Contrast-enhanced CT (**A**) and Gd-DTPA-enhanced fat-suppressed spin echo MR (**B**) images in a 58-year-old woman with ovarian cancer. Omental metastases (*long white arrow*) are well shown on CT and MR images. Peritoneum-based metastases are better appreciated on MR than on CT images (*short white arrow*). Reprinted with permission from ref. 17.

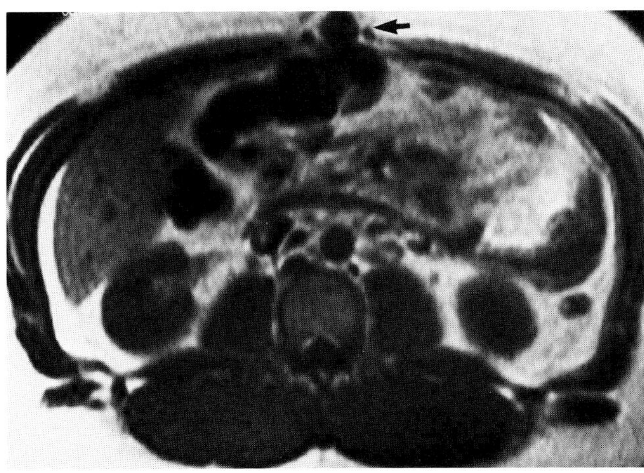

FIG. 6. Mesenteric lipodystrophy. A FLASH image in a 48-year-old man demonstrates prominent indistinct low-SI reticular tissue in the fat of the mesentery, findings consistent with mesenteric lipodystrophy. A small ventral hernia through the rectus sheath is also apparent (*arrow*).

suited for demonstrating this appearance (Fig. 7), as fat-suppressed images reduce the signal intensity difference between fat and fibrous tissue. The desmoplastic nature of this tissue renders negligible enhancement with Gd-DTPA.

INTRAPERITONEAL FLUID

Ascites

Ascites results from increased fluid production, leakage, or impaired removal. A variety of underlying conditions produce ascites. Common causes include hepatic cirrhosis, venous or lymphatic obstruction, inflammation, trauma, hypoproteinemia, and cancer.

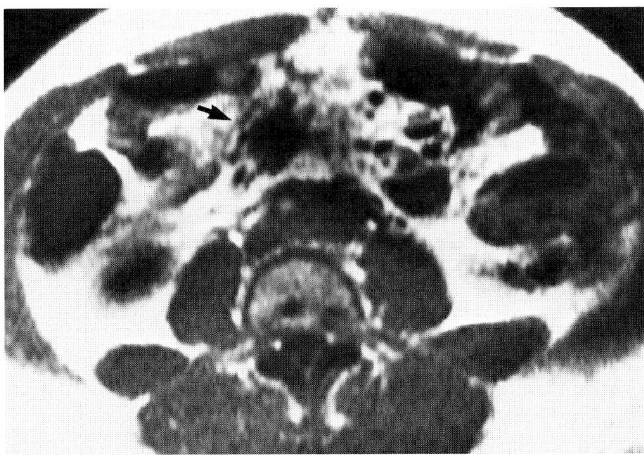

FIG. 7. Mesenteric fibrosis from carcinoid tumor. An irregular soft tissue mass with irregular radiating tissue strands is present in the root of the mesentery (*arrow*). This appearance is typical for mesenteric fibrosis caused by carcinoid tumor.

The SI of the fluid on T1-weighted images provides useful information in determining the nature of the fluid. This information is complementary to the distribution of ascites, which may suggest the underlying cause. T1-weighted images are particularly useful in distinguishing transudate from exudate or blood. Transudates are low in SI on T1-weighted images, whereas exudates are intermediate and subacute blood is high in SI (30–33).

Cirrhosis

Cirrhosis with portal hypertension is a common cause of ascites. Ascites occurs secondary to portal venous hypertension and on occasion hypoproteinemia. Ascites from hepatic cirrhosis is low in SI on T1-weighted images and high in SI on T2-weighted images (see Chapter 3 under "Cirrhosis").

Pancreatitis

Pancreatitis may result in fluid dissection into retroperitoneal and intraperitoneal spaces. Fluid related to pancreatitis has a great propensity to dissect along tissue planes, including the subcapsular location in the liver or spleen. Ascites associated with pancreatitis is usually low in SI on T1-weighted images. Fluid collection can, however, contain sufficient hemorrhage or protein to be high in SI.

Intraperitoneal Blood

Intraperitoneal blood most frequently occurs as a result of trauma. MRI is particularly well suited to detect blood and distinguish it from ascites because subacute blood is high in SI on T1-weighted images (34). T1-weighted fat suppression is particularly sensitive for the detection of blood (Fig. 8). As hematomas age, a rim of low SI develops, apparent on both T1- and T2-weighted images. This rim corresponds to peripherally deposited hemosiderin. Hematomas have a mixed high- and medium-SI internal fluid composition representing a combination of hemoglobin breakdown products and blood constituents. Not infrequently, a concentric ring of high-SI fluid surrounds a core of low-SI substance, which presumably represents extracellular methemoglobin surrounding the retracting clot (34).

Intraperitoneal Bile

Intraperitoneal bile accumulation (biloma) most frequently occurs as a result of surgery (35). The increasing performance of percutaneous cholecystectomies is associated with an increased occurrence of bilomas. Bilomas

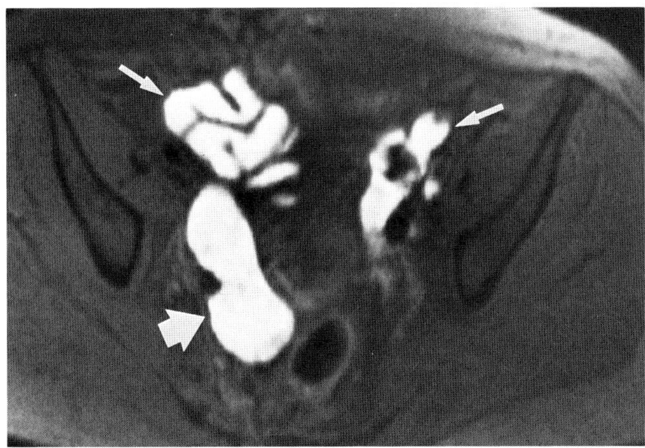

FIG. 8. Intraperitoneal blood. T1FS image in a 26-year-old woman obtained 1 week after hysterectomy demonstrates a high-SI fluid collection in the right pelvis consistent with subacute blood (*large arrow*). Bowel contents are frequently high in SI on T1FS images, presumably because of the presence of proteinaceous intraluminal material (*small arrows*).

tend to loculate in the right upper abdomen as bile elicits a mild inflammatory response, which results in the formation of a pseudocapsule and inflammatory adhesions. Since bile may be high in SI on T1-weighted images (see Chapter 4, Fig. 2), a biloma may be either low or high in SI on T1-weighted images and high on T2-weighted images.

Intraperitoneal Urine

Intraperitoneal urine most frequently occurs from traumatic rupture of the dome of the bladder. Contrast administration assists in making the diagnosis, as high-SI gadolinium may accumulate in the peritoneal cavity (see Chapter 8, Fig. 33).

ABSCESSES

Intraperitoneal abscesses are most commonly seen in the context of abdominal surgery, Crohn's disease, and diverticulitis (36). Abscesses frequently have a defined wall that enhances with Gd-DTPA (see Chapter 9, Figs. 41 and 42). The lack of features suggestive of bowel, such as haustral or valvular markings and tubular shape, and the presence of an irregular or oval shape suggest the diagnosis of an abscess. MRI is currently limited in its ability to assess abscesses because of the lack of routine use of oral contrast. In examination for an abscess, a positive oral contrast agent may be preferable to a negative agent to highlight the difference between high SI of intraluminal contrast and low SI of loculated abscess fluid on T1-weighted images.

REFERENCES

1. Cohen JM, Weinreb JC, Maravilla KP. Fluid collections in the intraperitoneal and extraperitoneal spaces: comparison of MR and CT. *Radiology* 1985;155:705–708.
2. Gore RM, Callen PW, Filly RA. Lesser sac fluid in predicting the etiology of ascites: CT findings. *AJR Am J Roentgenol* 1982;139:71–74.
3. Meyers MA. Roentgen significance of the phrenicocolic ligament. *Radiology* 1970;95:539–545.
4. Meyers MA. The spread and localization of acute intraperitoneal effusions. *Radiology* 1970;95:547–554.
5. Meyers MA. Distribution of intra-abdominal malignancy seeding: dependency on dynamic of flow of ascites fluid. *AJR Am J Roentgenol* 1973;119:198–206.
6. Meyers MA. *Dynamic Radiology of the Abdomen: Normal and Pathologic Anatomy*, 2nd ed. Springer-Verlag, New York, 1982.
7. Vanek VW, Phillips AK. Retroperitoneal, mesenteric, and omental cysts. *Arch Surg* 1984;119:838–842.
8. Haney PJ, Whitley NO. CT of benign cystic abdominal masses in children. *AJR Am J Roentgenol* 1984;142:1279–1281.
9. Naylor EW, Gardner EJ, Richards RC. Desmoid tumors and mesenteric fibromatosis in Gardner's syndrome. *Arch Surg* 1979;114:1181–1185.
10. Baron RL, Lee JKT. Mesenteric desmoid tumors: sonographic and computed-tomographic appearance. *Radiology* 1981;140: 777–779.
11. Magid D, Fishman EK, Jones B, Hoover HC, Feinstein R, Siegelman SS. Desmoid tumors in Gardner's syndrome: use of computed tomography. *AJR Am J Roentgenol* 1984;142:1141–1145.
12. McDonald AD, Harper A, El Attar OA, McDonald JC. Epidemiology of primary malignant mesothelial tumors in Canada. *Cancer* 1970;26:914–919.
13. Daniel O. The differential diagnosis of malignant disease of the peritoneum. *Br J Surg* 1951;39:147–156.
14. Meyers MA, McSweeney J. Secondary neoplasms of bowel. *Radiology* 1972;105:1–11.
15. Oliphant M, Berne AS. Computed tomography of the subperitoneal space: demonstration in direct spread of intraabdominal disease. *J Comput Assist Tomogr* 1982;6:1127–1137.
16. Meyers MA, Oliphant M, Berne AS, Feldberg MAM. The peritoneal ligament and mesenteries: pathways of intraabdominal spread of disease. *Radiology* 1987;163:593–604.
17. Semelka RC, Lawrence PH, Shoenut JP, Heywood M, Kroeker MA, Lotocki R. Primary malignant ovarian disease: prospective comparison of contrast enhanced CT and pre- and post intravenous Gd-DTPA enhanced fat suppressed and breath hold MRI with histological correlation. *JMRI* 1993;3:99–106.
18. Levitt RG, Sagel SS, Stanley RJ. Detection of neoplastic involvement of the mesentery and omentum by computed tomography. *AJR Am J Roentgenol* 1978;131:835–838.
19. Dachman AH, Lichtenstein JE, Friedman AC. Mucocele of the appendix and pseudomyxoma peritonei. *AJR Am J Roentgenol* 1985;144:923–929.
20. Mayes GB, Chuang VP, Fisher RG. CT of pseudomyxoma peritonei. *AJR Am J Roentgenol* 1981;136:807–808.
21. Novetsky GJ, Berlin L, Epstein AJ, Lobo N, Miller SH. Pseudomyxoma peritonei. *J Comput Assist Tomogr* 1982;6:398–399.
22. Seshul MB, Coulam CM. Pseudomyxoma peritonei: computed tomography and sonography. *AJR Am J Roentgenol* 1981;136: 803–806.
23. Yeh H-C, Shafir MK, Slater G, Meyer RJ, Cohen B, Geller SA. Ultrasonography and computed tomography of pseudomyxoma peritonei. *Radiology* 1984;153:507–510.
24. Goffinet DR, Castellino RA, Kim H, et al. Staging laparotomies in unselected previously untreated patients with non-Hodgkin's lymphoma. *Cancer* 1973;32:672–681.
25. Bernardino ME, Jing BS, Wallace S. Computed tomography diagnosis of mesenteric masses. *AJR Am J Roentgenol* 1979;32:33–36.
26. Whitley NO, Bohlman ME, Baker LP. CT patterns of mesenteric disease. *J Comput Assist Tomogr* 1982;6:490–496.
27. Kipfer RE, Moertel CG, Dahlin DC. Mesenteric lipodystrophy. *Ann Intern Med* 1974;80:582–588.

28. Picus D, Glazer HS, Levitt RG, Husband JE. Computed tomography of abdominal carcinoid tumors. *AJR Am J Roentgenol* 1984;143:581–584.

29. Cockey BM, Fishman EK, Jones B, Siegelman SS. Computed tomography of abdominal carcinoid tumor. *J Comput Assist Tomogr* 1985;9:38–42.

30. Terrier F, Revel D, Pajannen H, Richardson M, Hricak H, Higgins CB. MR imaging of body fluid collections. *J Comput Assist Tomogr* 1986;10:953–962.

31. Wall SD, Hricak H, Bailey GD, Kerlan RK Jr, Goldberg HI, Higgins CB. MR of pathologic abdominal fluid collections. *J Comput Assist Tomogr* 1986;10:746–750.

32. Dooms GC, Fisher MR, Hricak H, Higgins CB. MR of intramuscular hemorrhage. *J Comput Assist Tomogr* 1985;9:908–913.

33. Unger EC, Glazer HS, Lee JKT, Ling D. MRI of extracranial hematomas: preliminary observations. *AJR Am J Roentgenol* 1986;146:403–407.

34. Hahn PF, Saini S, Stark DD, Papanicolaou N, Ferrucci JT Jr. Intraabdominal hematoma: the concentric-ring sign in MR imaging. *AJR Am J Roentgenol* 1987;148:115–119.

35. Vazquez JL, Thorsen MK, Dodds WJ, et al. Evaluation and treatment of intraabdominal bilomas. *AJR Am J Roentgenol* 1985;144:933–938.

36. Wang SM, Wilson SE. Subphrenic abscess: the new epidemiology. *Arch Surg* 1977;112:934–936.

CHAPTER 11

The Retroperitoneum and the Abdominal Wall

Richard C. Semelka, J. Patrick Shoenut, and Mervyn A. Kroeker

THE RETROPERITONEUM

Normal Anatomy

The retroperitoneum extends from the diaphragm to the pelvic inlet, limited anteriorly by parietal peritoneum and posteriorly by the transversalis fascia. The important components of the retroperitoneum are the aorta, the inferior vena cava, lymph nodes, and the psoas muscles.

MR Technique

Several MR techniques are of value in assessing the retroperitoneum; however, an optimal approach has not been defined. T1-weighted sequences are routinely useful. It is not clear whether intravenous Gd-DTPA, conventional T2-weighted sequences, and fat-suppressed T1 or T2-weighted sequences are routinely necessary. MR angiography may also assume an important role in imaging the retroperitoneum. The multiplanar imaging capability of MRI allows image acquisition in the transverse, sagittal, and coronal planes, which permits direct evaluation of the extent of retroperitoneal disease.

R. C. Semelka: Department of Radiology and Magnetic Resonance Services, University of North Carolina at Chapel Hill, Chapel Hill, North Carolina 27599.

J. P. Shoenut: University of Manitoba and Department of Medicine, Saint Boniface General Hospital, Winnipeg, Manitoba R2H 2A6.

M. A. Kroeker: Department of Radiology, University of Manitoba, Winnipeg, Manitoba R2H 2A6.

Mass Lesions

Benign Mass Lesions

Retroperitoneal Fibrosis

Retroperitoneal fibrosis is most frequently idiopathic (1). Other causes of benign disease include drugs (classically methysergide) or aneurysms. The most important differential diagnosis is between idiopathic retroperitoneal fibrosis and malignant retroperitoneal fibrosis. The tomographic appearance of retroperitoneal fibrosis can vary from a focal region of fibrosis to dense infiltration of the retroperitoneum encasing the aorta, IVC, and ureters. The typical appearance is an oval, tubular tissue that encases the aorta. Early reports suggested that MRI might be a promising tool in the distinction between benign and malignant retroperitoneal fibrosis (2,3). Chronic benign retroperitoneal fibrosis is low in SI on T2-weighted images and demonstrates negligible contrast enhancement (Fig. 1). Acute benign retroperitoneal fibrosis can resemble malignant retroperitoneal fibrosis, since both may enhance substantially with contrast agent and may be bright on T2-weighted sequences (4,5) (Fig. 2). This enhancement pattern is due to the rich capillary network of acute benign granulation tissue, which eventually alters to a more fibrotic form after approximately 1 year of development.

Benign Retroperitoneal Tumors

Benign retroperitoneal tumors are much less common than their malignant counterparts. Therefore, any retroperitoneal tumor should be considered a malignant lesion.

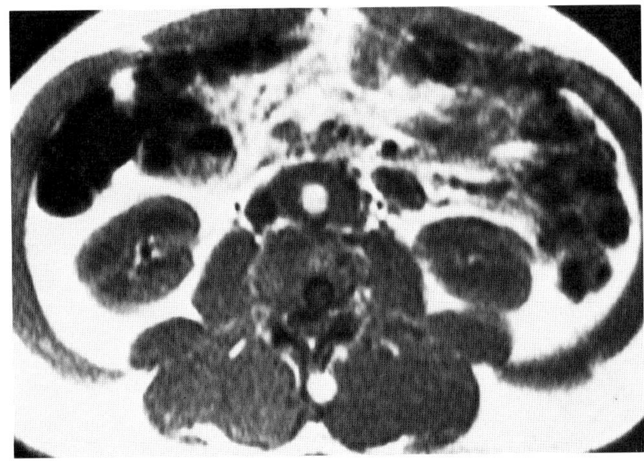
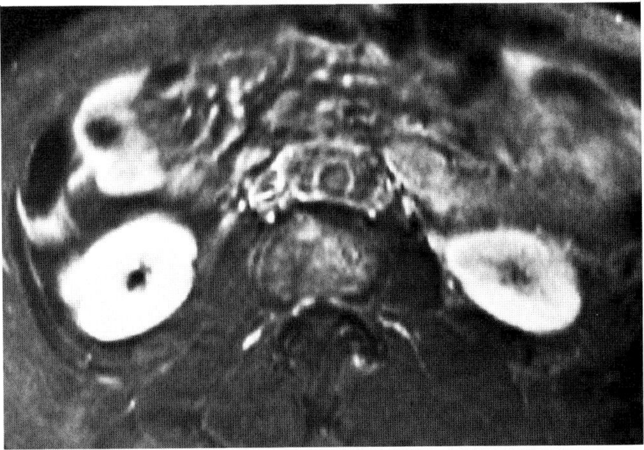

FIG. 1. Chronic benign retroperitoneal fibrosis. FLASH (**A**) and Gd-DTPA-enhanced T1FS (**B**) images in a 48-year-old man demonstrate low-SI oval tissue surrounding the aorta with an appearance typical of retroperitoneal fibrosis. High-SI blood in the aorta is from an inflow effect. Minimal enhancement of the tissue is present after Gd-DTPA administration, consistent with fibrotic tissue of greater than 1 year's duration.

Benign Lymphadenopathy

Benign lymphadenopathy may occur secondary to inflammatory or infectious disease. Castleman's disease is an unusual cause of benign lymphadenopathy which may be extensive and resemble malignant disease (Fig. 3).

Miscellaneous Benign Mass Lesions

Extramedullary hematopoiesis occurs in patients with chronic hemolytic anemias, usually of congenital origin. Masses of hematopoietic tissue develop in a paravertebral location, typically in the lower thorax and retrocrural space (Fig. 4).

Malignant Diseases

Malignant Retroperitoneal Fibrosis

Malignant retroperitoneal fibrosis is most commonly associated with cervical, bowel, or breast cancer (6). The tumor is usually high in SI on T2-weighted images and exhibits increased enhancement with Gd-DTPA (2–4).

Lymphoma

The most common malignant disease to affect the retroperitoneal space is lymphoma. Both Hodgkin's and non-Hodgkin's lymphoma affects the retroperitoneum (7–12). Intraabdominal Hodgkin's disease tends to be

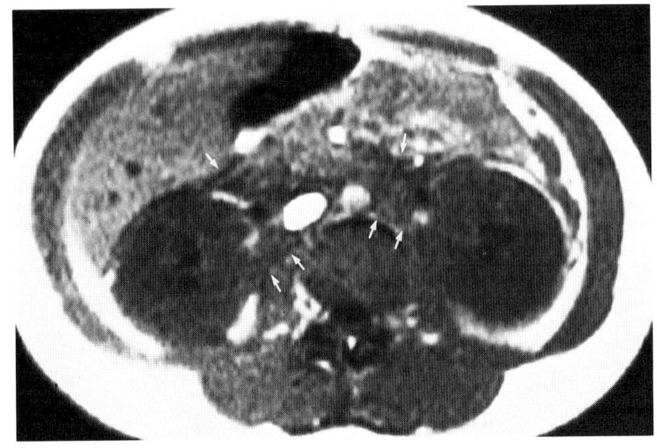
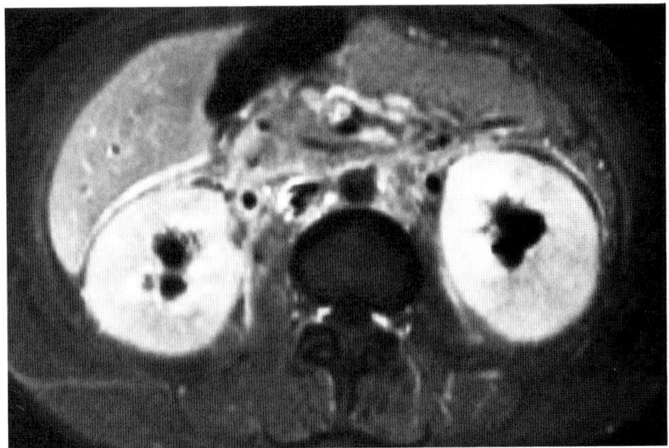

FIG. 2. Acute benign retroperitoneal fibrosis. FLASH (**A**) and Gd-DTPA-enhanced T1FS (**B**) images in a 17-year-old girl with acute benign retroperitoneal fibrosis. Extensive retroperitoneal tissue is present surrounding the aorta and IVC and extending to the kidneys, with involvement of the perirenal fascia (*small arrows*). The kidneys are noted to be swollen bilaterally, which may be related to compression of the renal veins. After Gd-DTPA administration, the retroperitoneal tissue enhances in a moderate, heterogeneous fashion.

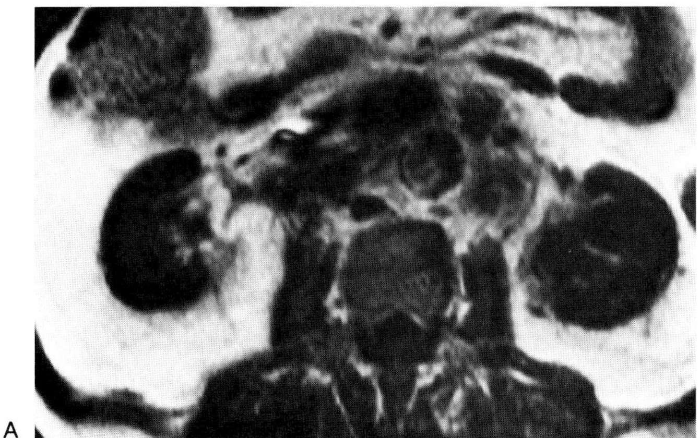
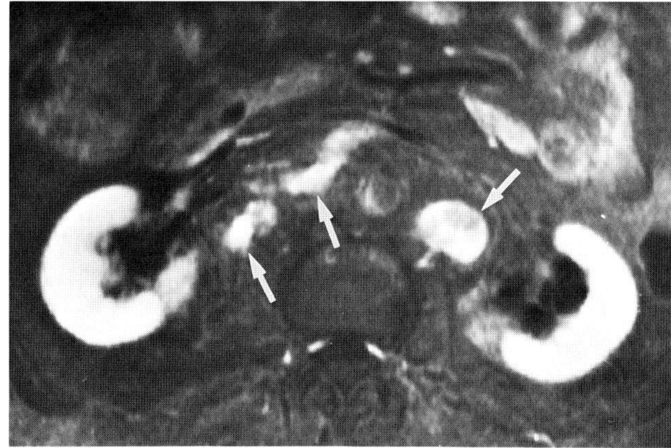

FIG. 3. Castleman's disease. Precontrast FLASH (**A**) and contrast enhanced T1FS (**B**) MR images in a 67-year-old man with Castleman's disease. Mulitple enlarged retroperitoneal nodes are apparent in the retroperitoneum, several of which demonstrate substantial contrast enhancement (*arrow*, B).

limited to the spleen and retroperitoneum (8) (Fig. 5). Non-Hodgkin's lymphoma has a greater tendency to affect a variety of nodal groups (in particular, mesenteric) and extranodal sites (12) (Fig. 6).

MRI and CT have similar abilities to demonstrate lymph nodes (13,14); however, MRI also has the potential to characterize persistent tissue after therapy as recurrent disease or fibrosis (15). After approximately 1 year, fibrotic tissue is low in SI on T2-weighted images, which permits distinction from recurrent disease, which is high or mixed in SI on T2-weighted images.

Testicular Cancer

Testicular cancer is the most common solid cancer in men between the ages of 15 to 34 years. The lymphatic drainage of the testes follows the course of testicular arteries and veins and drains into paraaortic and paracaval nodes at the level of the renal hila. The primary focus of tumor may arise in the retroperitoneum or mediastinum. MR and CT have comparable ability to detect lymphadenopathy associated with testicular cancer (16).

Malignant Retroperitoneal Lymphadenopathy

Common primary cancers associated with retroperitoneal lymphadenopathy are kidney, colon, pancreas, lung, and breast (13,17,18). There is a particular tendency for gastrointestinal cancer to involve lymph nodes without causing nodal enlargement, making the detection of malignant nodal disease difficult with current techniques.

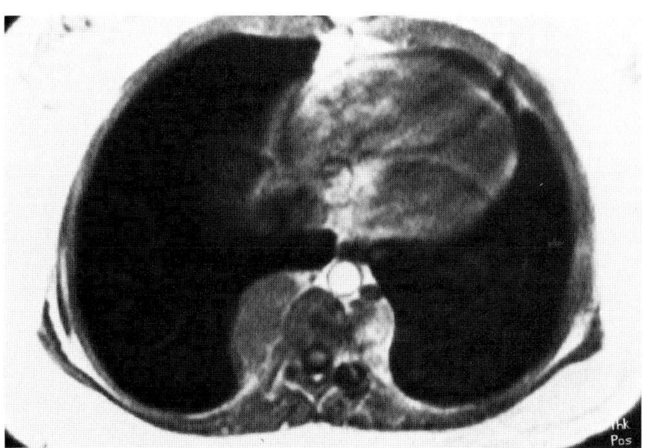
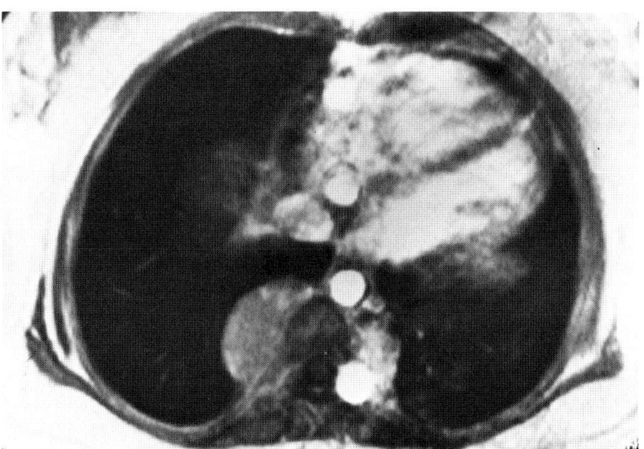

FIG. 4. Extramedullary hematopoiesis. FLASH (**A**) and 1-second postcontrast FLASH (**B**) images in a 34-year-old woman with thalassemia major and extramedullary hematopoiesis. Soft tissue masses in a paravertebral location in the lower thorax and upper abdomen are low in SI on T1-weighted images and enhance to a moderate degree after Gd-DTPA administration.

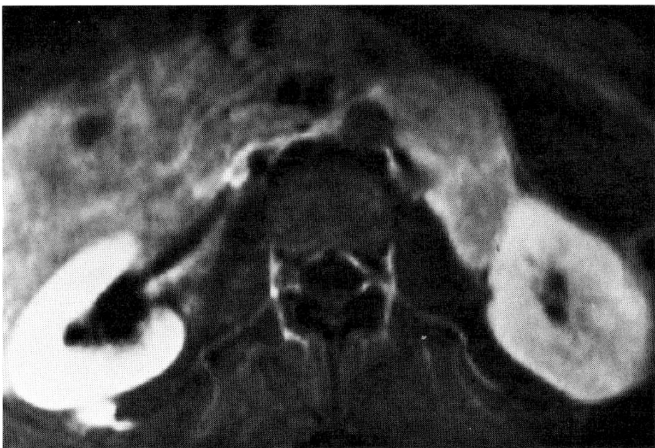

FIG. 5. Hodgkin's lymphoma. Gd-DTPA-enhanced T1FS image in a 16-year-old boy with splenic and retroperitoneal involvement with Hodgkin's disease. A 4-cm mass of nodal tissue is present in a left periaortic location at the level of the renal hilum.

Malignant Primary Retroperitoneal Tumors

Malignant primary retroperitoneal tumors are more common than their benign counterparts (19). The most common types are leiomyosarcoma, liposarcoma, and malignant fibrous histiocytoma. These tumors are typically large at presentation because they are clinically silent for a prolonged period due to their deep location. These tumors typically enhance in a heterogeneous fashion and demonstrate areas of necrosis. Imaging features usually cannot distinguish between them; uncommonly, however, liposarcomas are sufficiently well differentiated (lipogenic liposarcoma) to contain mature fat SI tissue. The multiplanar imaging capability of MRI adequately demonstrates the three-dimensional extent of tumor (Fig. 7).

The Aorta

The aorta is well evaluated by MRI because of the variety of techniques available to render flowing blood either signal void (black blood) or high in SI (bright blood). Black blood techniques usually use superior and inferior saturation radiofrequency pulses and include T1- and T2-weighted spin echo, fat-suppressed spin echo, and gradient echo techniques. Bright blood techniques often are sequences that refocus blood SI with gradient pulses and include cine gradient echo and MR angiography (Fig. 8). An alternative bright blood technique is the use of dynamic Gd-DTPA enhancement coupled with a fast imaging sequence such as FLASH or TurboFLASH. Blood velocity and flow volume can be determined by velocity-encoded MR techniques (Fig. 9).

Because of the vast array of sequences available, a standard protocol of sequences to evaluate aortic disease has not been agreed upon. As a rule, it may be of value to use both a bright blood and a black blood technique for studying the aorta. An attractive feature of MRI is the ability to image the aorta along its longitudinal length (Fig. 10), which has particular advantage in studying the length of a disease process such as aneurysm.

Aortic Aneurysms

Abdominal aortic aneurysm (AAA) is a common disease entity in North America. The incidence is 21.1/100,000, and men are 5 times more likely than women

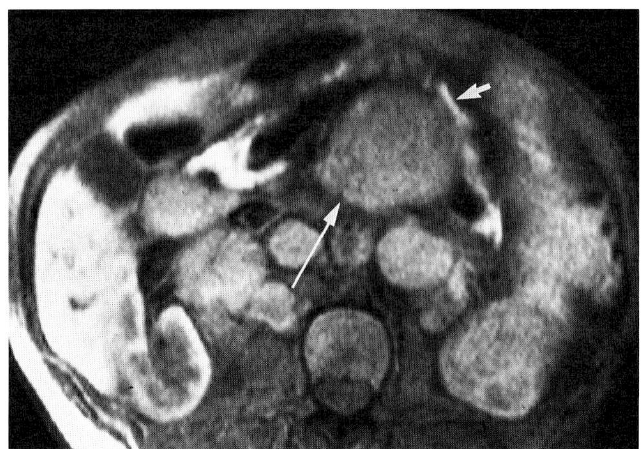
A

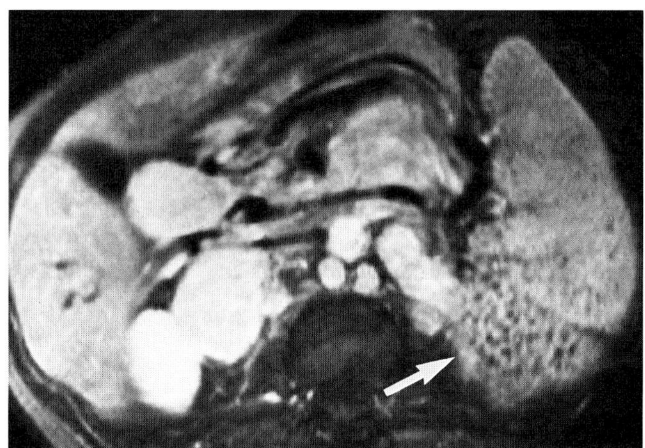
B

FIG. 6. Non-Hodgkin's lymphoma. T1FS (**A**) and postcontrast T1FS (**B**) images in a 68-year-old woman with non-Hodgkin's lymphoma. Extensive retroperitoneal and mesenteric lymph nodes are present. On the precontrast image there is excellent contrast resolution between high-SI pancreas (*short white arrow*) and intermediate-SI lymph nodes (*long white arrow*), demonstrating the extrapancreatic location of the large tumor mass. After Gd-DTPA administration the adenopathy enhances moderately to intensely. On this higher section, abnormal enhancement of the enlarged spleen is consistent with splenic infiltration (*arrow,* B).

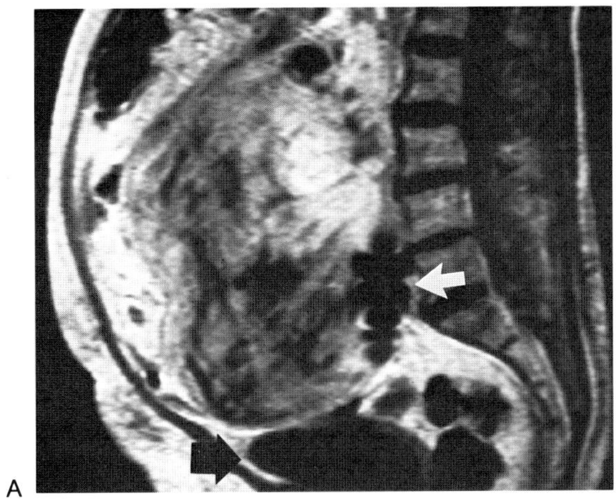
A

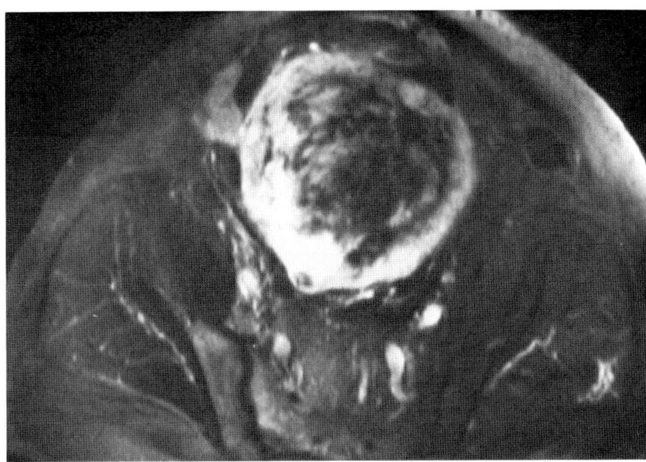
B

FIG. 7. Retroperitoneal leiomyosarcoma. One-second postcontrast sagittal FLASH (**A**) and postcontrast transverse T1FS (**B**) images in a 68-year-old woman with a recurrent retroperitoneal leiomyosarcoma. The longitudinal extent of the heterogeneously enhancing tumor is well shown on the sagittal image (*large black arrow* points to bladder, A). Susceptibility artifact from surgical clips placed during the initial resection is present (*white arrow*). The heterogeneous enhancement of the tumor is well shown on the T1FS image (B).

to be affected by AAA. The median age at diagnosis is 69 years for men and 78 years for women (20). Important diagnostic information for patient management includes the diameter of the aneurysm, the longitudinal length of the aneurysm, and its relationship to renal and common iliac arteries. Spontaneous rupture is a frequent complication of aneurysms 6 cm or more in diameter but is relatively uncommon for AAAs smaller than 5 cm (21,22). MR images with black blood and white blood techniques are successful at demonstrating aneurysms (23–27) (Fig. 11). Inflammatory aortitis is an uncommon entity in which an inflammatory reaction develops around an aortic aneurysm (28,29). This fibrosis is currently considered to result from an immune response to ceroid produced in atheromatous plaque (30).

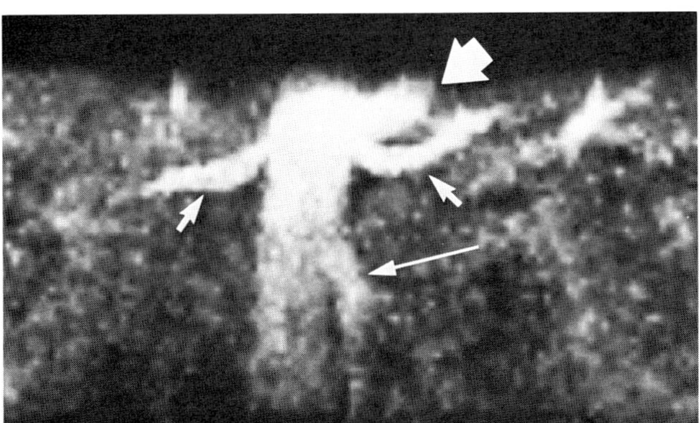

FIG. 8. Magnetic resonance angiography (MRA) of the normal abdominal aorta. Three-dimensional time-of-flight magnetic resonance angiogram of the abdominal aorta demonstrates the celiac axis (*large arrow*), renal arteries (*short arrows*), and superior mesenteric artery (*long arrow*).

Aortic Dissections

Aortic dissection usually originates in the thoracic aorta. MRI has been shown to be accurate in the detection of aortic dissection (31–33). A particular strength of MRI is the ability to demonstrate the intimal flap (31).

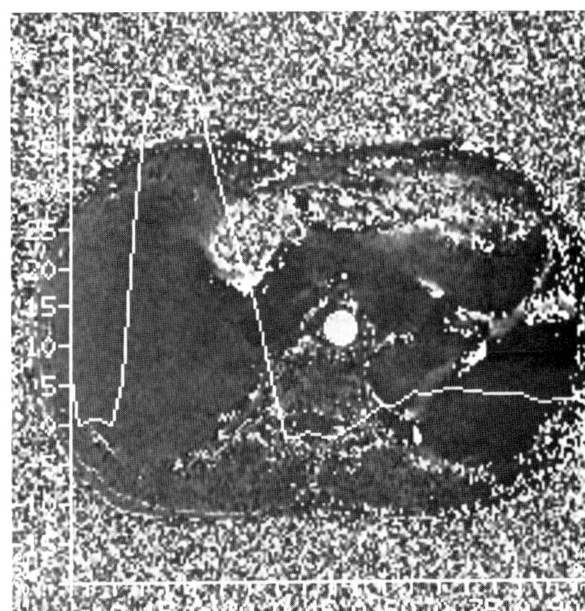

FIG. 9. Phase-map of the normal abdominal aorta. Phase map of the abdominal aorta demonstrates high SI of the abdominal aorta (*encircled*) in the systolic phase of antegrade blood flow. A blood velocity tracing obtained throughout the cardiac cycle is superimposed on the phase image, demonstrating the normal velocity profile of blood in the abdominal aorta.

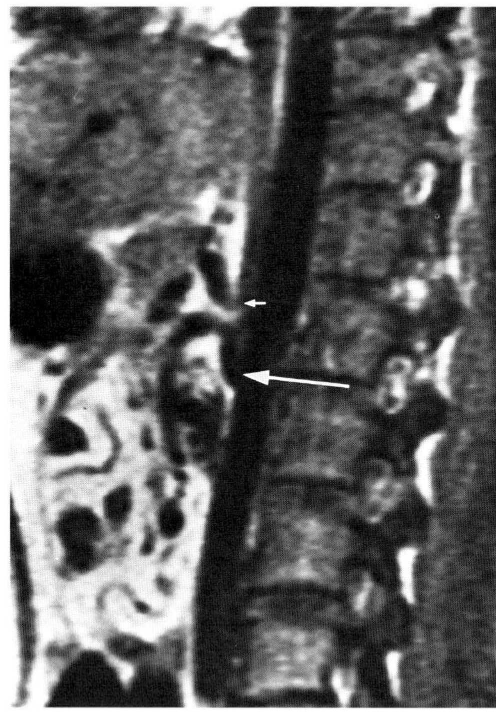

FIG. 10. Normal aorta. The longitudinal length of the aorta is well shown on this FLASH image. The celiac axis (*short arrow*) and the superior mesenteric artery (*long arrow*) are identified.

The noninvasive nature of the technique and the lack of nephrotoxicity are added advantages in the evaluation of patients with potential renal compromise. On spin echo images, flow in the true lumen is usually signal void whereas flow in the false lumen can be signal void or high in SI (Fig. 12). The SI of blood in the false lumen depends upon the velocity of blood flow. Fast flow is signal void, and slow flow is high in SI. Slow flow in the false lumen of a dissection can be difficult to differentiate from thrombosis. Image acquisition in a different plane or the employment of phase-sensitive MR sequences is useful to make this distinction.

Postoperative Aortic Graft Evaluation

Postoperative complications of abdominal aortic graft surgery include occlusion, hemorrhage with false aneurysm formation, infection, and aortoenteric fistula formation. Complications are well shown on MR images (34). Fluid is frequently present surrounding the graft within 2 to 3 months after surgery. Fluid surrounding the graft at >3 months or an increasing volume of perigraft fluid after 3 months on T1- and T2-weighted spin echo images is suggestive of infection (34–36). Although experience is preliminary, Gd-DTPA-enhanced fat-suppressed spin echo may also be an ideal technique for the evaluation of inflammatory enhancement in aortic graft infections.

The Inferior Vena Cava

The inferior vena cava is situated to the right of the aorta. The IVC is located in the retroperitoneum for the majority of its length and courses more anteriorly to be encased by the liver (intrahepatic IVC) in the upper abdomen (Fig. 13). As with the aorta, the IVC can be evaluated with bright blood and black blood techniques (37,38).

Congenital Abnormalities

Congenital abnormalities of the inferior vena cava and related veins are common (39–42). The most common venous anomaly is the retroaortic left renal vein (39,40) (see Chapter 8, Fig. 1). Right-sided vena cava, bilateral vena cava, and IVC interruptions with azygous/hemiazygous continuation are not uncommon anomalies.

Venous Thrombosis

Venous thrombosis is well evaluated by MRI (43,44). Gd-DTPA-enhanced T1-weighted conventional or fat-suppressed MRI permits distinction between tumor thrombus and blood thrombus. Tumor thrombus enhances, whereas blood thrombus does not enhance with Gd-DTPA (Fig. 14). SI measurements of thrombus pre- and postcontrast may be necessary because blood thrombus that is subacute or responding to anticoagulant therapy may be high in SI on precontrast images. Lack of increase in SI on postcontrast images would confirm the blood nature of the thrombus.

MRI is superior to CT in determining the presence and extent of tumor thrombus. Although administering Gd-DTPA for MR studies is useful, MRI does not rely on the administration of intravenous Gd-DTPA. This is an advantage over CT, which requires intravenous contrast to assess the presence of thrombus. Gd-DTPA may create difficulty in evaluating thrombus due to mixing of enhanced and nonenhanced blood.

The Psoas Muscles

The psoas muscles originate at the level of the 12th thoracic vertebra, parallel the lumbar vertebral bodies, and extend into the pelvis, joining the iliac muscles to form the iliopsoas muscles. Disease affecting the psoas muscle usually is due to extension from adjacent structures such as spine, kidney, bowel, pancreas, and retroperitoneal lymph nodes (see Chapter 7, Fig. 14) (45,46). Atrophy of the iliopsoas can occur from neuromuscular disease. Spontaneous hemorrhage may also occur in the iliopsoas muscle and is most frequently observed in patients on anticoagulant therapy. Hemorrhage is well

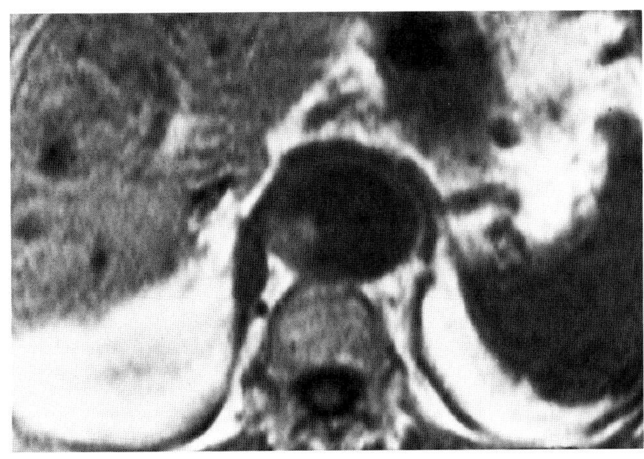

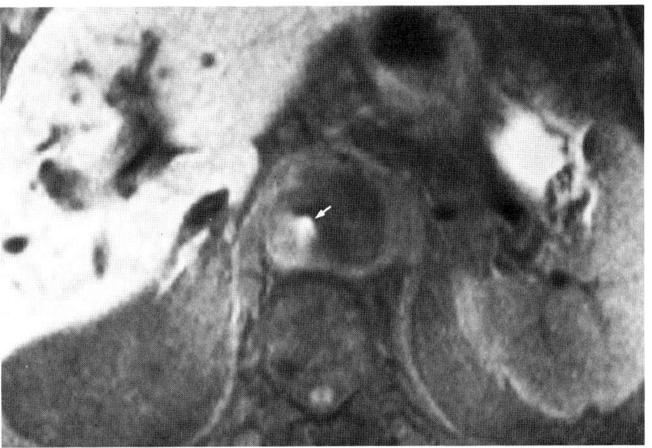

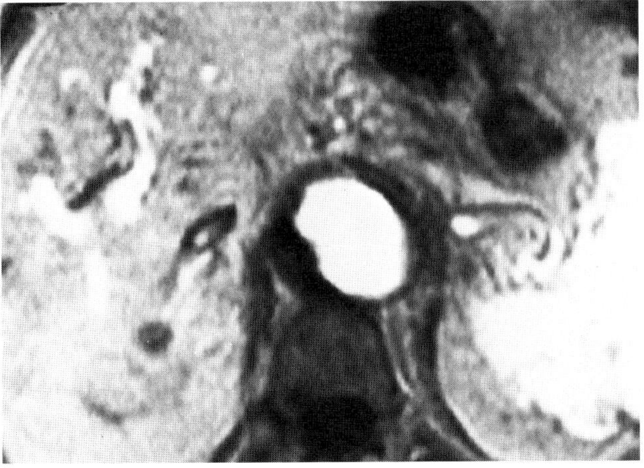

FIG. 11. Aortic aneurysm. FLASH (**A**), T1FS (**B**), and 1-second postcontrast FLASH (**C**) images in an 82-year-old man with a 3.5-cm-diameter aneurysm of the upper abdominal aorta. On the FLASH image (A) the flowing blood is black and an intermediate-SI atheromatous plaque is identified on the left posterior wall. On the T1FS image the thickness of the aortic wall is better appreciated because of suppression of surrounding retroperitoneal fat. A small, high-SI focus (*small arrow*) on the plaque is consistent with a blood clot. On the 1-second postcontrast FLASH image (C), flowing Gd-DTPA-containing blood is high in SI, demonstrating the luminal size and shape.

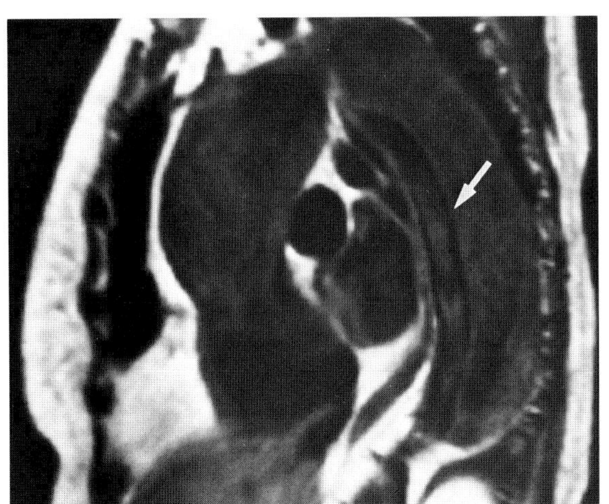

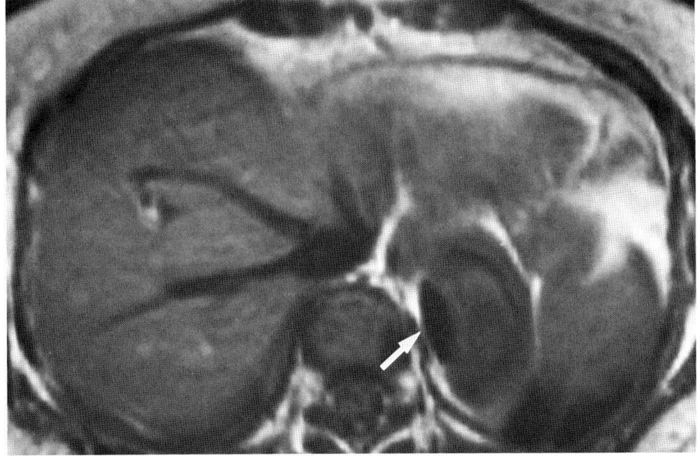

FIG. 12. Aortic dissection. Left anterior oblique parasagittal (**A**) and transverse (**B**) gated T1-weighted images of the thoracic and upper abdominal aorta. An intimal flap is clearly shown on the parasagittal image (*arrow*, A). On the transverse image the higher blood velocity in the true lumen results in a signal void (*arrow*, B), while slower flow in the false lumen is high in SI.

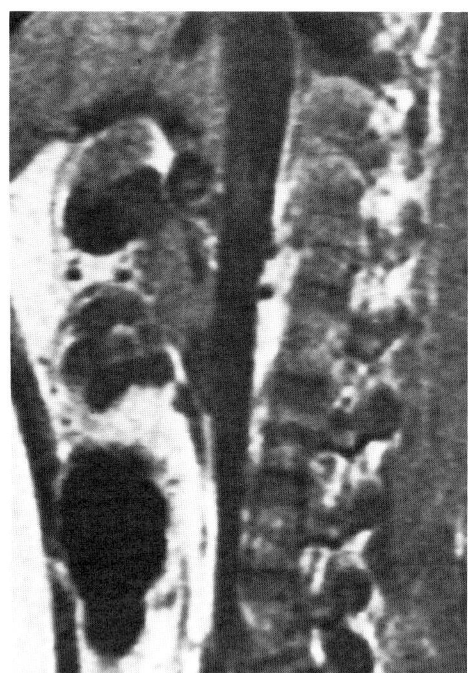

FIG. 13. Normal IVC. Sagittal FLASH image demonstrates the course of the normal IVC. Anterior curving of the IVC into the right atrium is well displayed.

shown on MR images because of the high SI of subacute blood on T1-weighted images (47–49).

THE ABDOMINAL WALL

Normal Anatomy

The abdominal wall is composed of skin, superficial fascia, subcutaneous fat, anterolateral muscles (external oblique, internal oblique, and transversus), rectus abdominis muscle, transversalis fascia, and extraperitoneal fat. The aponeuroses of the anterolateral muscles fuse along the medial margins of the muscles to form the Spigelian fascia, which more medially divides to form the anterior and posterior rectus sheath. These fascial sheaths reunite to form the midline fascial structure, the linea alba.

Neoplasms

Benign Tumors

Cysts and desmoid tumors are two common abdominal wall tumors (50). Desmoids are relatively avascular masses that are best shown on T1-weighted images (Fig. 15).

Malignant Tumors

Metastases, sarcomas, and lymphoma can involve the abdominal wall. Tumors are medium-SI masses that are well defined in the high SI of subcutaneous fat on T1-weighted images (Fig. 16).

Miscellaneous Diseases

A variety of disease processes involve the abdominal wall. They include hematomas, infections, arteriovenous malformations, and varices. Hematoma and vessels are well shown on MR images. Sequences should be selected to maximize contrast between diseased tissue and subcutaneous fat. Fibrous lesions are generally well shown on T1-weighted images. Malignant or vascular

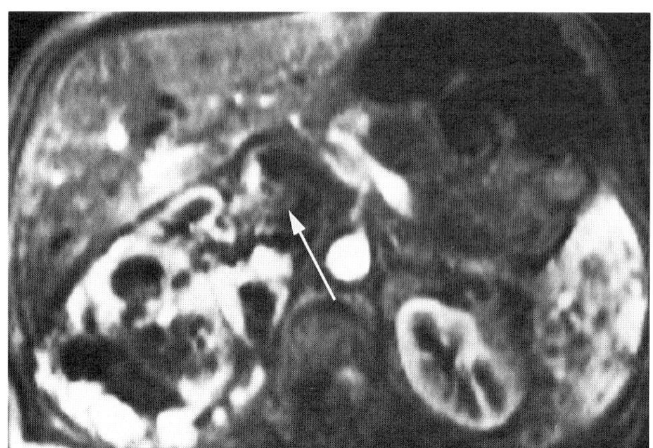

A

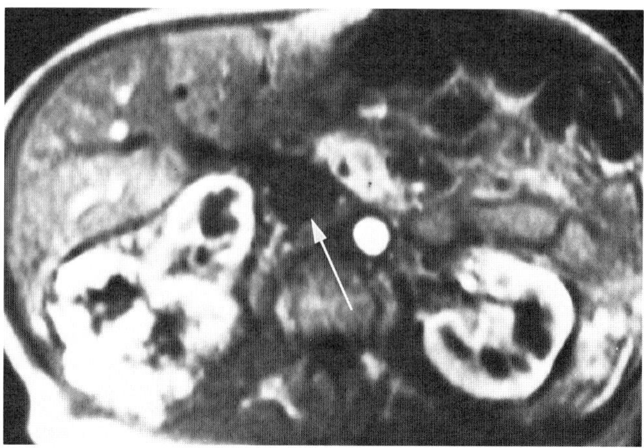

B

FIG. 14. Tumor and blood thrombus. One-second postcontrast FLASH images of the IVC obtained at the level of the renal vein (**A**) and below the renal vessels (**B**). Enhancing tumor thrombus extending from a large renal cancer is well shown (*arrow,* A). Blood thrombus in the IVC below the renal vessels does not enhance and is signal void (*arrow,* B).

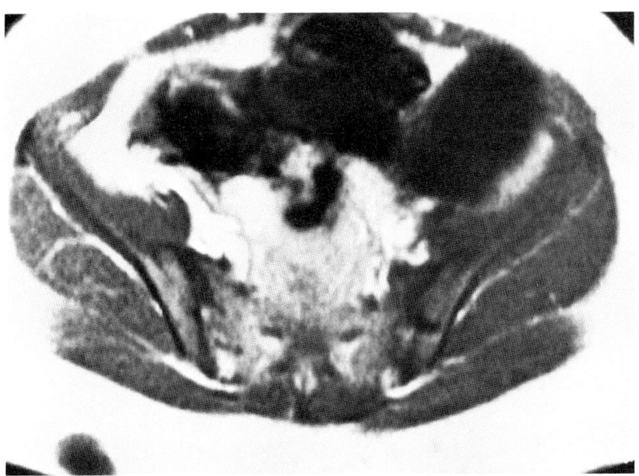

FIG. 15. Desmoid. FLASH image in a 48-year-old woman with Gardner's syndrome shows a low-SI, fibrous desmoid tumor set in the high SI of subcutaneous fat in the right gluteal region. T1-weighted images possess maximal contrast resolution for a fibrous tumor situated in fat.

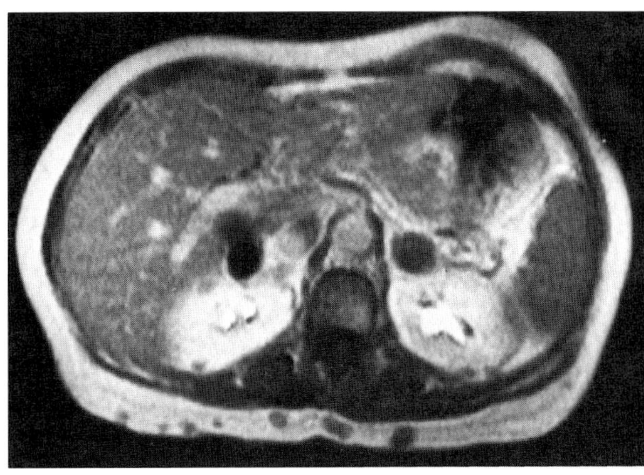

FIG. 16. Subcutaneous metastases. Ten-minute postcontrast FLASH image demonstrates subcutaneous metastases in a 56-year-old woman with diffuse metastatic disease from breast cancer.

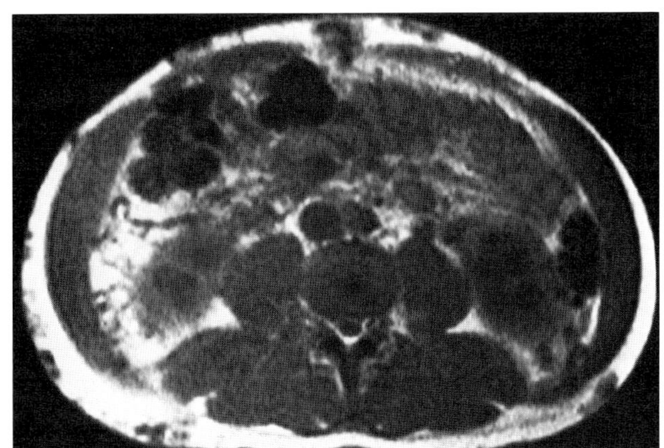

A

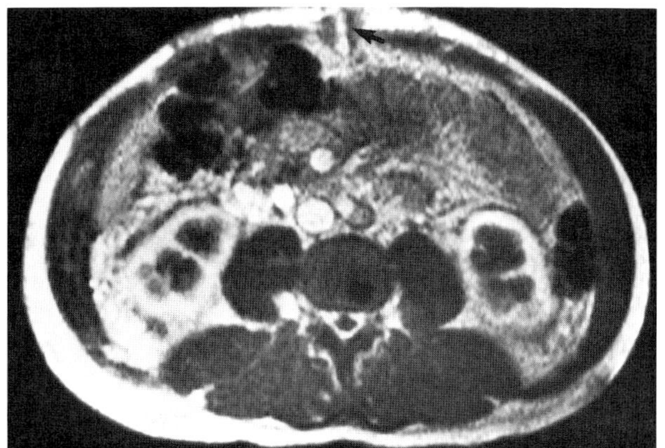

B

FIG. 17. Subcutaneous varices. Precontrast FLASH (**A**) and 1-second postcontrast FLASH (**B**) images in a 48-year-old man with Budd-Chiari syndrome and extensive varices. Multiple subcutaneous collaterals and perirenal collaterals are well seen on the precontrast FLASH images as low-SI serpiginous tubular structures in a background of high-SI fat. Immediately after Gd-DTPA injection the subcutaneous varies become obscured because of the increased SI of vessels caused by the presence of Gd-DTPA. A large recanalized umbilical vein is well visualized on the immediate postcontrast image (*arrow,* B) because of the presence of surrounding fibrous tissue.

lesions are well shown on T1-weighted images and fat-suppressed Gd-DTPA-enhanced images. Vessels are well shown on T1-weighted images, T2-weighted fat-suppressed images with gradient moment refocusing, and dynamic Gd-DTPA-enhanced images with or without fat suppression (Fig. 17). Distinction of cellulitis from abscess can be made on MR images by the demonstration of a signal-void center in an abscess.

REFERENCES

1. Lepor H, Walsh PC. Idiopathic retroperitoneal fibrosis. *J Urol* 1979;122:1–6.
2. Hricak H, Higgins CB, Williams RD, et al. Nuclear magnetic resonance imaging in retroperitoneal fibrosis. *AJR Am J Roentgenol* 1983;141:35–38.
3. Arrivé L, Hricak H, Tavares NJ, Miller TR. Malignant versus nonmalignant retroperitoneal fibrosis: differentiation with MR imaging. *Radiology* 1989;172:139–143.
4. Mulligan SA, Holley HC, Koehler RE, et al. CT and MR imaging in the evaluation of retroperitoneal fibrosis. *J Comput Assist Tomogr* 1989;13:277–281.
5. Rubenstein WA, Gray G, Auh YH, et al. CT of fibrous tissue and tumors with sonographic correlation. *AJR Am J Roentgenol* 1986;147:1067–1074.
6. Koep L, Zuidema GD. The clinical significance of retroperitoneal fibrosis. *Surgery* 1977;81:250–257.
7. Crowther D, Blackledge G, Best JJK. The role of computed tomography of the abdomen in the diagnosis and staging of patients with lymphoma. *Clin Hematol* 1979;83:567–591.
8. Blackledge G, Best JJK, Crowther F, Isherwood I. Computed tomography in the staging of patients with Hodgkin's disease: a report on 136 patients. *Clin Radiol* 1980;31:143–148.
9. Castellino RA, Marglin S, Blank N. Hodgkin disease, the non-Hodgkin lymphomas, and the leukemias in the retroperitoneum. *Semin Roentgenol* 1980;15:288–301.
10. Earl HM, Sutcliffe SBJ, Fry IK, et al. Computerized tomography (CT) abdominal scanning in Hodgkin's disease. *Clin Radiol* 1980;31:149–153.
11. Lee JKT, Balfe DM. Computed tomographic evaluation of lymphoma patients. *Crit Rev Diagn Imaging* 1981;18:1–28.
12. Neumann CH, Robert NJ, Canellos G, Rosenthal D. Computed tomography of the abdomen and pelvis in non-Hodgkin lymphoma. *J Comput Assist Tomogr* 1983;7:846–850.
13. Lee JKT, Heiken JP, Ling D, et al. Magnetic resonance imaging of abdominal and pelvic lymphadenopathy. *Radiology* 1984;153:181–188.
14. Dooms GC, Hricak H, Crooks LE, Higgins CB. Magnetic resonance imaging of the lymph nodes: comparison with CT. *Radiology* 1984;153:719–728.
15. Glazer HS, Lee JKT, Levitt RG, Heiken JP, Ling D, Totty WG. Radiation fibrosis: differentiation from recurrent tumor by MR imaging. *Radiology* 1985;156:721–726
16. Ellis JH, Bies JR, Kopecky KK, Klatte EC, Rowland RG, Donohue JP. Comparison of NMR and CT imaging in the evaluation of metastatic retroperitoneal lymphadenopathy from testicular carcinoma. *J Comput Assist Tomogr* 1984;87:709–719.
17. Hricak H, Demas BE, Williams RD, et al. Magnetic resonance imaging in the diagnosis and staging of renal and perirenal neoplasms. *Radiology* 1985;154:709–715.
18. Fein AB, Lee JKT, Balfe DM, et al. Diagnosis and staging of renal cell carcinoma: a comparison of MR imaging and CT. *AJR Am J Roentgenol* 1987;148:749–753.
19. McLeod AJ, Zornoza J, Shirkhoda A. Leiomyosarcoma: computed tomographic findings. *Radiology* 1984;152:133–136.
20. Bickerstaff LK, Hollier LH, Van Peenen HJ, Melton LJ III, Pairolero PC, Cherry KL. Abdominal aortic aneurysms: the changing natural history. *J Vasc Surg* 1984;1:6–12.
21. Szilagyi DE, Smith RF, DeRusso FJ, Elliott JP, Sherrin FW. Contribution of abdominal aortic aneurysmectomy to prolongation of life. *Ann Surg* 1966;164:678–699.
22. Szilagyi DE, Elliott JP, Smith RF. Clinical fate of the patient with asymptomatic abdominal aortic aneurysm and unfit for surgical treatment. *Arch Surg* 1972;104:600–606.
23. Herfkens RJ, Higgins CB, Hricak H, et al. Nuclear magnetic resonance imaging of atherosclerotic disease. *Radiology* 1983;148:161–166.
24. Lee JKT, Ling D, Heiken JP, et al. Magnetic resonance imaging of abdominal aortic aneurysms. *AJR Am J Roentgenol* 1984;143:1197–1202.
25. Flak B, Li DKB, Ho BYB, et al. Magnetic resonance imaging of aneurysms of the abdominal aorta. *AJR Am J Roentgenol* 1985;144:991–996.
26. Evancho AM, Osbakken M, Weidner W. Comparison of NMR imaging and aortography for preoperative evaluation of abdominal aortic aneurysm. *Magn Reson Med* 1985;2:41–55.
27. Amparo EG, Hoddick WK, Hricak H, et al. Comparison of magnetic resonance imaging and ultrasonography in the evaluation of abdominal aortic aneurysms. *Radiology* 1985;154:451–456.
28. Lindell OI, Sariola HV, Lehtonen TA. The occurrence of vasculitis in perianeurysmal fibrosis. *J Urol* 1987;138:727–729.
29. Cullenward MJ, Scanlan KA, Pozniak MA, et al. Inflammatory aortic aneurysm (periaortic fibrosis): radiologic imaging. *Radiology* 1986;159:75–82.
30. Mitchinson MJ. Retroperitoneal fibrosis revisited. *Arch Pathol Lab Med* 1986;110:784–786.
31. Amparo EG, Higgins CB, Hricak H, Sollitto R. Aortic dissection: magnetic resonance imaging. *Radiology* 1985;155:399–406.
32. Dinsmore RE, Wedeen VJ, Miller SW, et al. MRI of dissection of the aorta: recognition of the intimal tear and differential flow velocities. *AJR Am J Roentgenol* 1986;146:1286–1288.
33. Geisinger MA, Risius B, O'Donnell JA, et al. Thoracic aortic dissection: magnetic resonance imaging. *Radiology* 1985;155:407–412.
34. Auffermann W, Olofsson P, Stoney R, et al. MR imaging of complications of aortic surgery. *J Comput Assist Tomogr* 1987;11:982–989.
35. Justich E, Amparo EG, Hricak H, Higgins CB. Infected aortoiliofemoral grafts: magnetic resonance imaging. *Radiology* 1985;154:133–136.
36. Auffermann W, Olofsson P, Rabahie G, et al. Incorporation versus infection of retroperitoneal aortic grafts: MR imaging features. *Radiology* 1989;172:359–362.
37. Hricak H, Amparo E, Fisher MR, Crooks L, Higgins DB. Abdominal venous system: assessment using MR. *Radiology* 1985;156:415–422.
38. Colletti PM, Oide CT, Terk MR, Boswell WD Jr. Magnetic resonance of the inferior vena cava. *Magn Reson Imaging* 1992;10:177–185.
39. Royal SA, Callen PW. CT evaluation of anomalies of the inferior vena cava and left renal vein. *AJR Am J Roentgenol* 1979;132:759–763.
40. Cory DA, Ellis JH, Bies JR, Olson EW. Retroaortic left renal vein demonstrated by nuclear magnetic resonance imaging. *J Comput Assist Tomogr* 1984;8:339–340.
41. Schultz CL, Morrison S, Bryan PJ. Azygous continuation of the inferior vena cava: demonstration by NMR imaging. *J Comput Assist Tomogr* 1984;8:774–776.
42. Fisher MR, Hricak H, Higgins CB. Magnetic resonance imaging of developmental venous anomalies. *AJR Am J Roentgenol* 1985;145:705–709.
43. Erdman WA, Weinreb JC, Cohen JM, Buja LM, Chaney C, Peshock RM. Venous thrombosis: clinical and experimental MR imaging. *Radiology* 1986;161:233–238.
44. Higgins CB, Goldberg H, Hricak H, Crooks LE, Kaufman L, Brasch R. Nuclear magnetic resonance imaging of vasculature of abdominal viscera: normal and pathologic features. *AJR Am J Roentgenol* 1983;140:1217–1225.
45. Lee JKT, Glazer HS. Psoas muscle disorders: MR imaging. *Radiology* 1986;160:683–687.

46. Weinreb JC, Cohen JM, Maravilla KR. Iliopsoas muscles: MR study of normal anatomy and disease. *Radiology* 1985;156: 435–440.
47. Hahn PF, Saini S, Stark DD, Papanicolaou N, Ferrucci JT Jr. Intraabdominal hematoma: the concentric-ring sign in MR imaging. *AJR Am J Roentgenol* 1987;148:115–119.
48. Rubin JI, Gomori JM, Grossman RI, Gefter WB, Kressel HY. High-field MR imaging of extracranial hematomas. *AJR Am J Roentgenol* 1987;148:813–817.
49. Unger EC, Glazer HS, Lee JKT, Ling D. MRI of extracranial hematomas: preliminary observations. *AJR Am J Roentgenol* 1986;146:403–407.
50. Brasfield RD, Das Gupta TK. Desmoid tumors of the anterior abdominal wall. *Surgery* 1969;65:241–246.

Index*

* The bold numbers following entries in this list refer to figures. Bold, lower case "t" following a page number refers to a table on that page.

M

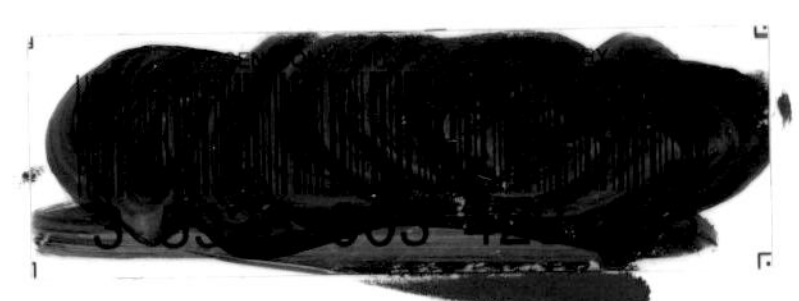